Management of Acute and Chronic Complications of Lysosomal Storage Diseases in Children and Adults: Current Practice and Future Opportunities

Management of Acute and Chronic Complications of Lysosomal Storage Diseases in Children and Adults: Current Practice and Future Opportunities

Editors

Karolina M. Stepien
Christian J. Hendriksz
Gregory M Pastores

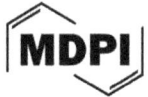

Basel • Beijing • Wuhan • Barcelona • Belgrade • Novi Sad • Cluj • Manchester

Editors

Karolina M. Stepien
Adult Inherited
Metabolic Department
Salford Royal NHS
Foundation Trust
Manchester, UK

Christian J. Hendriksz
Paediatrics and Child
Health Department
University of Pretoria
Pretoria, South Africa

Gregory M Pastores
Adult Inherited
Metabolic Diseases
The Mater Misericordiae
University Hospital
Dublin, Ireland

Editorial Office
MDPI
St. Alban-Anlage 66
4052 Basel, Switzerland

This is a reprint of articles from the Special Issue published online in the open access journal *Journal of Clinical Medicine* (ISSN 2077-0383) (available at: https://www.mdpi.com/journal/jcm/special_issues/Diseases_lysosomal).

For citation purposes, cite each article independently as indicated on the article page online and as indicated below:

Lastname, A.A.; Lastname, B.B. Article Title. *Journal Name* **Year**, *Volume Number*, Page Range.

ISBN 978-3-0365-9748-5 (Hbk)
ISBN 978-3-0365-9749-2 (PDF)
doi.org/10.3390/books978-3-0365-9749-2

© 2023 by the authors. Articles in this book are Open Access and distributed under the Creative Commons Attribution (CC BY) license. The book as a whole is distributed by MDPI under the terms and conditions of the Creative Commons Attribution-NonCommercial-NoDerivs (CC BY-NC-ND) license.

Contents

Jonathan Niranjan Rajan, Katharine Ireland, Richard Johnson and Karolina M. Stepien
Review of Mechanisms, Pharmacological Management, Psychosocial Implications, and Holistic Treatment of Pain in Fabry Disease
Reprinted from: *J. Clin. Med.* **2021**, *10*, 4168, doi:10.3390/jcm10184168 1

Chaitanya Gadepalli, Karolina M. Stepien, Reena Sharma, Ana Jovanovic, Govind Tol and Andrew Bentley
Airway Abnormalities in Adult Mucopolysaccharidosis and Development of Salford Mucopolysaccharidosis Airway Score
Reprinted from: *J. Clin. Med.* **2021**, *10*, 3275, doi:10.3390/jcm10153275 19

Alícia Dorneles Dornelles, Ana Paula Pedroso Junges, Tiago Veiga Pereira, Bárbara Corrêa Krug, Candice Beatriz Treter Gonçalves, Juan Clinton Llerena, Jr., et al.
A Systematic Review and Meta-Analysis of Enzyme Replacement Therapy in Late-Onset Pompe Disease
Reprinted from: *J. Clin. Med.* **2021**, *10*, 4828, doi:10.3390/jcm10214828 39

Moein Mobini, Shabnam Radbakhsh, Francyne Kubaski, Peyman Eshraghi, Saba Vakili, Rahim Vakili, et al.
Impact of Intravenous Trehalose Administration in Patients with Niemann–Pick Disease Types A and B
Reprinted from: *J. Clin. Med.* **2022**, *11*, 247, doi:10.3390/jcm11010247 59

Aditi Korlimarla, Jeong-A Lim, Paul McIntosh, Kanecia Zimmerman, Baodong D. Sun and Priya S. Kishnani
New Insights into Gastrointestinal Involvement in Late-Onset Pompe Disease: Lessons Learned from Bench and Bedside
Reprinted from: *J. Clin. Med.* **2021**, *10*, 3395, doi:10.3390/jcm10153395 71

Ewa Tobór-Świętek, Jolanta Sykut-Cegielska, Mirosław Bik-Multanowski, Mieczysław Walczak, Dariusz Rokicki, Łukasz Kałużny, et al.
COVID-19 Pandemic and Patients with Rare Inherited Metabolic Disorders and Rare Autoinflammatory Diseases—Organizational Challenges from the Point of View of Healthcare Providers
Reprinted from: *J. Clin. Med.* **2021**, *10*, 4862, doi:10.3390/jcm10214862 87

Andrea Dardis, Eleonora Pavan, Martina Fabris, Rosalia Maria Da Riol, Annalisa Sechi, Agata Fiumara, et al.
Plasma Neurofilament Light (NfL) in Patients Affected by Niemann–Pick Type C Disease (NPCD)
Reprinted from: *J. Clin. Med.* **2021**, *10*, 4796, doi:10.3390/jcm10204796 99

Ashwin Roy, Hamza Umar, Antonio Ochoa-Ferraro, Adrian Warfield, Nigel Lewis, Tarekegn Geberhiwot and Richard Steeds
Atherosclerosis in Fabry Disease—A Contemporary Review
Reprinted from: *J. Clin. Med.* **2021**, *10*, 4422, doi:10.3390/jcm10194422 109

Luise Sophie Ammer, Thorsten Dohrmann, Nicole Maria Muschol, Annika Lang, Sandra Rafaela Breyer, Ann-Kathrin Ozga and Martin Petzoldt
Disease Manifestations in Mucopolysaccharidoses and Their Impact on Anaesthesia-Related Complications—A Retrospective Analysis of 99 Patients
Reprinted from: *J. Clin. Med.* **2021**, *10*, 3518, doi:10.3390/jcm10163518 125

Fanny Thuriot, Elaine Gravel, Katherine Hodson, Jorge Ganopolsky, Bojana Rakic, Paula J. Waters, et al.
Molecular Diagnosis of Pompe Disease in the Genomic Era: Correlation with Acid Alpha-Glucosidase Activity in Dried Blood Spots
Reprinted from: *J. Clin. Med.* **2021**, *10*, 3868, doi:10.3390/jcm10173868 . . . . **141**

Orlaith McGrath, Leon Au and Jane Ashworth
Management of Corneal Clouding in Patients with Mucopolysaccharidosis
Reprinted from: *J. Clin. Med.* **2021**, *10*, 3263, doi:10.3390/jcm10153263 . . . . **153**

Sophie Thomas, Uma Ramaswami, Maureen Cleary, Medeah Yaqub and Eva M. Raebel
Gastrointestinal Manifestations in Mucopolysaccharidosis Type III: Review of Death Certificates and the Literature
Reprinted from: *J. Clin. Med.* **2021**, *10*, 4445, doi:10.3390/jcm10194445 . . . . **167**

Kelly D. Crisp, Amy T. Neel, Sathya Amarasekara, Jill Marcus, Gretchen Nichting, Aditi Korlimarla, et al.
Assessment of Dysphonia in Children with Pompe Disease Using Auditory-Perceptual and Acoustic/Physiologic Methods
Reprinted from: *J. Clin. Med.* **2021**, *10*, 3617, doi:10.3390/jcm10163617 . . . . **177**

Ritma Boruah, Ahmad Ardeshir Monavari, Tracey Conlon, Nuala Murphy, Andreea Stroiescu, Stephanie Ryan, et al.
Secondary Hyperparathyroidism in Children with Mucolipidosis Type II (I-Cell Disease): Irish Experience
Reprinted from: *J. Clin. Med.* **2022**, *11*, 1366, doi:10.3390/jcm11051366 . . . . **193**

Nadia Ali, Amanda Caceres, Eric W. Hall and Dawn Laney
Attention Deficits and ADHD Symptoms in Adults with Fabry Disease—A Pilot Investigation
Reprinted from: *J. Clin. Med.* **2021**, *10*, 3367, doi:10.3390/jcm10153367 . . . . **205**

Chaitanya Gadepalli, Karolina M. Stepien and Govind Tol
Hyo-Mental Angle and Distance: An Important Adjunct in Airway Assessment of Adult Mucopolysaccharidosis
Reprinted from: *J. Clin. Med.* **2021**, *10*, 4924, doi:10.3390/jcm10214924 . . . . **215**

Aleksandra Jezela-Stanek, Grazina Kleinotiene, Karolina Chwialkowska and Anna Tylki-Szymańska
Do Not Miss the (Genetic) Diagnosis of Gaucher Syndrome: A Narrative Review on Diagnostic Clues and Management in Severe Prenatal and Perinatal-Lethal Sporadic Cases
Reprinted from: *J. Clin. Med.* **2021**, *10*, 4890, doi:10.3390/jcm10214890 . . . . **227**

Luise Sophie Ammer, Nicole Maria Muschol, René Santer, Annika Lang, Sandra Rafaela Breyer, Phillip Brenya Sasu, et al.
Anaesthesia-Relevant Disease Manifestations and Perianaesthetic Complications in Patients with Mucolipidosis—A Retrospective Analysis of 44 Anaesthetic Cases in 12 Patients
Reprinted from: *J. Clin. Med.* **2022**, *11*, 3650, doi:10.3390/jcm11133650 . . . . **237**

Jessica I. Gold and Karolina M. Stepien
Healthcare Transition in Inherited Metabolic Disorders—Is a Collaborative Approach between US and European Centers Possible?
Reprinted from: *J. Clin. Med.* **2022**, *11*, 5805, doi:10.3390/jcm11195805 . . . . **253**

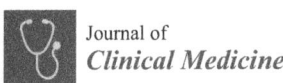

Review

Review of Mechanisms, Pharmacological Management, Psychosocial Implications, and Holistic Treatment of Pain in Fabry Disease

Jonathan Niranjan Rajan [1,*], Katharine Ireland [1], Richard Johnson [2] and Karolina M. Stepien [3,4]

1. Pain Medicine and Anaesthesia Department, Salford Royal NHS Foundation Trust, Stott Lane, Salford M6 8HD, UK; katharine.ireland@btinternet.com
2. Manchester & Salford Pain Centre, Salford Royal NHS Foundation Trust, Stott Lane, Salford M6 8HD, UK; richard.johnson@srft.nhs.uk
3. Adult Inherited Metabolic Diseases, Salford Royal NHS Foundation Trust, Stott Lane, Salford M6 8HD, UK; Karolina.Stepien@srft.nhs.uk
4. Division of Diabetes, Endocrinology & Gastroenterology, University of Manchester, Manchester M13 9PL, UK
* Correspondence: jonathan.rajan@srft.nhs.uk

Abstract: Fabry disease is a progressive X-linked lysosomal storage disease caused by a mutation in the *GLA* gene, encoding the lysosomal hydrolase α-galactosidase A. The consequent reduced enzyme activity results in the toxic accumulation of glycosphingolipids, particularly globortriaosylceramide (Gb3 or GL_3), in blood vessels, renal epithelia, myocardium, peripheral nervous system, cornea and skin. Neuropathic pain is the most common manifestation of Fabry disease and can be extremely debilitating. This often develops during childhood and presents with episodes of burning and sharp pain in the hands and feet, especially during exercise and it is worse with increased heat or fever. It is thought to be due to ischaemic injury and metabolic failure, leading to the disruption of neuronal membranes and small fibre neuropathy, caused by a reduced density of myelinated Aδ and unmyelinated C-fibres and alterations in the function of ion channels, mediated by Gb3 and lyso Gb3. It is important to confirm small fibre neuropathy before any Fabry disease treatment modality is considered. There is a clinical need for novel techniques for assessing small fibre function to improve detection of small fibre neuropathy and expand the role of available therapies. The current Fabry disease guidelines are in favour of pharmacological management as the first-line treatment for pain associated with Fabry disease. Refractory cases would benefit from a rehabilitation approach with interdisciplinary input, including medical, physiotherapy and psychological disciplines and including a Pain Management Programme.

Keywords: fabry disease; neuropathic pain; depression

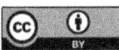

1. Introduction

Fabry (sometimes referred to as Anderson–Fabry) disease is a progressive X-linked lysosomal storage disorder caused by a mutation in the *GLA* gene, encoding the lysosomal hydrolase α-galactosidase A (α-Gal A) [1]. This results in the toxic accumulation of glycosphingolipids, particularly globortriaosylceramide (Gb3 or GL_3), and lyso-Gb3, the decylated form of Gb3 in blood vessels, renal epithelia, myocardium, peripheral nervous system, cornea and skin [1].

The estimated prevalence of Fabry disease is 1:40,000–170,000 [2]. The systemic manifestations of Fabry disease can be divided into early manifestations occurring in childhood and those occurring in a second phase in early adulthood and later life. The implications on organ function are wide ranging and progressive (Table 1).

Table 1. Systemic manifestation of Fabry disease at early and advanced staged of the disease. Early phase systemic manifestations, excluding bradycardia, affect only those with classical Fabry disease [3].

Phase	System Involved	Manifestations
Early Phase	Neurological	Acroparesthesia, Neuropathic-type pain
	Gastrointestinal	Irritable bowel disease like symptoms; diarrhoea, abdominal pain, cramps nausea, vomiting
	Psychological	Behavioural issues Anxiety Depression Vascular dementia
	Ophthalmic	Corneal opacities, corneal verticillata
	Cardiovascular	Bradycardia–T wave inversion increased increased PR interval (other cardiovascular complications unusual in early phase) [2,4,5]
	Autonomic	Hyporhidrosis
	Dermatological	Angiokeratomas corporis diffusum Lymphedema
Second Phase	Ear Nose and Throat	Impaired hearing
	Nephrological	Proteinuria and microalbuminuria
	Reproductive	Azoospermia
	Musculoskeletal	Reduced bone mineral density and disuse atrophy Secondary mitochondrial changes
Late Phase	Cardiac	Diastolic and systolic dysfunction, arrhythmias including atrial fibrillation, atrial flutter and sinus node disease Ischaemia, myocardial fibrosis, left ventricular hypertrophy valvular regurgitation Sudden cardiac death
	Cerebrovascular	White and grey matter changes Transient ischaemic attacks, strokes Vascular dementia

The PR is the interval between the start of the P wave and the start of the QRS complex. A normal interval is between 0.12 s to 0.2 s.

In untreated males, the median life expectancy is approximately 50 years [6,7]. Mortality is related to cardiac hypertrophy, arrhythmias, cerebral infarction and renal failure if renal replacement therapy is not utilised [1].

Pain is a hallmark of classical Fabry disease and is a significant feature particularly within the first two decades of life. This has implications for normal childhood development, academic progress and family life. Pain has a significant impact on both male and female patients and leads to a significant reduction in quality of life compared to the general population. This appears to coincide with depression, anxiety and chronic fatigue in a significant percentage of people living with Fabry disease [8]. Neuropathic pain and Fabry crisis are typical of the classical phenotype of Fabry in males with no residual enzymatic activity, rather than the non-classical phenotype [9].

This review presents the pathophysiology and investigations of pain in adults with Fabry disease, with a focus on the multidisciplinary team (MDT) management of different types of pain.

1.1. Epidemiology of Pain

Acroparesthesiae (neuropathic pain) is the most common manifestation of Fabry disease, occurring in up to 62–80% of classical hemizygous male patients and 30–65.3% of heterozygous female patients [10–12]. Long-term observational studies confirmed that a mean onset of pain is 14.8 years for men and 19.8 years for females [12]. The rate of Fabry-specific small fibre neuropathy has been documented in 78% [13] and 50–75% [14] of females affected with this condition.

Although Fabry disease is an X-linked disorder, it is becoming clearer that heterozygote females develop acroparaesthesiae at rates in excess to that seen in the general population [15,16]. However, a significant heterogeneity among individuals with the same mutation in the *GLA* gene makes it difficult to predict which patients will experience pain [17].

Pain in Fabry disease is dependent on the amount of residual enzymatic activity. Hence, pain is a hallmark of disease in the classical phenotype with no residual enzymatic activity. However, there may be a wide spectrum of phenotypes ranging from classical to later onset type in males [18], and a wide variation in pain experienced by heterozygous female [19]. In females this can occur by two mechanisms. The first being lionisation, whereby a copy of the X chromosome is inactivated during the embryonic stage. The second being X chromosome skewing, where the mutant form is expressed to a high degree in certain key tissues. Hence, variability in pain can occur in females with either of these X-linked inheritance patterns [20–22].

1.2. Types of Pain

Pain often develops during childhood and presents with episodes of burning, sharp, stabbing and shooting pains in the hands and feet, especially during exercise and it is worse with increased heat or fever [23]. Patients often report heat and cold intolerance, intense intermittent pain, hypersensitivity to mechanical stimuli and gastrointestinal pain [17,24].

In females with classic Fabry disease, small nerve fibre dysfunction remains largely restricted to the calf. However, males with classical Fabry disease, show additional involvement of the thigh with disease progression [14,17]. Small fibre neuropathy starts at a distal site at a young age, in both females and males with Fabry disease ascending more proximally only in males with the classical form of the disease at a later stage [14,17].

Evoked pain, triggered by stimuli including brushing, pressure or cold, has been reported in 31–45% of patients [25]. While evoked pain is frequently experienced by Fabry disease patients, pain crises are the most debilitating acute pain experienced by them [17]. Severe episodes of acute limb pain known as 'Fabry crises' can last from minutes to weeks and are thought to be caused by small fibre involvement in peripheral nerves. These crises are thought to be triggered by several factors including exercise, changes in ambient temperature, stress, over exertion, concurrent illness, alcohol and heat [23]. These typically occur distally in the hands and feet with pain and acroparesthesia radiating proximally, as the crisis progresses [17]. Pain crises occur weekly to once a year, lasting minutes to weeks [17].

Significant heterogeneity in thermal and mechanical responses among Fabry disease patients depends on severity and progression of the disease.

Additional information is required to determine whether small fibre neuropathy is Fabry disease related or caused by other conditions giving rise to damage to small nerve fibres. Other symptoms and signs of Fabry disease crises include hypohydrosis, reduced cerebrovascular reactivity and labile blood pressure. Post-prandial abdominal pain with alterations in gastrointestinal motility and early satiety have been also described [23]. Many Fabry patients experience severe gastrointestinal pain, both chronic pain between meals and intermittent pain after eating, that is often followed by diarrhoea, bloating, and early satiety [25].

Chronic pain, lasting over 3 months, is reported by 12–40% of patients and affects joints in the legs, shoulders, back, but also abdomen and head [17,26]. It is unclear whether acute pain progresses into chronic pain over time.

2. Pathophysiology of Pain

The processes involved in the development of pain in Fabry disease are complex and are thought to be mainly neuropathic in nature, due to the involvement of Lyso-globotriaosylceramide (Gb_3) on dorsal root ganglia and the peripheral nervous system which lead to cell swelling [27,28].

Gb3 gradually accumulates within the dorsal root ganglia, causing change in its structure, while peripheral nerve morphology is changed to a minimal degree. Gb3 content within dorsal root ganglia neurons has also been documented ex vivo [28] and has been found to be 10-fold higher than in the brain [27]. Abundant Gb3 deposits were documented in perineurial, endothelial and smooth muscle cells but not within peripheral axons potentially relating to an indirect effect of Gb3 deposits on peripheral nerves causing damage due to vasa nervorum obstruction with a subsequent peripheral nerve ischaemia [29]. Gb3 accumulation was documented in all classical Fabry disease patients, with lower skin innervation as compared to Fabry disease patients with late-onset variants or polymorphisms [30].

In one study, exogenous lyso-Gb3 was administered into dorsal root ganglia, and resulted in an increase in cytoplasmic Ca^{2+} levels within the sensory neurons, suggesting a direct effect of lyso-Gb3 on sensory neuron altering nociception and ultimately pain production [31].

In addition, a decreased blood supply in dorsal root ganglia and a hypoxic environment may result in neuronal apoptosis and/or a decreased microvascular supply of the distal nerve segments [32]. The progressive Gb3 accumulation in dorsal root ganglia was also observable both an α-Gal A mouse model and rat model [33,34].

2.1. Types of Fibres

Fabry disease neuropathy it is largely thought to be due to ischaemic injury and metabolic failure, leading to the disruption of neuronal membranes and small fibre neuropathy caused by a reduced density of myelinated Aδ and unmyelinated C-fibres [35,36]. This leads to impaired temperature and pain transmission. The remarkable small fibre loss is most pronounced in the distal long axons of the lower extremities. The fibre loss has been found to be substantially higher in the skin than in the peripheral nerve trunk [37].

While there is minimal impact on nerve conduction in large-diameter, myelinated Aβ-type fibres, there is impaired function and loss of cutaneous Aδ- and C-sensory neurons [26,38].

Cold sensation can be transmitted through polymodal C-fibres and Aδ thinly myelinated fibres, and harmful heat and gentle touch is transduced though mechanically sensitive C-fibres [39]. Therefore, small fibre neuropathy results in hyposensitivity to warmth, cold and touch. The presence of Fabry-specific small fibre neuropathy features should be obligatory to confirm diagnosis and start therapeutic interventions.

2.2. Ion Channels

Several ion channels have been associated with pain including, voltage-gated sodium, potassium, and calcium channels, transient receptor potential (TRP), acid sensing (ASIC), and hyperpolarisation-activated cyclic nucleotide-gated (HCN) ion channels. In Fabry disease, the slowing of action potential generation from nerve fibres, which is commonly related to sodium channel dysfunction, was not affected, indicating that sodium channel function and expression is normal in C fibres from Fabry disease patients [39,40]. In another study, potassium channel abnormalities and increased sensory neuron depolarisation correlated with pain severity [41].

Further changes in voltage-dependent sodium channel (including Nav1.3, Nav1.8, and Nav1.9) [33,39], voltage-gated potassium channels (including KCNB2) [39,42], voltage-gated calcium channels (including CACNA1H) [31,42], and transient receptor potential (TRP) channels in Fabry rodents (including TRPV1 and TRPA1) [33,42] have been observed in animal models that displayed pain behaviour [43].

2.3. Reduced Perfusion

The characteristic pathophysiological vasculopathy seen in Fabry patients causing an alteration of nitric oxide liberation, leading to an abnormal vascular response and reduced perfusion, could be linked to pain conditions associated with physical stress in Fabry. Politei et al. (2016) suggested that the application of capsaicin cream or lidocaine may reduce physical stress induced pain in Fabry patients [44]. In particular, capsaicin leads to a distinct increase in blood perfusion and thereby could attenuate these specific pain conditions [36,45]. It has also been reported that p75 neurotrophin receptor (p75^{NTR}) plays a critical role in nerve growth factor (NGF)-induced sensitisation of capsaicin-sensitive small-diameter sensory neurons [46,47] and that the majority of capsaicin-responsive neurons respond to globotriasylsphingosine, a deacylated form of Gb3 [31].

2.4. Inflammation

Inflammation has been postulated as a potential pathomechanisms of Fabry disease [48] with NGF being the key molecule mediating pain [49–52]. In experimental studies, treatment with a neutralising antibody against a precursor of NGF (proNGF) or its receptor, p75^{NTR}, led to the improvement in Gb3-induced allodynia [52]. It has been suggested that toxic concentration of Gb3 activates the pain pathway mediated through functional upregulation of proNGF–p75^{NTR} signalling [52].

In addition, in vivo studies have shown involvement of pro-inflammatory cytokine mediators in the immune system, including TNF-alpha, IL-1beta, TLR4, and IL-6, suggesting that pain, apart from being neuropathic, may also encompass inflammatory components [53,54].

2.5. Oxidative Stress

Lysosomes degrade and recycle organelles in a process known as autophagy. The degradation of mitochondria is known as mitophagy. Mitophagy prevents the build-up of reactive oxygen species (ROS) in cells including neurons [25]. The effects of ROS may lead to a reduction in the ability to produce ATP in cells which have a limited scope to increase glycolytic production of ATP. As such, it may not then be possible for the ATP-dependent proton pump to maintain acidity in the lumen of lysosomes, which may have a role to play in neuronal dysfunction and pain in FD [55]. GB3 has been shown to increase the production of ROS in Fabry disease patients. Since this effect is maintained in the plasma of Fabry disease patients despite reductions in intracellular GB3 other factors in the plasma may be contributing to the production of ROS [56].

The effect of GB3 on inflammation and ROS is complex. The intracellular accumulation of GB3 leads to a reauction in eNOS and a concomitant increase in the iNOS, leading to NO production and increased ROS. Furthermore, ROS reduced glutathione (GSH) levels. GSH is the key non-enzymatic antioxidant, which preferentially oxidises key reactive species thus preserving more important biomolecules [57,58].

ROS lead to an alteration in superoxide dismustase:catalase activity ratio (SOD), which is a key antioxidant within mitochondria [55]. Its downregulation may allow for greater ROS effects on the mitochondrial respiratory chain. (MRC) Whilst evidence for the contribution of ROS comes mainly form studies in cardiac cells, vascular endothelium and renal disease, it raises the question as to whether such effects in neuronal cells, are integral to pain in Fabry disease [59].

2.6. Additional Mechanisms

There is some evidence that cholinergic nerve fibre dysfunction contributes to the altered nitric oxide metabolism in Fabry disease [36]. Moreover, a dysfunctional cholinergic response may explain the characteristic general heat intolerance observed in Fabry patients [60], due to its co-regulation in response to whole-body heating [61].

Central sensitisation and altered pain modulation are also likely involved in patients with Fabry disease [44]. Intermittent peripheral neuropathic pain in individuals sensitive to multiple stress factors may sensitise the central neural pain system, resulting in amplification of pain in the body. It has been postulated that central sensitisation of pain may also contribute to fatigue, sleep disorders and mood fluctuations in patients with Fabry disease [44].

Pain in Fabry disease also consists of nociceptive or inflammatory components, as demonstrated by its responsiveness to non-steroidal anti-inflammatory drugs (NSAIDs), in many Fabry disease patients [15–17]. It has been postulated that some of the spontaneous types of pain in patients with Fabry disease may be associated with hyperexcitability of peripheral nociceptive neurons affected by upregulation of sodium ion channels (Nav1.8) [33], TRPV1 [45], or an increase in calcium (Ca^{2+}) influx which is lyso-Gb3 dependent [31].

3. Investigation of Pain

In heterozygote females, in the absence of other manifestations of Fabry disease, confirmation of small fibre neuropathy using insensitive traditional techniques (e.g., quantitative sensory testing, quantitative sudomotor axon reflex test, skin biopsy and assessment of intraepidermal nerve fibre density) is usually required before commencement of enzyme replacement therapy (ERT) or any other treatment modality is considered [44].

The severity of neuropathy closely correlates with plasma levels of Gb3 or its metabolites [35,44]. Unfortunately, small nerve fibre function (A-δ and C-fibres) is difficult to accurately quantify using current techniques (e.g., quantitative sensory testing) as high levels of patient cooperation are required, making it inherently difficult to minimise subjectivity.

The advantage of skin biopsy is its effectiveness in assessing small fibre neuropathy when compared to electromyography and nerve conduction studies. It can be also repeated multiple times to monitor disease progression or treatment efficacy [62].

In such cases, however, it is also likely that improvements in response to ERT or chaperone therapy will be difficult to detect given the level of structural nerve fibre damage that has already occurred.

There is a clinical need for novel techniques for assessing small fibre function to improve detection of small fibre neuropathy and expand the role for the available therapies [35] (Table 2).

Microneurography is a minimally invasive technique which involves using a microelectrode (fine electrical recording needle) to record nerve activity in a superficial nerve [63,64]. The method is technically demanding and lasts many hours hence it is not suitable as a routine diagnostic tool to diagnose small fibre neuropathy. A key advantage of microneurography is the ability to detect different profiles of neural activity corresponding to different subpopulations of sensory neurons and peripheral nociceptors. Microneurography has only been previously performed in some studies of patients with Fabry disease heterozygote females [49]. By detecting evidence of small fibre dysfunction (i.e., hyperexcitability of C-nociceptors) prior to the onset of significant structural nerve damage, microneurography has the potential to improve the ability to detect small fibre neuropathy in patients with Fabry disease and in manifesting heterozygote females. As has been demonstrated for renal and heart disease in Fabry disease, it is thought that improved detection, and hence early treatment, of small fibre neuropathy in patients with Fabry disease and heterozygote females will be associated with improved clinical outcomes, reducing or delaying permanent nerve damage [65].

Table 2. Summary Systematic Guide to diagnosing and investigating the pain in Fabry disease [44].

Investigation of Pain	Diagnostic Cues and Tools
History	Burning pain in hands and feet ('glove and socks' distribution) Pain preventing sporting activities Symmetrical distribution Pain gets worse in high or low temperatures Family history of similar complaints History of pain crisis Pain does not respond to analgesic agents
Differentials	Diabetic polyneuropathy Post-herpetic neuralgia, radicular pain Autoimmune neuropathy Amyloidosis Complex regional pain syndrome Eryromelagia Idiopathic small fibre neuropathy
Neuropathic Pain Screening tools	Neuropathic pain symptom inventory (NPSI) Neuropathic pain questionnaire (NPQ) Doleur neuropathique 4 (DN4) Pain DETECT Leeds assessment of neuropathic signs and symptoms questionnaire (LANNS)
Screening specific to pain	Fabry-specific paediatric health questionnaire (paediatric patients only) Fabry scan questionnaire Wurzburg Fabry pain questionnaire (pain history, character, triggers, impact on quality of life) BPI SF36
Somatosensory Testing Specialist Tests	Quantitative sensory testing Nociceptive evoked potentials Skin biopsy for intraepidermal nerve fibre density nerve conduction studies (to assess for associated carpal tunnel syndrome)
Somatosensory Testing bedside tests	Thermal perception tests Cold perception tests Tests of sensation to pinprick and soft touch Vibration testing

4. Available Therapies for Fabry Disease

The recent development of enzyme replacement therapy (ERT) for Fabry disease has revolutionised outcomes and has become the standard of care in affected patients [66]. Other options include pharmacological chaperone therapy (Migalastat) [67] as well as novel emerging therapies including Lucerastat [67] and gene therapy [68,69].

ERT has been shown to not only prevent major organ complications, but also to reduce neuropathic pain. Although ERT did not impact intra-epidermal nerve fibre density [15], small nerve fibre function improved as a result of ERT [12,70], with differences from baseline detected after 18 months treatment [12].

Whilst pain-related quality of life has been shown to improve in response to ERT, a significant proportion of patients respond incompletely, presumably because of the presence of irreversible nerve damage [71]. In children, ERT has also been shown to have a positive effect on pain [72].

Several studies investigated treatment response to ERT. In one placebo-controlled trial, Gb3 clearance in skin from the back was observed 20 weeks after the initiation of ERT [73]. Another study assessed skin Gb3 under ERT and showed its partial clearance after 3 years of the therapy [74]. However, the study by Uceyler et al. (2014) did not observe any difference in the Gb3 load of patients on ERT compared to treatment naïve group [75].

Migalastat is an oral pharmacological chaperon therapy (daily tablet), which stabilises amenable mutant forms of α-Gal A in the endoplasmic reticulum, thus facilitating passage to the lysosomes and enzymatic breakdown of Gb-3. The pain severity component of the Brief Pain Inventory (BPI) showed that patients had mild pain at baseline and it remained stable over the 18 month treatment period, when patients were treated with Migalastat [76]. Whilst Migalastat shows promise in cardiac outcomes in patients with Fabry disease, its effect on pain and quality of life are still to be determined.

Lucerastat, an iminosugar, is currently under investigation in a phase 3 study of Fabry disease with neuropathic pain as the primary end point (MODIFY study: CLinicalTrials.gov Identifier: NCT03425539).

Gene therapy is the delivery of a therapeutic gene for cellular expression to alter a disease phenotype. Recombinant lentivirus base gene therapy and adeno-associated virus therapy have begun in Fabry disease [69]. Gene editing including repairing disease-related mutant genes may also have a role in slowing the disease progression in Fabry patients in future [69]. Trials on gene therapy in Fabry disease are open for recruitment around the world (ClinicalTrials.gov Identifier: NCT04519749; NCT04046224; NCT04040049; NCT04455230; NCT03454893).

5. Analgesic Agents
Treatment Goals in Fabry Disease

Pain therapy in Fabry disease remains an unmet need. When considering therapeutic goals with respect to pain in Fabry, patients can be divided into two groups, namely, patients with pain and significant associated distress, and those with predominantly neuropathic pain without overt distress. The priority in the first group is to optimise their analgesics and implement holistic support, whilst in the second group a largely medical approach is employed. Patients should be encouraged to adopt pain diaries and the BPI and SF36 (Short form 36) or EQ5D uses as quality of life scores on a 6 monthly basis [44,77].

Despite clarity with respect to therapeutic goals, there appears to be a limited consensus on how best to effectively manage pain in this cohort of Fabry disease patients. Further to recent European recommendations on the pain management in Fabry disease [43], a systematic review by Schuller et.al (2016) analysed 731 articles and found a range of different therapies being offered with no clear guidance [78]. Amalgamating recent expert guidance and our own experience we present an analgesic ladder suitable for Fabry disease [44,77] (Table 3).

Table 3. Analgesic ladder for the treatment of Fabry disease [77,79–82].

Agent	Mechanism of Action	Dose	Side Effects	Cardiac Caveats	Renal Caveats
		First Line			
Tricyclic antidepressant - Amitriptyline - Nortriptyline	5HT and NA reuptake Inhibition. Action on dopaminergic pathways and locus coeruleus.	12.5–150 mg/day	Dry mouth, sedation, arrythmias, urinary retention Diarrhoea, cognitive disturbance, worsening of autonomic instability		Reduce dose in renal impairment
Serotonin and noradrenaline reuptake inhibitors - Duloxetine - Venlafaxine	5HT and NA reuptake Inhibition.	60–120 mg/day 150–225 mg/day	Serotonergic syndrome Gastrointestinal discomfort diarrhoea, anxiety, dizziness	Caution: arrhythmogenic Monitor QTc interval	Reduced dose if eGFR < 30 Reduce dose in renal impairment
Carbamazepine	Reduced Na + channel conductance. Reduction in ectopic discharges.	250–800 mg/day in two divided doses	Associated with blood dyscrasias, Steven's Johnson's syndrome, toxic epidermal necrolysis and hyponatraemia		None
Gabapentin	Inhibit calcium mediated neurotransmitter release through effects on $\alpha_2 \delta$-1 subunits. NMDA receptor antagonism.	Titrated from 100 mg/day to 3600 mg/day in three divided doses	Weight gain, cognitive dysfunction, lethologica		Reduce dose in graduated fashion with renal impairment
Pregabalin	As Gabapentin.	Starting dose 50 mg bd up to 300 mg bd	As Gabapentin		Reduce dose in renal impairment
		Second Line			
Intravenous lidocaine	Local anaesthetic causing sodium channel blockade.	2–5 mg/kg			None
Topical capsaicin	Depletion in substance P.	0.0125% applied topically for 12 h daily	Burning, pruritus		None
Tramadol	Noradrenaline and serotonin reuptake inhibitor. Mu (μ) opioid receptor agonist.	100–400 mg/day	May lower seizure threshold		Caution in renal insufficiency

Table 3. Cont.

Agent	Mechanism of Action	Dose	Side Effects	Cardiac Caveats	Renal Caveats
		Third Line			
Strong opioids Morphine oxycodone	Opioid receptor agonists.	30–120 mg 12 hourly 20–60 mg 12 hourly	Nausea, constipation, itch, respiratory depression, osteoporosis, reduced immunity, endocrine dysfunction		Caution in renal insufficiency
Cannabinoids	Stimulation of CB1 and CB2 receptors, action on serotoninergic receptors.		Decreased appetite, nausea, vomiting, fatigue, mood changes, suicidal ideation		
		Fourth Line			
Methadone	NMDA antagonist activity Noradrenaline reuptake inhibition and mu-opioid receptor agonist.	50 mg BD maximum 500 mg daily	As per strong opioids	Risk of QTc prolongation	
Tapentadol	Sodium channel blockade and supressed release of glutamate.	25 mg once daily for 2 weeks up to 400 mg daily.	Anxiety; anorexia asthenia; diarrhoea; heat or cold intolerance, gastrointestinal discomfort; muscle spasms; sleep disorders; tremor	May cause Brugada syndrome	
Less efficacious anti-convulsants (Lamotrigine)			Aggression; agitation; arthralgia; diarrhoea; dizziness; drowsiness; dry mouth; fatigue; headache; irritability; nausea; pain; rash; sleep disorders; tremor; vomiting		

Gastrointestinal symptoms and abdominal discomfort can be managed with dietetic recommendations regarding meal content, portion sizes and frequency. Nausea and vomiting can be treated with metoclopramide and domperidone, with motilin receptor agonists added in case of severe symptoms [44]. Frequent bowel motions can be managed with loperamide. There is increasing evidence from the phase 3 FACETS trial that Migalastat reduces diarrhoea in patients with Fabry disease [83,84].

A multidisciplinary approach is important when forming an analgesic care plan involving not just metabolic and pain specialists, but also specialist pharmacists, pain psychologists and physiotherapists in the service. The management of pain in Fabry disease is challenging as a result of the unique interplay between a number of factors. Neuropathic pain, which is normally challenging to treat, is combined with a presentation in patients with multiorgan dysfunction, often limiting pharmacological management. In addition, the most severe symptoms are often found in males starting in their youth at a time of great flux in their psychosocial development. Fabry disease may be well recognised within the family unit but poorly recognised and understood by the medical community as a whole.

6. Psychology Support in Pain Management
6.1. Mental Health and Pain in Fabry Disease

High rates of depression have been reported in patients with Fabry disease. Pain is a significant contributory factor to depression [85] and anxiety [8,23]. However, biopsychosocial factors may also contribute to the mood disorder in Fabry disease [86]. Overall, it is estimated that Fabry patients experience higher rates of depression (27–57% of patients) compared to the general population (7–27%) [23,85]. A recent study found that as many as 46% of patients have depression and 28% could be classified as having severe clinical depression [87].

Given the range of developmental, physical, and neurological challenges associated with Fabry disease, its association with depression is unsurprising. However, faced with this context, both patients and clinicians are at risk of viewing such negative psychological associations as an inevitable consequence of Fabry disease. Indeed, this perception is consistent with the finding that the magnitude of decrement in social adaptive functioning correlates with anxiety and depression [60]. However, Laney et al. (2010) also note that in their study, decreased social adaptive functioning was not significantly associated with disease severity, pain, or level of vitality [88]. This finding implies that other variables are involved in the mediation of Fabry disease and negative social, functional, and psychological outcomes. Candidates include modifiable factors such as coping behaviours which can therefore form treatment targets of psychological and rehabilitative approaches, as in other pain conditions, such as chronic low back pain [89].

In Fabry disease, examples of such modifiable factors include behavioural and psychological moderators (such as overexertion and stress) of physical symptoms such as pain. The cognitive model underpinning cognitive behavioural therapy [90] emphasises the role of cognitions (e.g., appraisals, perceptions) in shaping behavioural, emotional and concomitant physiological responses. Psychological intervention with such moderators of symptoms in Fabry disease may therefore involve helping patients to identify and manage environmental, cognitive and emotional factors which can drive unhelpful behaviours such as overexertion; or unhelpful physiological states such as stress.

Psychological treatment in the form of cognitive behavioural therapy has been used in the treatment of anxiety and depression for several decades [91,92], and continues to be a mainstay of treatment presently [93,94]. Similarly, the approach has been shown to be effective in improving psychological status, function, and health outcomes in a range of physical health conditions [95]. Similarly, a recent study, Ali et al. (2018) demonstrated the utility of psychological treatment in improving depression and quality of life in participants with Fabry disease [25].

Depressive symptoms have a significant impact on neuropsychological functioning in up to 16% of patients [96]. Therefore, there is a clinical need for future psychological treatment tailored to coping styles.

6.2. Pain Management Programme

The best evidenced rehabilitation treatment for patients with persistent pain and disability is the group Pain Management Programme. These programmes are an interdisciplinary treatment approach including medical, physiotherapy and psychological input and are based on Cognitive Behavioural Therapy, typically providing around 36 h of rehabilitation treatment [97].

Whilst the majority of patients attending Pain Management Programmes have musculoskeletal pain, the British Pain Society (2013) notes that "a minority have visceral, neuropathic, phantom or central pain, and/or pain from identified disease such as osteoarthritis and rheumatoid arthritis". Therefore, Pain Management Programmes are effectively used in our tertiary Adult Metabolic Centre for patients with Fabry disease.

6.3. MDT in a Tertiary Metabolic Centre

Our model of working with Fabry disease (along with other metabolic conditions) has evolved to encompass joint metabolic and pain clinics, involving both patients and their carers. We see on average 4–5 Fabry patients per joint clinic, the majority of whom are male and with moderate to high psychometric scores. This allows a combination of expertise in metabolic and pain medicine and the involvement of a selected number of the rehabilitative interdisciplinary team, featuring psychologists, pain physiotherapists and occupational therapists.

At our institution, pain in Fabry disease patients is managed in a holistic manner. Adult and transitional patients with pain first have access to the pain clinic in a joint clinic often with parents and carers. As part of this assessment, routine care with involvement of other specialties is initiated and a range of psychometric scores are completed by the patient, to act as a baseline and help inform the next steps in holistic control and management of pain and quality of life. These psychometric scores include, the PHQ-9 score, GAD-7 score, TSK and PCS scores, to assess for depression, anxiety, kinsesiophobia and catastrophisation, respectively. Specific Fabry questionnaires such as the Fabry scan questionnaire may also be employed [25]. This is a 15-item questionnaire with bedside sensory function tests of both small and large fibres. It may help distinguish Fabry disease from other chronic neuropathic pain. Alternatives include the Fabry-specific paediatric pain questionnaire and the Würzburg Fabry pain questionnaire which consists of 22 open questions addressing the four main types of pain in Fabry disease [44]. More generic neuropathic pain questionnaires, such as the Pain DETECT questionnaire may also help establish a baseline but are not validated for Fabry disease.

Physiotherapy and psychology colleagues work collaboratively to address issues such as pacing, exercise and activity medication, passive cooling strategies, sleep hygiene, goal setting, flare up management, confidence, and identity. Pharmaceutical agents are used alongside this where appropriate.

The interdisciplinary team must be mindful of the impact of Fabry disease on educational attainment, marital status, social support and employment which are significantly affected by the effects of the disease [6].

As an example, a 45-year-old female patient with Fabry disease benefited from this treatment at our institution. The preliminary assessment identified that stressors often aggravated her pain symptoms, and this in turn led to avoidance of potentially stressful situations, which then contributed to increased disability. Activity cycling was also a feature. This pattern involves determined efforts to undertake activities, which fuels overexertion and is then followed by an increase in pain and reduction in activities. Treatment goals developed with the Pain Management Programme Team included (i) increasing understanding and effective management of anxiety to reduce the impact of stress on pain, (ii) improved stress management skills to enable a reduction in avoidant coping and thereby to reduce disability, (iii) problem-solving skills to manage work demands and avoid activity cycling, and (iv) improved activity pacing skills to enable a return to leisure activities. Standard physical outcome measures showed significant gains in physical function after the Pain Management Programme. Psychometric outcome measures at 12 months post-programme showed substantial improvements in depression, anxiety, and pain catastrophising.

7. Avoiding Precipitating Factors

In addition it is recommended that activities that may trigger painful crises such as emotional stress, physical exertion and temperature changes are minimised [77].

Patients are advised to monitor when painful crises occur and to try to avoid anything which may precipitate a crisis. Passive cooling strategies can be utilised to improve tolerance to exercise and heat induced pain. Gastrointestinal pain can be managed with smaller meals, low-fat diets and motility agents whilst the use of antianginal agents may also be helpful for ischaemia angina pectoris-related pain.

8. Conclusions

The management of pain in Fabry disease is challenging as a result of the unique interplay between a number of factors. Pain in Fabry disease may affect patients from childhood. Novel techniques in detecting small fibre neuropathy are needed, whilst traditional disease modifying treatments have a limited impact on pain.

Neuropathic pain, which is not normally easy to treat, is further complicated by patients with multiorgan dysfunction, often limiting pharmacological management. In addition, the most severe symptoms are often found in males starting in their youth, at a time of great flux in their psychosocial development.

Ultimately, patients may derive great benefit from interdisciplinary rehabilitation. A multimodal pharmacological approach using a combination of neuropathic agents such as the gabapentinoids and duloxetine may facilitate a reduction in neuropathic pain whilst achieving an opioid-sparing effect. In turn, a reduction in neuropathic pain may also facilitate greater engagement with interdisciplinary rehabilitation to achieve a better quality of life.

Author Contributions: J.N.R., K.M.S., R.J. and K.I. were involved in designing the concept of the review and oversight, contributed to the literature review. All authors contributed to the overall writing and reviewing of the manuscript. All authors have read and agreed to the published version of the manuscript.

Funding: N/AGL3 This research received no external funding.

Institutional Review Board Statement: Not applicable.

Informed Consent Statement: Not applicable.

Data Availability Statement: Data available on request due to restrictions e.g., privacy or ethical. The data presented in this study are available on request from the corresponding author. The data are not publicly available due to protecting the privacy of subjects.

Conflicts of Interest: The authors declare no conflict of interest.

Abbreviations

Abbreviations	
ASIC	Acid-Sensing Ion Channels
BPI	Brief Pain Inventory
ERT	Enzyme Replacement Therapy
GAD-7	Generalised Anxiety Disorder-7
HCN	Hyperpolarisation-Activated Cyclic Nucleotide-Gated
Lyso-Gb3/Lyso-GL3	Globotriaosylsphingosine
NGF	Nerve Growth Factor
NSAIDs	Non-Steroidal Anti-Inflammatory Drugs
PCS	Pain Catastrophising Scale
PHQ-9	Patient Health Questionaire-9
SF-36	Short Form 36
TLR4	Toll-Like Receptor 4
TRP	Transient Receptor Potential
TSK	Tampa Scale of Kinesiophobia

References

1. Brady, R.O.; Gal, A.E.; Bradley, R.M.; Martensson, E.; Warshaw, A.L.; Laster, L. Enzymatic defect in Fabry's disease. *N. Engl. J. Med.* **1967**, *276*, 1163–1167. [CrossRef] [PubMed]
2. Zarate, Y.A.; Hopkin, R.J. Fabry's disease. *Lancet* **2008**, *372*, 1427–1435. [CrossRef]
3. Ortiz, A.; Germain, D.P.; Desnick, R.J.; Politei, J.; Mauer, M.; Burlina, A.; Eng, C.; Hopkin, R.J.; Laney, D.; Linhart, A.; et al. Fabry disease revisited: Management and treatment recommendations for adult patients. *Mol. Genet. Metab.* **2018**, *123*, 416–427. [CrossRef] [PubMed]
4. Seino, Y.; Takahashi, H.; Fukumoto, H.; Utsumi, K.; Hirai, Y. Cardiovascular manifestations of Fabry disease and the novel therapeutic strategies. *J. Nippon. Med. Sch.* **2005**, *72*, 254–261. [CrossRef]
5. Havranek, S.; Linhart, A.; Urbanová, Z.; Ramaswami, U.; Zschocke, J.; Gibson, K.M. Early cardiac changes in children with anderson-fabry disease. *JIMD Rep.* **2013**, *11*, 53–64.
6. MacDermot, K.D.; Holmes, A.; Miners, A.H. Anderson-Fabry disease: Clinical manifestations and impact of disease in a cohort of 60 obligate carrier females. *J. Med. Genet.* **2001**, *38*, 769–775. [CrossRef]
7. Meikle, P.J.; Hopwood, J.J.; Clague, A.E.; Carey, W.F. Prevalence of lysosomal storage disorders. *JAMA* **1999**, *281*, 249–254. [CrossRef]
8. Pihlstrøm, H.K.; Weedon-Fekjær, M.S.; Bjerkely, B.L.; von der Lippe, C.; Ørstavik, K.; Mathisen, P.; Heimdal, K.; Jenssen, T.G.; Dahle, D.O.; Solberg, O.K. Health-related quality of life in Norwegian adults with Fabry disease: Disease severity, pain, fatigue and psychological distress. *JIMD Rep.* **2021**. [CrossRef]
9. Arends, M.; Wanner, C.; Hughes, D.; Mehta, A.; Oder, D.; Watkinson, O.T.; Elliott, P.; Linthorst, G.E.; Wijburg, F.A.; Biegstraaten, M.; et al. Characterization of classical and nonclassical Fabry disease: A multicenter study. *J. Am. Soc. Nephrol.* **2017**, *28*, 1631–1641. [CrossRef] [PubMed]
10. Moller, A.T.; Jensen, T.S. Neurological manifestations in Fabry's disease. *Nat. Clin. Pract. Neurol.* **2007**, *3*, 95–106. [CrossRef]
11. Hoffmann, B.; Beck, M.; Sunder-Plassmann, G.; Borsini, W.; Ricci, R.; Mehta, A. Nature and prevalence of pain in Fabry disease and its response to enzyme replacement therapy—A retrospective analysis from the Fabry Outcome Survey. *Clin. J. Pain.* **2007**, *23*, 535–542. [CrossRef]
12. Hilz, M.J.; Brys, M.; Marthol, H.; Stemper, B.; Dütsch, M. Enzyme replacement therapy improves function of C-, Adelta-, and Abeta-nerve fibers in Fabry neuropathy. *Neurology* **2004**, *62*, 1066–1072. [CrossRef] [PubMed]
13. von Cossel, K.; Muschol, N.; Friedrich, R.E.; Glatzel, M.; Ammer, L.; Lohmöller, B.; Bendszus, M.; Mautner, V.F.; Godel, T. Assessment of small fiber neuropathy in patients carrying the non-classical Fabry variant p.D313Y. *Muscle Nerve* **2021**, *63*, 745–750. [CrossRef] [PubMed]
14. Biegstraaten, M.; Hollak, C.E.; Bakkers, M.; Faber, C.G.; Aerts, J.; van Schaik, I.N. Small fiber neuropathy in Fabry disease. *Mol. Genet. Metab.* **2012**, *106*, 135–141. [CrossRef] [PubMed]
15. Schiffmann, R. Neuropathy and Fabry disease: Pathogenesis and enzyme replacement therapy. *Acta Neurol. Belg.* **2006**, *106*, 61–65. [PubMed]
16. Bouwman, M.G.; Rombach, S.M.; Schenk, E.; Sweeb, A.; Wijburg, F.A.; Hollak, C.E.M.; Linthorst, G.E. Prevalence of symptoms in female Fabry disease patients: A case-control survey. *J. Inherit. Metab. Dis.* **2012**, *35*, 891–898. [CrossRef] [PubMed]
17. Üçeyler, N.; Ganendiran, S.; Kramer, D.; Sommer, C. Characterization of pain in Fabry disease. *Clin. J. Pain* **2014**, *30*, 915–920. [CrossRef] [PubMed]
18. Matern, D.; Gavrilov, D.; Oglesbee, D.; Raymond, K.; Rinaldo, P.; Tortorelli, S. Newborn screening for lysosomal storage disorders. *Semin. Perinatol.* **2015**, *39*, 206–216. [CrossRef]

19. Echevarria, L.; Benistan, K.; Toussaint, A.; Dubourg, O.; Hagege, A.; Eladari, D.; Jabbour, F.; Beldjord, C.; De Mazancourt, P.; Germain, D. X-chromosome inactivation in female patients with Fabry disease. *Clin. Genet.* **2016**, *89*, 44–54. [CrossRef]
20. Germain, D.P. Fabry disease. *Orphanet. J. Rare Dis.* **2010**, *5*, 30. [CrossRef]
21. Lyon, M.F. Gene action in the X-chromosome of the mouse (*Mus musculus* L.). *Nature* **1961**, *190*, 372–373. [CrossRef]
22. Dobyns, W.B.; Filauro, A.; Tomson, B.N.; Chan, A.S.; Ho, A.; Ting, N.T.; Oosterwijk, J.C.; Ober, C. Inheritance of most X-linked traits is not dominant or recessive, just X-linked. *Am. J. Med. Genet. A* **2004**, *129A*, 136–143. [CrossRef]
23. Arends, M.; Körver, S.; Hughes, D.; Mehta, A.; Hollak, C.E.M.; Biegstraaten, M. Phenotype, disease severity and pain are major determinants of quality of life in Fabry disease: Results from a large multicenter cohort study. *J. Inherit. Metab. Dis.* **2018**, *41*, 141–149. [CrossRef]
24. Rickert, V.; Kramer, D.; Schubert, A.-L.; Sommer, C.; Wischmeyer, E.; Üçeyler, N. Globotriaosylceramide-induced reduction of KCa1.1 channel activity and activation of the Notch1 signaling pathway in skin fibroblasts of male Fabry patients with pain. *Exp. Neurol.* **2020**, *324*, 113134. [CrossRef] [PubMed]
25. Ali, N.; Gillespie, S.; Laney, D. Treatment of Depression in Adults with Fabry Disease. *JIMD Rep.* **2018**, *38*, 13–21.
26. Siedler, G.; Káhn, A.-K.; Weidemann, F.; Wanner, C.; Sommer, C.; Üçeyler, N. Dyshidrosis is associated with reduced amplitudes in electrically evoked pain-related potentials in women with Fabry disease. *Clin. Neurophysiol.* **2019**, *130*, 528–536. [CrossRef] [PubMed]
27. Tabira, T.; Goto, I.; Kuroiwa, Y.; Kikuchi, M. Neuropathological and biochemical studies in Fabry's disease. *Acta Neuropathol.* **1974**, *30*, 345–354. [CrossRef]
28. Gadoth, N.; Sandbank, U. Involvement of dorsal root ganglia in Fabry's disease. *J. Med. Genet.* **1983**, *20*, 309–312. [CrossRef]
29. Lacomis, D.; Roeske-Anderson, L.; Mathie, L. Neuropathy and Fabry's disease. *Muscle Nerve* **2005**, *31*, 102–107. [CrossRef]
30. Liguori, R.; Incensi, A.; De Pasqua, S.; Mignani, R.; Fileccia, E.; Santostefano, M.; Biagini, E.; Rapezzi, C.; Palmieri, S.; Romani, I.; et al. Skin globotriaosylceramide 3 deposits are specific to Fabry disease with classical mutations and associated with small fibre neuropathy. *PLoS ONE* **2017**, *12*, e0180581. [CrossRef] [PubMed]
31. Choi, L.; Vernon, J.; Kopach, O.; Minett, M.; Mills, K.; Clayton, P.; Meert, T.; Wood, J. The Fabry disease-associated lipid Lyso-Gb3 enhances voltage-gated calcium currents in sensory neurons and causes pain. *Neurosci. Lett.* **2015**, *594*, 163–168. [CrossRef]
32. Godel, T.; Köhn, A.; Muschol, N.; Kronlage, M.; Schwarz, D.; Kollmer, J.; Heiland, S.; Bendszus, M.; Mautner, V.-F.; Bäumer, P. Dorsal root ganglia in vivo morphometry and perfusion in female patients with Fabry disease. *J. Neurol.* **2018**, *265*, 2723–2729. [CrossRef]
33. Lakoma, J.; Rimondini, R.; Donadio, V.; Liguori, R.; Caprini, M. Pain related channels are differentially expressed in neuronal and non-neuronal cells of glabrous skin of fabry knockout male mice. *PLoS ONE* **2014**, *9*, e108641.
34. Miller, J.J.; Aoki, K.; Moehring, F.; Murphy, C.A.; O'Hara, C.L.; Tiemeyer, M.; Stucky, C.L.; Dahms, N.M. Neuropathic pain in a Fabry disease rat model. *JCI Insight* **2018**, *3*, 1–20. [CrossRef]
35. Üçeyler, N.; Kahn, A.-K.; Kramer, D.; Zeller, D.; Casanova-Molla, J.; Wanner, C.; Weidemann, F.; Katsarava, Z.; Sommer, C. Impaired small fiber conduction in patients with Fabry disease: A neurophysiological case-control study. *BMC Neurol.* **2013**, *13*, 47. [CrossRef] [PubMed]
36. Forstenpointner, J.; Sendel, M.; Moeller, P.; Reimer, M.; Canaan-Kühl, S.; Gaedeke, J.; Rehm, S.; Hüllemann, P.; Gierthmühlen, J.; Baron, R. Bridging the Gap Between Vessels and Nerves in Fabry Disease. *Front. Neurosci.* **2020**, *14*, 448. [CrossRef] [PubMed]
37. Scott, L.J.C.; Griffin, J.W.; Luciano, C.; Barton, N.W.; Banerjee, T.; Crawford, T.; McArthur, J.C.; Tournay, A.; Schiffmann, R. Quantitative analysis of epidermal innervation in Fabry disease. *Neurology* **1999**, *52*, 1249–1254. [CrossRef] [PubMed]
38. Valeriani, M.; Mariotti, P.; Le Pera, D.; Restuccia, D.; De Armas, L.; Maiese, T.; Vigevano, F.; Antuzzi, D.; Zampino, G.; Ricci, R.; et al. Functional assessment of A delta and C fibers in patients with Fabry's disease. *Muscle Nerve* **2004**, *30*, 708–713. [CrossRef]
39. Namer, B.; Ørstavik, K.; Schmidt, R.; Mair, N.; Kleggetveit, I.P.; Zeidler, M.; Martha, T.; Jorum, E.; Schmelz, M.; Kalpachidou, T.; et al. Changes in Ionic Conductance Signature of Nociceptive Neurons Underlying Fabry Disease Phenotype. *Front. Neurol.* **2017**, *8*, 335. [CrossRef]
40. Serra, J.; Campero, M.; Ochoa, J.; Bostock, H. Activity-dependent slowing of conduction differentiates functional subtypes of C fibres innervating human skin. *J. Physiol.* **1999**, *515*, 799–811. [CrossRef] [PubMed]
41. Geevasinga, N.; Tchan, M.; Sillence, D.; Vucic, S. Upregulation of inward rectifying currents and Fabry disease neuropathy. *J. Peripher. Nerv. Syst.* **2012**, *17*, 399–406. [CrossRef]
42. Kummer, K.K.; Kalpachidou, T.; Kress, M.; Langeslag, M. Signatures of Altered Gene Expression in Dorsal Root Ganglia of a Fabry Disease Mouse Model. *Front. Mol. Neurosci.* **2018**, *10*, 449. [CrossRef]
43. Biegstraaten, M.; Arngrímsson, R.; Barbey, F.; Boks, L.; Cecchi, F.; Deegan, P.B.; Feldt-Rasmussen, U.; Geberhiwot, T.; Germain, D.P.; Hendriksz, C.; et al. Recommendations for initiation and cessation of enzyme replacement therapy in patients with Fabry disease: The European Fabry Working Group consensus document. *Orphanet. J. Rare Dis.* **2015**, *10*, 36. [CrossRef] [PubMed]
44. Politei, J.M.; Bouhassira, D.; Germain, D.; Goizet, C.; Sola, A.G.; Hilz, M.J.; Hutton, E.; Karaa, A.; Liguori, R.; Üçeyler, N.; et al. Pain in Fabry Disease: Practical Recommendations for Diagnosis and Treatment. *CNS Neurosci. Ther.* **2016**, *22*, 568–576. [CrossRef] [PubMed]
45. Geber, C.; Fondel, R.; Krämer, H.H.; Rolke, R.; Treede, R.-D.; Sommer, C.; Birklein, F. Psychophysics, flare, and neurosecretory function in human pain models: Capsaicin versus electrically evoked pain. *J. Pain* **2007**, *8*, 503–514. [CrossRef] [PubMed]

46. Zhang, Y.H.; Khanna, R.; Nicol, G.D. Nerve growth factor/p75 neurotrophin receptor-mediated sensitization of rat sensory neurons depends on membrane cholesterol. *Neuroscience* **2013**, *248*, 562–570. [CrossRef]
47. Zhang, Y.H.; Nicol, G.D. NGF-mediated sensitization of the excitability of rat sensory neurons is prevented by a blocking antibody to the p75 neurotrophin receptor. *Neurosci. Lett.* **2004**, *366*, 187–192. [CrossRef]
48. Rozenfeld, P.; Feriozzi, S. Contribution of inflammatory pathways to Fabry disease pathogenesis. *Mol. Genet. Metab.* **2017**, *122*, 19–27. [CrossRef] [PubMed]
49. Aarão, T.L.D.S.; De Sousa, J.R.; Falcão, A.S.C.; Falcão, L.F.M.; Quaresma, J.A.S. Nerve Growth Factor and Pathogenesis of Leprosy: Review and Update. *Front. Immunol.* **2018**, *9*, 939. [CrossRef]
50. McKelvey, L.; Shorten, G.D.; O'Keeffe, G.W. Nerve growth factor-mediated regulation of pain signalling and proposed new intervention strategies in clinical pain management. *J. Neurochem.* **2013**, *124*, 276–289. [CrossRef]
51. Khodorova, A.; Nicol, G.D.; Strichartz, G. The TrkA receptor mediates experimental thermal hyperalgesia produced by nerve growth factor: Modulation by the p75 neurotrophin receptor. *Neuroscience* **2017**, *340*, 384–397. [CrossRef]
52. Sugimoto, J.; Satoyoshi, H.; Takahata, K.; Muraoka, S. Fabry disease-associated globotriaosylceramide induces mechanical allodynia via activation of signaling through proNGF-p75(NTR) but not mature NGF-TrkA. *Eur. J. Pharmacol.* **2021**, *895*, 173882. [CrossRef]
53. Üçeyler, N.; Urlaub, D.; Mayer, C.; Uehlein, S.; Held, M.; Sommer, C. Tumor necrosis factor-alpha links heat and inflammation with Fabry pain. *Mol. Genet. Metab.* **2019**, *127*, 200–206. [CrossRef]
54. De Francesco, P.N.; Mucci, J.M.; Ceci, R.; Fossati, C.A.; Rozenfeld, P.A. Fabry disease peripheral blood immune cells release inflammatory cytokines: Role of globotriaosylceramide. *Mol. Genet. Metab.* **2013**, *109*, 93–99. [CrossRef]
55. Stepien, K.M.; Roncaroli, F.; Turton, N.; Hendriksz, C.J.; Roberts, M.; Heaton, R.A.; Hargreaves, I. Mechanisms of Mitochondrial Dysfunction in Lysosomal Storage Disorders: A review. *J. Clin. Med.* **2020**, *9*, 2596. [CrossRef] [PubMed]
56. Shen, J.-S.; Meng, X.-L.; Moore, D.F.; Quirk, J.M.; Shayman, J.A.; Schiffmann, R.; Kaneski, C.R. Globotriaosylceramide induces oxidative stress and up-regulates cell adhesion molecule expression in Fabry disease endothelial cells. *Mol. Genet. Metab.* **2008**, *95*, 163–168. [CrossRef] [PubMed]
57. Halliwell, B. Reactive species and antioxidants. Redox biology is a fundamental theme of aerobic life. *Plant Physiol.* **2006**, *141*, 312–322. [CrossRef] [PubMed]
58. Biancini, G.B.; Vanzin, C.S.; Rodrigues, D.B.; Deon, M.; Ribas, G.S.; Barschak, A.; Manfredini, V.; Netto, C.B.; Jardim, L.B.; Giugliani, R.; et al. Globotriaosylceramide is correlated with oxidative stress and inflammation in Fabry patients treated with enzyme replacement therapy. *Biochim. Biophys. Acta* **2012**, *1822*, 226–232. [CrossRef] [PubMed]
59. Chung, S.; Son, M.; Chae, Y.; Oh, S.; Koh, E.S.; Kim, Y.K.; Shin, S.J.; Park, C.W.; Jung, S.-C.; Kim, H.-S. Fabry disease exacerbates renal interstitial fibrosis after unilateral ureteral obstruction via impaired autophagy and enhanced apoptosis. *Kidney Res. Clin. Pract.* **2021**, *40*, 208–219. [CrossRef] [PubMed]
60. Mehta, A.; Beck, M.; Eyskens, F.; Feliciani, C.; Kantola, I.; Ramaswami, U.; Rolfs, A.; Rivera, A.; Waldek, S.; Germain, D. Fabry disease: A review of current management strategies. *QJM* **2010**, *103*, 641–659. [CrossRef]
61. Johnson, J.M.; Minson, C.T.; Kellogg, D.L., Jr. Cutaneous vasodilator and vasoconstrictor mechanisms in temperature regulation. *Compr. Physiol.* **2014**, *4*, 33–89. [PubMed]
62. Lauria, G.; Hsieh, S.-T.; Johansson, O.; Kennedy, W.R.; Leger, J.M.; Mellgren, S.I.; Nolano, M.; Merkies, I.S.J.; Polydefkis, M.; Smith, A.G.; et al. European Federation of Neurological Societies/Peripheral Nerve Society Guideline on the use of skin biopsy in the diagnosis of small fiber neuropathy. Report of a joint task force of the European Federation of Neurological Societies and the Peripheral Nerve Society. *Eur. J. Neurol.* **2010**, *17*, 903–912, e44–e49.
63. Serra, J. Re-emerging microneurography. *J. Physiol.* **2009**, *587*, 295–296. [CrossRef]
64. Gasparotti, R.; Padua, L.; Briani, C.; Lauria, G. New technologies for the assessment of neuropathies. *Nat. Rev. Neurol.* **2017**, *13*, 203–216. [CrossRef] [PubMed]
65. Germain, D.P.; Charrow, J.; Desnick, R.J.; Guffon, N.; Kempf, J.; Lachmann, R.; Lemay, R.; Linthorst, G.E.; Packman, S.; Scott, C.R.; et al. Ten-year outcome of enzyme replacement therapy with agalsidase beta in patients with Fabry disease. *J. Med. Genet.* **2015**, *52*, 353–358. [CrossRef] [PubMed]
66. El Dib, R.; Gomaa, H.; Carvalho, R.P.; Camargo, S.E.A.; Bazan, R.; Barretti, P.; Barreto, F.C. Enzyme replacement therapy for Anderson-Fabry disease. *Cochrane Database Syst. Rev.* **2016**, *7*, CD006663. [CrossRef]
67. Nowak, A.; Huynh-Do, U.; Krayenbuehl, P.; Beuschlein, F.; Schiffmann, R.; Barbey, F. Fabry disease genotype, phenotype, and migalastat amenability: Insights from a national cohort. *J. Inherit. Metab. Dis.* **2020**, *43*, 326–333. [CrossRef] [PubMed]
68. Guérard, N.; Oder, D.; Nordbeck, P.; Zwingelstein, C.; Morand, O.; Welford, R.W.; Dingemanse, J.; Wanner, C. Lucerastat, an Iminosugar for Substrate Reduction Therapy: Tolerability, Pharmacodynamics, and Pharmacokinetics in Patients with Fabry Disease on Enzyme Replacement. *Clin. Pharmacol. Ther.* **2018**, *103*, 703–711. [CrossRef]
69. Domm, J.M.; Wootton, S.K.; Medin, J.A.; West, M.L. Gene therapy for Fabry disease: Progress, challenges, and outlooks on gene-editing. *Mol. Genet. Metab.* **2021**. [CrossRef]
70. Schiffmann, R.; Floeter, M.K.; Dambrosia, J.M.; Gupta, S.; Moore, D.F.; Sharabi, Y.; Khurana, R.K.; Brady, R.O. Enzyme replacement therapy improves peripheral nerve and sweat function in Fabry disease. *Muscle Nerve* **2003**, *28*, 703–710. [CrossRef]
71. Burand, A.J., Jr.; Stucky, C.L. Fabry disease pain: Patient and preclinical parallels. *Pain* **2021**, *162*, 1305–1321. [CrossRef] [PubMed]

72. Ramaswami, U.; Wendt, S.; Pintos-Morell, G.; Parini, R.; Whybra, C.; Leal, J.A.L.; Santus, F.; Beck, M. Enzyme replacement therapy with agalsidase alfa in children with Fabry disease. *Acta Paediatr.* **2007**, *96*, 122–127. [CrossRef] [PubMed]
73. Eng, C.M.; Banikazemi, M.; Gordon, R.E.; Goldman, M.; Phelps, R.; Kim, L.; Gass, A.; Winston, J.; Dikman, S.; Fallon, J.T.; et al. A phase 1/2 clinical trial of enzyme replacement in fabry disease: Pharmacokinetic, substrate clearance, and safety studies. *Am. J. Hum. Genet.* **2001**, *68*, 711–722. [CrossRef]
74. Thurberg, B.L.; Byers, H.R.; Granter, S.R.; Phelps, R.G.; Gordon, R.E.; O'Callaghan, M. Monitoring the 3-year efficacy of enzyme replacement therapy in fabry disease by repeated skin biopsies. *J. Investig. Dermatol.* **2004**, *122*, 900–908. [CrossRef]
75. Üçeyler, N.; Schröter, N.; Kafke, W.; Kramer, D.; Wanner, C.; Weidemann, F.; Sommer, C. Skin Globotriaosylceramide 3 Load Is Increased in Men with Advanced Fabry Disease. *PLoS ONE* **2016**, *11*, e0166484. [CrossRef]
76. NICE. *Migalastat for Treating Fabry Disease*; National Institute for Clinical Excellence: London, UK, 2017.
77. Hiwot, D.H.T.; Ramaswami, U. Guidelines for the Treatment of Fabry Disease. 2020. Available online: https://bimdg.org.uk/store/lsd//FabryGuide_LSDSS_Jan2020_700523_11032020.pdf (accessed on 13 September 2021).
78. Schuller, Y.; Linthorst, G.E.; Hollak, C.E.M.; Van Schaik, I.N.; Biegstraaten, M. Pain management strategies for neuropathic pain in Fabry disease—A systematic review. *BMC Neurol.* **2016**, *16*, 25.
79. Chincholkar, M. Analgesic mechanisms of gabapentinoids and effects in experimental pain models: A narrative review. *Br. J. Anaesth.* **2018**, *120*, 1315–1334. [CrossRef]
80. Tremont-Lukats, I.W.; Megeff, C.; Backonja, M.M. Anticonvulsants for neuropathic pain syndromes: Mechanisms of action and place in therapy. *Drugs* **2000**, *60*, 1029–1052. [CrossRef]
81. Obata, H. Analgesic Mechanisms of Antidepressants for Neuropathic Pain. *Int. J. Mol. Sci.* **2017**, *18*, 2483. [CrossRef] [PubMed]
82. Vučković, S.; Srebro, D.; Vujović, K.S.; Vučetić, C.; Prostran, M. Cannabinoids and Pain: New Insights from Old Molecules. *Front. Pharmacol.* **2018**, *9*, 1259. [CrossRef]
83. Germain, D.P.; Nicholls, K.; Giugliani, R.; Bichet, D.G.; Hughes, D.A.; Barisoni, L.M.; Colvin, R.B.; Jennette, J.C.; Skuban, N.; Castelli, J.P.; et al. Efficacy of the pharmacologic chaperone migalastat in a subset of male patients with the classic phenotype of Fabry disease and migalastat-amenable variants: Data from the phase 3 randomized, multicenter, double-blind clinical trial and extension study. *Genet. Med.* **2019**, *21*, 1987–1997. [CrossRef]
84. Schiffmann, R.; Bichet, D.G.; Jovanovic, A.; Hughes, D.A.; Giugliani, R.; Feldt-Rasmussen, U.; Shankar, S.P.; Barisoni, L.; Colvin, R.B.; Jennette, J.C.; et al. Migalastat improves diarrhea in patients with Fabry disease: Clinical-biomarker correlations from the phase 3 FACETS trial. *Orphanet. J. Rare Dis.* **2018**, *13*, 68. [CrossRef]
85. Rosa Neto, N.S.; Bento, J.C.B.; Pereira, R.M.R. Depression, sleep disturbances, pain, disability and quality of LIFE in Brazilian Fabry disease patients. *Mol. Genet. Metab. Rep.* **2020**, *22*, 100547. [CrossRef]
86. Forshaw-Hulme, S.; Gorton, J.; Mcgrae, T.; Thompson, L.; Chen, C.; Roberts, M.; Jovanovic, A.J.; Sharma, R.; Wilcox, G.; Adrees, F.; et al. Understanding the biopsychosocial factors contributing to mental health issues in Fabry disease: One tertiary centre experience. *Mol. Genet. Metab.* **2019**, *129*, S58. [CrossRef]
87. Cole, A.L.; Lee, P.J.; Hughes, D.; Deegan, P.; Waldek, S.; Lachmann, R. Depression in adults with Fabry disease: A common and under-diagnosed problem. *J. Inherit. Metab. Dis.* **2007**, *30*, 943–951. [CrossRef]
88. Laney, D.A.; Gruskin, D.J.; Fernhoff, P.M.; Cubells, J.F.; Ousley, O.Y.; Hipp, H.; Mehta, A.J. Social-adaptive and psychological functioning of patients affected by Fabry disease. *J. Inherit. Metab. Dis.* **2010**, *33*, S73–S81. [CrossRef]
89. Marshall, P.W.M.; Schabrun, S.; Knox, M.F. Physical activity and the mediating effect of fear, depression, anxiety, and catastrophizing on pain related disability in people with chronic low back pain. *PLoS ONE* **2017**, *12*, e0180788. [CrossRef] [PubMed]
90. Winterowd, C.; Beck, A.T.; Gruener, D. Cognitive Therapy with Chronic Pain Patients. *Pain Pract.* **2004**, *4*, 67. [CrossRef]
91. Clark, D.A. *Cognitive Therapy of Anxiety Disorders: Science and Practice*; Guilford Press: New York, NY, USA, 2011.
92. Young, J.E.; Weinberger, A.D.; Beck, A.T. Cognitive Therapy for Depression. In *Clinical Handbook of Psychological Disorders: A Step by Step Treatment Manual*; Guilford Press: New York, NY, USA, 2014.
93. NICE. Depression in Adults: Recognition and Management. 2009. Available online: https://www.nice.org.uk/guidance/cg90 (accessed on 10 September 2021).
94. NICE. Common Mental Health Problems: Identification and Pathways to Care. 2011. Available online: https://www.nice.org.uk/guidance/cg123 (accessed on 3 July 2021).
95. Llewellyn, S.S.P.K. *Handbook of Clinical Health Psychology*; Wiley: Hoboken, NJ, USA, 2003.
96. Körver, S.; Geurtsen, G.J.; Hollak, C.E.M.; Van Schaik, I.N.; Longo, M.G.F.; Lima, M.R.; Vedolin, L.; Dijkgraaf, M.G.W.; Langeveld, M. Depressive symptoms in Fabry disease: The importance of coping, subjective health perception and pain. *Orphanet. J. Rare. Dis.* **2020**, *15*, 28. [CrossRef] [PubMed]
97. The British Pain Society. *Guidelines for Pain Management Programmes for Adults*; The British Pain Society: London, UK, 2013.

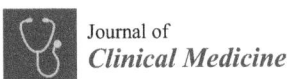

Review

Airway Abnormalities in Adult Mucopolysaccharidosis and Development of Salford Mucopolysaccharidosis Airway Score

Chaitanya Gadepalli [1,*], Karolina M. Stepien [2], Reena Sharma [2], Ana Jovanovic [2], Govind Tol [3] and Andrew Bentley [4]

[1] Ear Nose and Throat Department, Salford Royal NHS Foundation Trust, Manchester M6 8HD, UK
[2] Adult Inherited Metabolic Department, Salford Royal NHS Foundation Trust, Manchester M6 8HD, UK; karolina.stepien@srft.nhs.uk (K.M.S.); reena.sharma@srft.nhs.uk (R.S.); ana.jovanovic@srft.nhs.uk (A.J.)
[3] Anaesthetics Department, Salford Royal NHS Foundation Trust, Manchester M6 8HD, UK; govind.tol@srft.nhs.uk
[4] Intensive Care & Respiratory Medicine, Manchester University NHS Foundation Trust, Wythenshawe Hospital, Manchester M23 9LT, UK; andrew.bentley@mft.nhs.uk
* Correspondence: chaitanya.gadepalli@srft.nhs.uk; Tel.: +44-1612-0647-60

Abstract: (1) Background: Mucopolysaccharidoses (MPS) are a heterogeneous group of lysosomal storage disorders caused by the absence of enzymes required for degradation of glycosaminoglycans (GAGs). GAGs deposition in tissues leads to progressive airway narrowing and/or tortuosity. Increased longevity of patients has posed newer problems, especially the airway. This study aims to characterise various airway abnormalities in adult MPS from a regional centre and proposes a method to quantify the severity of the airway disease. (2) Methods: Retrospective analysis by case notes review, clinical examination, endoscopy, cross-sectional imaging, 3-dimensional reconstruction, and physiological investigations were used to assess the airway abnormalities. Quantitative assessment of the airway severity was performed a validated questionnaire of 15 parameters to derive Salford Mucopolysaccharidosis Airway Score (SMAS). (3) Results: Thirty-one adult MPS patients (21M/ 9F; median 26.7 years; range 19–42 years) were reviewed. There were 9 MPS I, 12 MPS II, 2 MPS III, 5 MPS IV, 2 MPS VI, and 1 MPS VII. Airway abnormalities in each MPS type are described. Patients scoring more than 35 on SMAS had some form of airway intervention. The area under curve of 0.9 was noted at a score of 25, so SMAS more than 25 may predict a difficult airway and potential to have complications. Pearson's correlation between SMAS and height, weight, BMI were poor ($p < 0.05$). (4) Conclusions: Airway abnormalities in adult MPS are varied and complex. Assessment of the airway should be holistic and include multiple parameters. An objective multidimensional score such as SMAS may help to predict and manage difficult airways warranting further investigation and validation.

Keywords: mucopolysaccharidoses; airway; obstruction; management

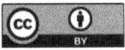

1. Introduction

Mucopolysaccharidoses (MPS) are rare, inherited, lysosomal storage diseases with a combined incidence of 1 in 22,000 [1]. Lysosomal hydrolase enzyme deficiencies result in accumulation of glycosaminoglycans (GAGs), leading to structural abnormalities and organ dysfunction that can increase the risk of anaesthesia complications [2]. Depending on the type of MPS, glycosaminoglycan accumulations can occur in various organs, resulting in cardiovascular, pulmonary, gastrointestinal, neurologic, and musculoskeletal dysfunction (Table 1) [3]. MPS can be grouped into four broad categories according to their dominant clinical features: (1) MPS I, II, and VII affect soft tissue storage and the skeleton with or without intracranial involvement; (2) MPS VI affects both soft tissues and the skeleton; (3) MPS IVA and IVB are primarily associated with skeletal disorders; and (4) MPS III A–D primarily affects the central nervous system [4].

Table 1. Various types of MPS; reproduced with permission from Braunlin et al. [5], who compiled data from Neufeld et al. [2] and Valayannopoulos et al. [6].

MPS Type (Eponym)	Incidence per 10^5 Live Births; Inheritance Pattern	Typical Age at Diagnosis	Typical Life Expectancy If Untreated	Enzyme Deficiency	GAG
MPS I Hurler (H) MPS I Hurler–Scheie (H-S) MPS I Scheie (S)	0.11–1.67; AR	H: <1 year H-S: 3–8 years S: 10–20 years	H: death in childhood H-S: death in teens or early adulthood S: normal to slightly reduced lifespan	α-L-iduronidase	DS, HS
MPS II (Hunter)	0.1–1.07; XR	1–2 years when rapidly progressing	rapidly progressing: death < 15 years slowly progressing: death in adulthood	iduronate-2-sulfatase	DS, HS
MPS III (Sanfilippo) A-B-C-D	0.39–1.89; AR	4–6 years	death in puberty or early adulthood	heparan sulfamidase (A) N-acetyl-α-D-glucosaminidase (B) acetyl-CoA-α-glucosaminidase N-acetyltransferase (C) N-acetylglucosamine-6-sulfatase (D)	HS
MPS IV (Morquio) A-B	0.15–0.47; AR	1–3 years	death in childhood- middle age	N-acetylgalactosamine-6-sulfatase (A) β-galactosidase (B)	CS, KS (A) KS (B)
MPS VI (Maroteaux-Lamy)	0–0.38; AR	rapidly progressing: 1–9 years slowly progressing: >5 years	rapidly progressing: death in 2nd–3rd decade slowly progressing: death in 4–5th decade	N-acetylgalactosamine-4-sulfatase	DS
tblMPS VII (Sly)	0–0.29; AR	neonatal to adulthood	death in infancy- 4th decade **	β-D-glucuronidase	CS, DS, HS
MPS IX (Natowicz) *	unknown	adolescence	unknown	hyaluronidase	CS

AR—autosomal recessive, CS—chondroitin sulphate, DS—dermatan sulphate, GAG—glycosaminoglycan, H—Hurler syndrome, HS—heparan sulphate, H-S—Hurler-Scheie syndrome, KS—keratan sulphate, S—Scheie syndrome, XR—X-linked recessive. * Only 1 patient reported in literature (Natowicz et al. 1996); ** death can occur in utero with hydrops fetalis.

GAG accumulation in the upper airway results in hypertrophy of soft tissues, including adenoids, tonsils, tongue, and laryngopharynx, which may all cause airway problems and pose difficulty in anaesthetic airway management due to bulky airways. This is especially important because MPS patients frequently require surgical interventions requiring anaesthesia [4]. Airway complications are a common feature of MPS I, II, IV, and VI and considerably contribute to morbidity and premature mortality [7,8]. The bulky airways can predispose to breathing related problems, which may worsen during sleep. These include snoring, upper airway resistance syndrome, obstructive sleep apnoea [9]. A multidimensional assessment by Dalewski et al. [10], which incorporates modified Mallampati score [11], upper airway volume measurements using CT scan, Berlin questionnaire [12], is useful. Measures of airway obstruction and pulmonary function have frequently been used as primary or secondary outcomes in interventional trials [3,13–15]. Current therapeutic modalities, such as enzyme replacement therapy (ERT) in MPS I Hurler–Scheie (HS) and Scheie, II, IVA, and VI, and haemopoietic stem cell transplantation (HSCT) in MPS I Hurler (H), have demonstrated organ specific and systemic metabolic correction [16–19]. Despite the positive outcomes, airway disease continues to cause significant complications resulting from structural rather than inflammatory abnormalities [20–22]. Current treatment with ERT fails to fully reverse adenotonsillar storage pathology in MPS type I, III, IV, and VI, manifesting with ongoing clinical disease [21]. It has been previously shown that pathological changes in tonsils and adenoids are responsible for not only the increased incidence of hypertrophy causing obstruction, but also the high regrowth rate in adenoid tissue commonly necessitating revision surgery later in adolescence and possibly adulthood [20,21]. Airway problems in MPS are multifactorial as evidenced by limited relief from adenotonsillectomy [8]. By the time an MPS patient has transitioned from paediatric to adult care, issues such as adenoids and tonsils may have already been addressed, and the airway problems shift towards other aspects of upper and lower airways.

We aim to evaluate and characterise airway abnormalities in adult MPS patients. The purpose of this study is to identify various airway abnormalities in our cohort of adult MPS and quantify the degree of airway problems for prognosis and planning. We have used various parameters that can adversely affect the airway and developed Salford MPS Airway Score (SMAS) as a novel tool in assessing the severity of airway disease in adult MPS disorders.

2. Materials and Methods

2.1. Study Design

Retrospective review of case notes of adult MPS patients attending airway assessment was performed. Ethical approval from the Research and Innovation department, Salford Royal NHS Foundation Trust, Northern Care Alliance NHS, United Kingdom was obtained, reference: S20HIP40.

2.2. Patients

All patients were assessed in airway multi-disciplinary team clinic by the same anaesthetic and ear, nose, and throat consultant with special interest in adult MPS airways. In our cohort, the specific modalities of treatment for MPS patients were enzyme replacement therapy (ERT), haematopoietic stem cell transplant (HSCT), or none.

2.3. Assessment

Apart from clinical examination, investigative tools such as nasendoscopy, computer tomography scans, pulmonary function tests, three-dimensional imaging, and virtual endoscopy were sought where possible. Nasendoscopy is performed by passing a fibre optic camera via the nasal cavity and examination of the nasal cavities, oropharynx, and larynx under a local anaesthetic.

2.4. SMAS

Fifteen parameters were chosen that can holistically assess both upper and lower airway. The parameters and method to calculate the SMAS are depicted in Table 2. Each of these parameters are graded in an ordinal score from zero to three: zero corresponding to normal, one—mild abnormality, two—moderate abnormality, and three—severe abnormality. Adding the score for each of the 15 parameters will provide a final score, which will quantify the degree of airway severity. A high score corresponds to a complex airway. The range of the score can be from 0 to 45. Parameters one to six are calculated using clinical examination. Protrusion of teeth and bulkiness of the tongue can be assessed on clinical examination and CT scans. Parameters 7 to 10 are calculated using nasendoscopy. Parameters 11 to 13 are calculated using cross-sectional imaging such as CT scans. Parameters 14 and 15 are calculated using pulmonary function tests. Certain parameters such as pulmonary function tests cannot be carried out in patients who lack capacity or would not comply with the assessment. Likewise, nasendoscopy cannot be carried without a patient's co-operation. This will limit the maximal score that can be attained. The content, criterion validity, and clinical use of the questionnaire was assessed by distributing the questionnaire to 15 senior anaesthetists to be used in their daily practice. To assess the impact of body habitus on the airway, Pearson's correlation was used to assess the relationship between height, weight, body mass index, and SMAS. To assess the usefulness of the SMAS score in clinical application, a receiver operating curve (ROC) curve was plotted.

Table 2. Salford Mucopolysaccharidosis Airway Score (SMAS).

S. No.	Parameter	Measure	Score	Final Score
1	MPS Type Mouth opening	>5 cm	0	
		4–5 cm	1	
		3–4 cm	2	
		<3 cm	3	
2	Teeth protrusion on clinical exam and scans	Non-protruding	0	
		Mild	1	
		Moderate	2	
		Severe	3	
3	Cervical spine mobility, stability	unrestricted	0	
		60–90 degrees flexion	1	
		30–60 degrees flexion	2	
		<30 degrees or unstable	3	
4	Tongue bulkiness on examination and Scan	Normal	0	
		Mild (filling less than 1/3 of floor mouth)	1	
		Moderate (filling 1/3 to 1/2 of oral cavity)	2	
		Severe (filling more than 1/2 of oral cavity)	3	
5	Modified Mallampati grade [11]	1	0	
		2	1	
		3	2	
		4	3	
6	Thyromental distance	>6 cm	0	
		5–6 cm	1	
		4–5 cm	2	
		<4 cm	3	
7	Larynx height epiglottis to soft palate	>4 cm	0	
		3–4 cm	1	
		2–3 cm	2	
		<2 cm	3	
8	Epiglottis bulkiness	Normal (filling less than 1/3 of oropharynx)	0	
		Mild (filling 1/3 to 1/2 of oropharynx)	1	
		Moderate (filling 1/2 to complete oropharynx)	2	
		Severe (Filling entire oropharynx)	3	
9	Supraglottis bulkiness	Normal (filling less than 1/3 of laryngopharynx)	0	
		Mild (filling 1/3 to 1/2 of laryngopharynx)	1	
		Moderate (filling $\frac{1}{2}$ to complete laryngopharynx)	2	
		Severe (filling entire oropharynx)	3	
10	Glottis bulkiness	Normal (filling less than 1/3 of glottis)	0	
		Mild (filling 1/3 to 1/2 of glottis)	1	
		Moderate (filling 1/2 to complete glottis)	2	
		Severe (filling entire glottis)	3	
11	Subglottis diameter at cricoid level	>7 mm	0	
		6–7 mm	1	
		5–6 mm	2	
		<5 mm	3	

Table 2. Cont.

S. No.	Parameter	Measure	Score	Final Score
12	Tracheomalacia or tracheal stenosis (degree of narrowing)	No narrowing	0	
		50–75% lumen narrowing	1	
		75–99% lumen narrowing	2	
		100% lumen narrowing	3	
13	Tracheal tortuosity	None	0	
		present	3	
14	FEV1%	>80%	0	
		60–79%	1	
		40–59%	2	
		<40%	3	
15	FVC%	>80%	0	
		60–79%	1	
		40–59%	2	
		<40%	3	

3. Results

Thirty-one adult MPS patients were reviewed, there were 21 males and 10 females. The age range was 19–43 years. The mean age was 28 years, and the median age was 26.7 years. Table 3 shows the demographics in each type of MPS.

Table 3. Demographics of all adult MPS patients.

MPS Type	Number	Age in Years and Number of Patients	Sex
1	9	23–27 = 5 31–32 = 2 39 = 1 43 = 1	Females = 3 Males = 6
2	12	20–27 = 7 29–33 = 5	All males
3	2	19–21 = 2	Both females
4	5	19, 21, 23, 33, 41	Females = 4 Male = 1
6	2	27, 38	Female = 1, Male = 1
7	1	31	Male

Various airway abnormalities were noted in the MPS patients. The modified Mallampati grade was either three or four in all patients. There was a pattern of macroglossia, high larynx, and large epiglottis noted in almost all patients in the cohort. MPS I and MPS III had the least severe airway abnormalities. In both these groups, learning difficulties and/or blindness was a relevant challenge. Common airway abnormalities and relevant airway challenges in each type of MPS are depicted in Table 4.

3.1. Nasendoscopy

This outpatient procedure helped us to assess which nasal cavity was wider to plan nasal intubation, assess the height and bulk of epiglottis, bulk of posterior two-thirds of the tongue, appearance of supraglottis, and vocal cord mobility. It also provided information on oropharyngeal or supraglottic collapse on valsalva manoeuvre. A bulky supraglottis made use of supraglottic airway devices such as laryngeal mask airway or trans nasal humidified rapid insufflation ventilatory exchange (THRIVE) difficult. Figures 1–4 shows a nasendoscopy appearances in various types of MPS.

Table 4. Common airway abnormalities and relevant airway challenges in each type of adult MPS.

MPS Type	Airway Findings	Relevant Airway Challenges
1	Protruding teeth, large tongue, high larynx, moderately bulky supraglottis, narrow subglottis	Learning difficulties, poor vision
2	Protruding teeth, large tongue, high larynx, very bulky supraglottis, narrow subglottis, tracheobronchomalacia	Cervical spine instability, short neck
3	Large tongue, malacia of supraglottis	Learning difficulties
4	Large tongue, protruding teeth, large jaw, moderately bulky supraglottis, large epiglottis, tortuous trachea with tracheomalacia	Short neck, hypermobility
6	Large tongue, protruding teeth, large jaw, large epiglottis, tortuous trachea with tracheomalacia	Short neck, c-spine problems, kyphoscoliosis
7	Slightly protruding teeth, high larynx, narrow subglottis, tortuous trachea	Kyphoscoliosis

MPS—mucopolysacharridosis.

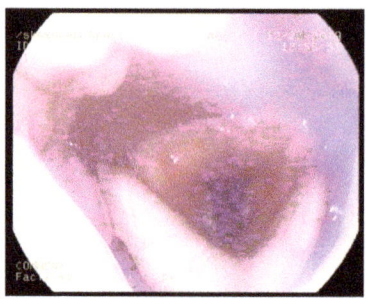

Figure 1. High anterior larynx in mucopolysacharridosis I.

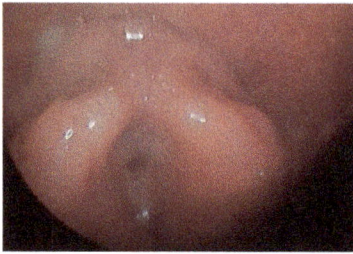

Figure 2. Bulky supraglottis in mucopolysacharridosis II.

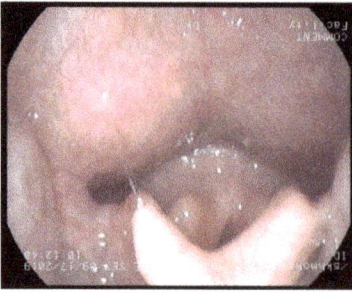

Figure 3. Large overhanging epiglottis, high larynx in mucopolysacharridosis IV.

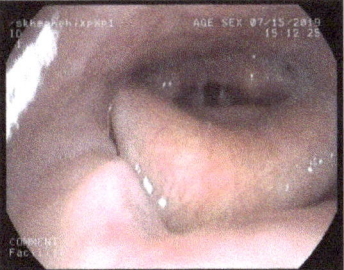

Figure 4. Large epiglottis almost touching soft palate in mucopolysacharridosis VI.

3.2. Cross-Sectional Imaging

Computer tomography (CT) and magnetic resonance imaging (MRI) are very helpful in assessing both upper and lower airway. In the upper airway, the bulky soft tissue of the tongue and supraglottis can be assessed using MRI scans. In the lower airway, the calibre of the airway, tracheomalacia, tracheal stenosis, and tracheal tortuosity can be assessed using CT scans. Figures 5–8 shows cross-sectional imaging in various types of MPS.

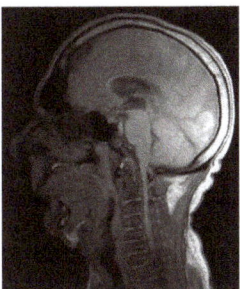

Figure 5. MRI scan of MPS I showing large tongue and high, anterior larynx, and absence of cervical lordosis.

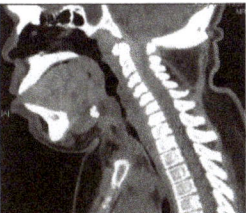

Figure 6. CT scan of MPS II, showing large bulky tongue, flat palate, prominent teeth, short neck, and absence of cervical lordosis.

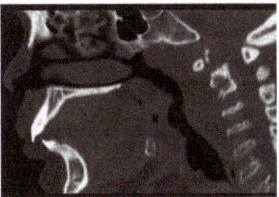

Figure 7. CT scan of MPS IV showing contracted nasopharynx, large tongue, prominent teeth, and high larynx.

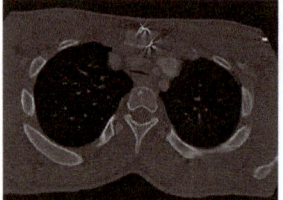

Figure 8. CT scan of MPS II showing collapsed trachea, suggestive of tracheomalacia.

3.3. 3-Dimensional Reconstruction (3D) and Virtual Endoscopy (VE)

Using information from the cross-sectional imaging, 3-dimensional reconstruction and virtual endoscopy of the airway can be performed. Figures 9–13 shows 3D appearances in various types of MPS.

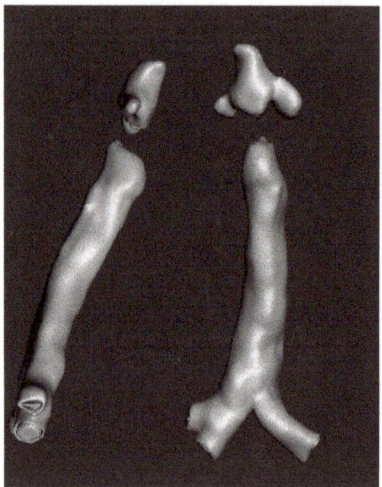

Figure 9. 3-Dimensional reconstruction of MPS I showing normal trachea.

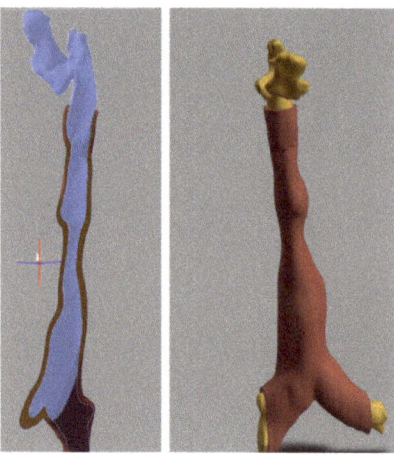

Figure 10. 3-Dimensional reconstruction of MPS II showing tracheomalacia.

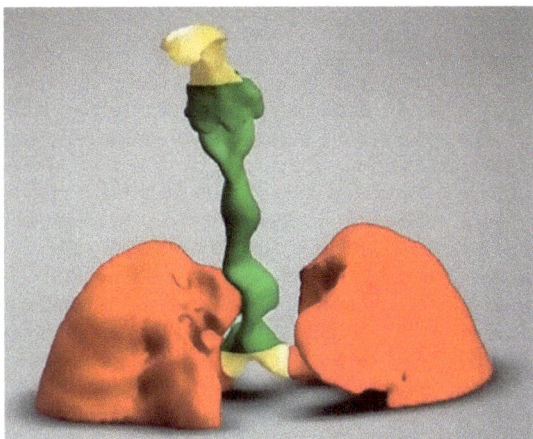

Figure 11. 3-Dimensional reconstruction of MPS IV showing tortuous trachea and tracheomalacia.

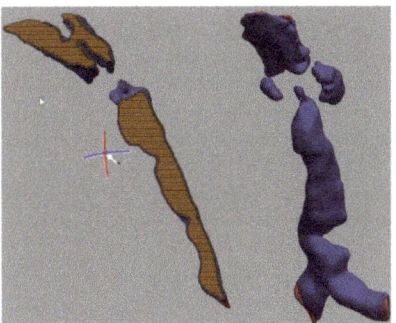

Figure 12. 3-Dimensional reconstruction of MPS VI showing tortuous trachea and tracheomalacia.

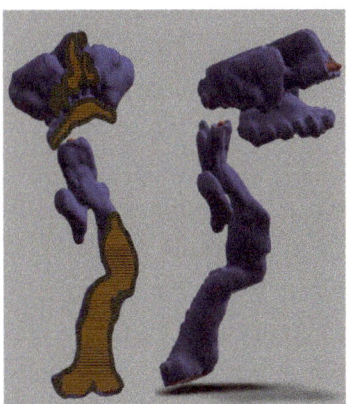

Figure 13. 3-Dimensional reconstruction of MPS VII showing tortuous trachea and tracheomalacia.

3.4. Salford Mucopolysaccharidosis Airway Score (SMAS)

The questionnaire looked at various aspects of the airway. Questions 1–10 in Table 2 reflect the upper airway, which is access. Questions 11–13 reflect mid airway, and questions 14 and 15 reflect the lower airways, which is the lung physiological functions.

Validation and Usefulness of SMAS

The scores were distributed to 25 senior anaesthetists in a tertiary hospital and were asked to use it in their daily practice. All the anaesthetists were requested to fill a questionnaire (Appendix A) that addressed content, criterion validity, and internal consistency. Following responses from the anaesthetic colleagues, we felt comfortable to use this in our study.

All the 15 parameters were used in 21 patients. In four patients (MPS I = 1, MPS II = 1, MPS III = 2) pulmonary functions could not be done due to learning difficulties. In six patients (MPS I = 1, MPS II = 2, MPS IV = 2, MPS VII = 1), pulmonary functions were not considered as they were more than one year old. In the MPS III group (n = 2), cross-sectional imaging, 3D, and VE were not performed as they had no clinical symptoms of airway problems so they could only be assessed for 10 parameters. Table 5 summarises SMAS scores and percentages for all 31 adult MPS patients. It can be deduced that scores 0–15 (33%) correspond to mild airway abnormality, 15–30 (33–66.7%) to moderate abnormality, and 30–45 (66.8–100%) to severe abnormality. It was noted that patients in MPS II, MPS IV, and MPS VI groups have high scores. Patients who have scored more than 35 have had some form of airway intervention. Patient number 10, 14, and 30 needed tracheostomy to improve breathing. Patient number 11, 24, and 26 needed hospital admission for difficulty in breathing following a viral infection. All patients scoring more than 25 had obstructive sleep apnoea. Hypothetically, we can say that a score more than 25 should be considered a difficult airway and may have potential complications. To assess the sensitivity of this hypothesis, the receiver operating characteristic (ROC) was calculated. Patients who needed any airway intervention was the measurable outcome and the SMAS being the predictor. The sensitivity at score 25 is 1 and 0.9 at score 26. Figure 14 shows the ROC curve.

Table 5. Summary of the SMAS scores for all patients, mutation type, and therapy.

Patient Number	MPS Type	Sex	Age in Years	SMAS	Score Percentage	Associated Abnormality	Therapy	Mutation
1	I	M	39.1	20	51.3		HSCT	p.(Trp402Ter), p.(Leu218Pro)
2	I	M	31.3	15	33.3		HSCT	p.(Leu490Pro), p.(Leu490Pro)
3	I	M	25.9	23	51.1		HSCT	p.(Trp402Ter), p.(Trp402Ter)
4	I	M	25.7	10	22.2		HSCT	p.(Gln70Ter), p.(Gln70Ter)
5	I	M	32.2	24	53.3		HSCT	p.(Trp402Ter), p.(Ser633Leu)
6	I	M	26.7	31	68.9	OSA	ERT	hom L490P, exon 10 IDUA gene
7	I	F	23.0	10	22.2		ERT	N/A
8	I	F	43.0	29	64.4	OSA	ERT	N/A
9	I	F	24.0	20	48.7		ERT	N/A
10	II	M	30.1	40	88.9	TRACH	ERT	c.1152delT, exon 8 IDS gene
11	II	M	31.7	36	80	OSA	ERT	N/A
12	II	M	29.1	35	77.8	OSA	ERT	N/A
13	II	M	20.7	32	82.1	OSA	ERT	c.1528insT
14	II	M	33.0	40	88.9	TRACH	ERT STOPPED	N/A
15	II	M	32.9	34	75.6	OSA	ERT	N/A
16	II	M	25.2	32	82.1	OSA	ERT	N/A

Table 5. Cont.

Patient Number	MPS Type	Sex	Age in Years	SMAS	Score Percentage	Associated Abnormality	Therapy	Mutation
17	II	M	26.3	11	24.4		ERT	T14gT, exon4 IDS gene
18	II	M	23.7	21	46.7		ERT	N/A
19	II	M	20.9	31	79.5	OSA	ERT	N/A
20	II	M	26.9	29	64.4	OSA	ERT	missense mutation in N63D, exon 2, IDS gene
21	II	M	23.3	14	31.1		ERT	N/A
22	III	F	19.6	9	30		none	N/A
23	III	F	20.3	2	6.7		none	hom c.234+1G>T, HGSNAT gene
24	IV	F	23.0	32	82.1	OSA	none	N/A
25	IV	F	21.1	28	71.7	OSA	ERT?	N/A
26	IV	F	41.1	38	84.4	OSA	ERT STOPPED	hom c.871G>A p.(Ala291Thr) GALNS gene
27	IV	M	33.5	27	60	OSA	none	N/A
28	IV	M	19.3	26	57.8	OSA	ERT	N/A
29	VI	F	27.3	30	66.7	OSA	ERT	T442R/245delT
30	VI	M	38.1	41	91.1	TRACH	ERT paused	N/A
31	VII	M	31.0	16	41.1		none	c.526C>T p.(Leu176Phe), c.1820G>C p.(Gly607Ala)

MPS—mucopolysacharridosis, M—male, F—female, HSCT—haematopoetic stem cell transplantation, ERT—enzyme replacement therapy, SMAS—Salford Metabolic Airway Score, TRACH—tracheostomy, OSA—obstructive sleep apnoea.

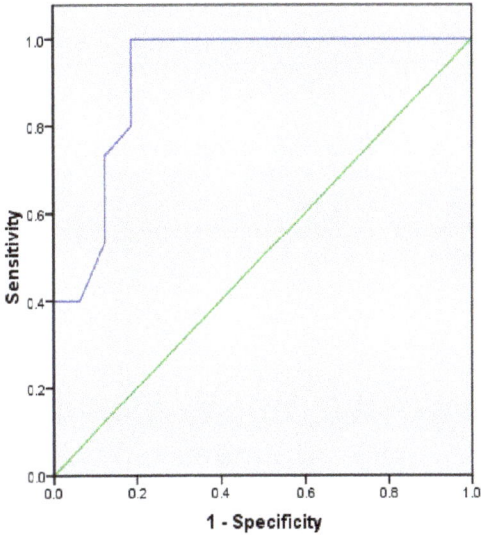

Figure 14. ROC curve to assess usefulness of SMAS as a predictor of complex airway.

ROC—receiver operating characteristic, SMAS—Salford Mucopolysaccharidosis Airway Score.

It could be argued that a bulky airway may be secondary to body habitus. So Pearson's correlation was used to assess the impact of height and body mass index on SMAS. It was noted that there was no statistically significant correlation noted. Table 6 summarises the correlation values.

Table 6. Pearson's correlation between Salford Metabolic Airway Score and height, weight, and body mass index.

Subtitle	Subtitle	Total Score
Height	Correlation coefficient	−0.438
	p-value	0.014
Weight	Correlation coefficient	−0.168
	p-value	0.367
Body Mass Index	Correlation coefficient	0.340
	p-value	0.061

4. Discussion

Holistic assessment of a difficult airway is key to successful management. It is important to assess and identify various abnormalities in a difficult airway; failure to identify these and failure to act on abnormal findings in the management of difficult airway can lead to poor outcomes [23]. The airway in MPS patients has a complex anatomy due to MPS deposits, skeletal, and soft tissue abnormalities. Adult MPS airway is complicated not just by age-related changes on the soft tissue and skeletal structures but also due to associated comorbidities. All the patients in our cohort had short stature, short necks, and restricted neck mobility, making access to the airway difficult. Large lower jaw in the MPS IV and MPS VI groups made access to the larynx difficult. The American Society of Anesthesiologists (ASA) [24] has considered the following outcomes as difficult airway—difficult facemask ventilation, difficult laryngoscopy, difficult tracheal intubation, failed intubation, and difficulty in placing and using supraglottic devices. In our experience, we have observed all of these in our adult MPS cohort in some form or other; all patients needed a smaller sized tube. We have found use of the microcuffed endotracheal tube produced by Avanos® very useful in adult MPS airways. All of the difficult airway parameters pointed by ASA were noted in our MPS II group. MPS I tolerated supraglottic airway device, as the supraglottis was not bulky. In MPS IV and MPS VI groups, use of the supraglottic airway device was not considered due to large epiglottis and high anterior larynx. Roth et al. [25] reviewed 133 studies involving 844,206 participants to assess the diagnostic accuracy bedside tests for assessment of difficult airway. The common bedside tests to assess the difficult airway include Mallampati score [26], modified Mallampati score [11], Wilson score [27], thyromental distance, sternomental distance, mouth opening, and upper lip bite.

There is no one perfect tool for airway assessment; however, a combination of various tools is a better predictor of complex airway, and this is better than a single test used in isolation [28]. Cattano et al. [29] addressed the impact airway assessment by using 11 ASA's airway risk factors by residents. The authors observed there was a better documentation of difficult airway but did not significantly impact the assessment of difficult airways. However, in the study group, there were only 17% of patients with difficult airways. It is not clear from the paper if the group had patients with a background of metabolic diseases, and the study used only bedside tests. By contrast, our group includes all patients with difficult airways with multiple comorbidities. In this new SMAS score developed by our team, not all parameters can be assessed in all patients, such as nasendoscopy and spirometry, which need the patient's co-operation. This was the case in some MPS I and both MPS III patients with learning difficulties. In the same way, if the patient did not have any breathing or respiratory issues, such as MPS III, performing investigations will add undue discomfort to the patient. So, they should be only considered if the investigations change the way we manage our patients. Cross-sectional imaging using CT or MR scans are very useful. We have found assessment of the supraglottis is better with an MRI scan, as it shows the soft tissues better. The infraglottis, trachea, and lungs are better assessed by CT scans, as they show cartilaginous structures better and help in assessing the airway calibre, tortuosity, and malacia. Studies by Wittenborg et al. [30] in the 1960s suggested that a decrease in the diameter of 50% of the lumen of the trachea should be considered tracheomalacia. Tracheomalacia can be classified according to the reduction tracheal lumen into mild (50–75%), moderate (75–100%), and severe (100%), which is complete collapse [31].

Boiselle et al. [32] showed that tracheal collapse can be noted in expiration in healthy population; hence, tracheomalacia should be diagnosed in conjunction with clinical symptoms, signs, and lung functions. Although a CT scan may indicate changes suggestive of tracheomalacia, a dynamic expiratory CT scan demonstrates malacia better [33]. In our cohort of patients, tracheomalacia was also noted in CT scans taken in inspiration; hence, the actual problem of tracheomalacia in adult MPS may be underestimated. Symptomatic tracheomalacia can be conservatively managed by airway splinting using continuous positive air way pressure and surgically treated by stenting inside or outside the lumen of trachea, tracheostomy, and resection of the diseased segment of trachea [34] and tracheopexy [35]. Extrinsic compression of trachea by an anomalous innominate artery in a 16-year-old male with MPS IVa has been reported by Pizarro et al. [36]. The authors describe the surgical technique of tracheal and vascular reconstruction and have reported successful outcome without the need for tracheostomy. Any extensive thoracic surgery has to be carefully considered in adult MPS due to chest wall deformities, difficult airways, and associated comorbidities. Given the progressive nature of the disease, we managed our patients with a tracheostomy and positive pressure non-invasive ventilation rather than stenting and surgical splinting of the airway. We found the Bivona® uncuffed adult tracheostomy tube from Smith medical® very useful in our MPS II patient (patient number 14) with tracheomalacia. In one of our MPS VI patients (patient number 30), we managed tracheomalacia with tracheostomy and the paediatric Montgomery® Safe-T-Tube™. The indication for tracheostomy in both these patients was worsening upper and lower airway obstruction, leading to obstructive sleep apnoea and dyspnoea at rest with resultant worsening quality of life. Tracheostomy was performed under a general anaesthetic following the securing of the upper airway with an endotracheal tube. Recovery following the tracheostomy in both these patients was protracted. Both were discharged following tracheostoma. There were no immediate complications, but stoma granulations were delayed complications needing topical corticosteroid ointments.

Respiratory function testing using spirometry is very useful in quantifying the lung physiology. However, obtaining a normalised value for the MPS patients will be difficult and will have to be interpreted carefully. Input from a respiratory physician with special interest in pulmonary physiology is important. It is important to consider that MPS are associated with both obstructive and restrictive airway disease. The use of spirometry is the most objective way of identifying these problems accepting practical limitations of use in certain situations. A six-minute walk test has been used as a surrogate of pulmonary function but is an overall functional assessment of combined cardiopulmonary status and therefore not specifically related to the airway's disease. It is clear that in conditions associated with growth abnormalities that absolute values of FEV and FVC will be reduced. Therefore, the FEV and FVC percentages predicted are defined as the percentage predicted values based on age, sex, and height. The definition of obstruction is an FEV1 < 80% predicted and a FEV1/FVC ratio of <0.7. Conversely, a restrictive disease is reflected in a greater reduction in FVC compared with FEV1 resulting in a FEV1/FVC ration > 0.7. In the context of MPS, we have the obvious difficulty of the validity of height and age normalised curves in this group of patients. In the absence of alternatives, however, FEV1 and FVC will remain the mainstay of our monitoring of pulmonary functions. The value of spirometry is the ability to detect changes overtime, and it has been shown that there is a correlation with identification of sleep disordered breathing identified by the ODI 3% in MPS IVA [37]. A flow volume loop may help to assess intra- and extra thoracic obstruction, which will in turn aid in the management of the complex airway. However, in the absence of a normalised value, it may be difficult to interpret. We may also falsely interpret intra- and extra thoracic obstruction.

The SMAS was designed to quantify the degree of airway abnormality with an aim to assess all airway and breathing factors together. The aim was to use this score when adult MPS patients are planned for a general anaesthetic. Prominent teeth, mouth opening, neck movements, and modified Mallampati grade [26] are all important factors to access the airway. The thyromental angle and nasendoscopic findings help to decide if the larynx is high and/or anterior. Once the airway is accessed, the supraglottic, glottic, and subglottic bulkiness due to GAG deposits will dictate the size of the endotracheal tube. Once the airway is secured, the degree of tracheobronchomalacia and tracheal tortuosity will govern the oxygen delivery to lungs. We have scored tortuous trachea as 3, as this will have a big impact on securing the airway and ventilation. The pulmonary function tests will help us understand the physiological state of the lungs. In our experience, a score more than 25 indicates a complex airway. This information obtained during pre-operative assessment can be used to explain the patients, family members, and other health professionals to make a decision for general anaesthetic. We feel that a combination of parameters rather than a single parameter is useful in assessing the complex MPS airway. The limitations in our study are a small cohort of adult MPS patients; this is due to the rarity of the disease and reduced longevity. However, given the small cohort, extensive airway assessment has been performed. Secondly, SMAS cannot be scored for all parameters, especially in patients with learning difficulties; in this situation, percentage scores may be useful. Thirdly, the validation of the scores can be improved by performing on a larger cohort via a multicentre collaboration and perhaps assessing its usefulness in paediatric MPS. Haematopoietic stem cell transplantation (HSCT) [38] and enzyme replacement therapy (ERT) [39] have been shown to be effective therapeutic options for various types of MPS; they will reduce the deformities in adulthood, which in turn may lead to less complex airways. Future studies comparing patients who received therapy and those who did not will be helpful to understand the impact on skeletal and soft tissue abnormalities contributing to airway issues. Similarly, mutations of certain types may help us to prognosticate the severity of the airways. Unfortunately, both these could not be investigated in our study due to a small number of patients. A multicentre collaboration involving patients from various geographical regions may help in better understanding of the airway issues in this complex metabolic disease with multisystem involvement.

5. Conclusions

Adult MPS airway is challenging. With the advancements of treatment modalities, patients present with varying degrees of abnormalities in the airway. Given the rarity of the disease, mutations, and varying treatments in patients, it may be difficult to construe a specific airway pattern for each MPS. In our experience, we have noted that MPS I and III patients have milder airway abnormalities; MPS II patients have the most difficult airways; and MPS IV, VI, VII patients have both complex upper airway and tortuous trachea. Various factors have to be taken into consideration in assessing the complex airway with a multidisciplinary team. We have found use of the SMAS very helpful in assessing and quantifying the severity of airway problems. Adult MPS patients have complications associated with comorbidities, and communication issues due to vision and hearing. All these factors have to be carefully considered in assessing the complex airway. Nasendoscopy, cross-sectional imaging, 3D, VE, and respiratory functions are important tools apart from clinical examination in airway assessment. We recommend a joint ENT, anaesthetic, respiratory, and metabolic team with special interest in MPS for the assessment of adult MPS airway.

Author Contributions: The authors come from different specialties with common interest in adult mucopolysaccharidosis (MPS). The otolaryngologist C.G., anaesthetist G.T. and respiratory physician A.B., who have special interest in airway diseases, came up with the conceptualisation of the idea of holistic airway assessment in MPS. The methodology of the study was devised by C.G. and K.M.S. The validation of the SMAS questionnaire was done by C.G. and G.T. Formal analysis of the data was performed by C.G. and K.M.S. Investigation into each aspect was conducted by C.G., K.M.S. and R.S. The resources and data curation was performed by C.G. and K.M.S.; the original draft was prepared by C.G. and A.B. and it was reviewed and edited by C.G., K.M.S. and A.B. Visualisation of the project was planned by C.G. and A.J. The project was supervised by C.G. and A.B. All authors contributed towards project administration. All authors have read and agreed to the published version of the manuscript.

Funding: This research received no external funding.

Institutional Review Board Statement: The study was conducted according to the guidelines of the Declaration of Helsinki, and ethical approval from the local research and development department of the Salford Royal NHS Foundation Trust, Manchester, UK, was obtained, reference: S20HIP40. The study did not involve any animals. This study was a retrospective case notes review of adult MPS patients.

Informed Consent Statement: Informed consent was obtained from all subjects involved in the study. However, no personal identifiable information has been used in this study.

Data Availability Statement: All the necessary medical information has been provided in the study. Any further data presented in this study are available on request from the corresponding author. The data are not publicly available due to privacy.

Acknowledgments: We would like to thank Stuart Watson and Prawin Samraj for helping with 3-dimensional reconstruction of the airways. We would also like to thank Karen Tylee and Heather Church for helping us with the information regarding mutations.

Conflicts of Interest: The authors declare no conflict of interest.

Appendix A Difficult Airway Assessment Questionnaire

Dear Colleague,
Your feedback is very important to us.
Can you please give your opinion (agree or disagree) on 15 parameters which can be used to assess a difficult airway, breathing, respiration assuming you have all investigations such as clinical examination, nasendoscopy, and CT scans available.
There are only 16 questions, which will take less than 5 min to answer.
Many thanks for your opinion.
Chai Gadepalli

1. Mouth opening.

More than 5 cm = 0 score
4–5 cm = 1
3–4 cm = 2
Less than 3 cm = 3

Strongly agree
Agree
Neutral
Disagree
Strongly disagree

2. Teeth protrusion.

Non-protruding = 0 score
Mild protrusion = 1
Moderate protrusion = 2
Severe protrusion = 3 *

Strongly agree
Agree
Neutral
Disagree
Strongly disagree

3. Cervical spine mobility, stability on clinical examination.

Unrestricted = 0 score
60–90 degrees flexion = 1
30–60 degrees flexion = 2
Less than 30 degrees flexion or unstable or fixed = 3 *

Strongly agree
Agree
Neutral
Disagree
Strongly disagree

4. Tongue bulkiness on examination and scan.

Normal = 0 score
Mild = 1 (tongue fills floor of the mouth)
Moderate = 2 (tongue fills between 1/3 to 1/2 of oral cavity)
Severe = 3 (tongue fills more than 1/2 of oral cavity) *

Strongly agree
Agree
Neutral
Disagree
Strongly disagree

5. Modified Mallampati grade.

Grade 1 = 0 score
Grade 2 = 1
Grade 3 = 2
Grade 4 = 3 *

Strongly agree
Agree
Neutral
Disagree
Strongly disagree

6. Thyromental distance on clinical examination.

More than 6 cm = 0 score
5–6 cm = 1
4-5 cm = 2
Less than 4 cm = 3 *

Strongly agree
Agree
Neutral
Disagree
Strongly disagree

7. Larynx height-distance between epiglottis and soft palate on nasendoscopy/scan.

More than 4 cm = 0 score
3–4 cm = 1
2–3 cm = 2
Less than 2 cm = 3

Strongly agree
Agree
Neutral
Disagree
Strongly disagree

8. Epiglottis bulkiness on nasendoscopy / scan.

Normal= 0 score (filling less than less than 1/3 of oropharynx)
Mild bulkiness = 1 (filling 1/3–1/2 of oropharynx)
Moderate bulkiness = 2 (filling 1/2 to complete oropharynx)
Severe bulkiness = 3 (filling the entire oropharynx) *

Strongly agree
Agree
Neutral
Disagree
Strongly disagree

9. Supraglottis bulkiness on nasendoscopy/scan.

Normal= 0 score (filling less than less than 1/3 of supraglottis)
Mild bulkiness = 1 (filling 1/3–1/2 of supraglottis)
Moderate bulkiness = 2 (filling 1/2 to complete supraglottis)
Severe bulkiness = 3 (filling the entire supraglottis) *

Strongly agree
Agree
Neutral
Disagree
Strongly disagree

10. Glottis bulkiness on nasendoscopy.

Normal = 0 score (filling less than less than 1/3 of glottis)
Mild bulkiness = 1 (filling 1/3–1/2 of glottis)
Moderate bulkiness = 2 (filling 1/2 to complete glottis)
Severe bulkiness = 3 (filling the entire glottis) *

Strongly agree
Agree
Neutral
Disagree
Strongly disagree

11. Subglottis diameter at cricoid level on CT scan.

More than 7 mm = 0 score
6–7 mm = 1
5–6 mm = 2
Less than 5 mm = 3 *

Strongly agree
Agree
Neutral
Disagree
Strongly disagree

12. Tracheomalacia or stenosis (degree of lumen collapse) on CT scan.

No malacia = 0 score
50–75% lumen collapse = 1
75–99% lumen collapse = 2
100% lumen collapse = 3 *

Strongly agree
Agree
Neutral
Disagree
Strongly disagree

13. Tracheal tortuosity on CT scan.

None = 0 score
Tortuosity present = 3

Strongly agree
Agree
Neutral
Disagree
Strongly disagree

14. FEV1% in last one year.

More than > 80% = 0 score
60–79% = 1
40–59% = 2
Less than 40% = 3

Strongly agree
Agree
Neutral
Disagree
Strongly disagree

15. FVC% in last one year.

More than 80% = 0 score
60–79% = 1
40–59% = 2
Less than 40% = 3 *

Strongly agree
Agree
Neutral
Disagree
Strongly disagree

16. The above questions helps me in holistic airway assessment (contains all criteria to assess a difficult airway) *

Strongly agree
Agree
Neutral
Disagree
Strongly disagree

17. Please use the space below to make any comments

————————————End of questionnaire————————————

References

1. Mehta, A.B.; Winchester, B. *Lysosomal Storage Disorders: A Practical Guide*; Wiley-Blackwell: Chicester, UK, 2012.
2. Neufeld, E.; Muenzer, J. The Mucopolysaccharidoses. In *The Metabolic and Molecular Bases of Inherited Diseases*, 8th ed.; Scriver, C.R., Beaudet, A.L., Sly, W.S., Valle, D., Childs, R., Kinzler, K.W., Eds.; McGraw-Hill: New York, NY, USA, 2001; pp. 3421–3452.
3. Muenzer, J. Overview of the mucopolysaccharidoses. *Rheumatology* **2011**, *50*, v4–v12. [CrossRef] [PubMed]
4. Clark, B.M.; Sprung, J.; Weingarten, T.N.; Warner, M.E. Anesthesia for patients with mucopolysaccharidoses: Comprehensive review of the literature with emphasis on airway management. *Bosn. J. Basic Med. Sci.* **2018**, *18*, 1. [CrossRef]
5. Braunlin, E.A.; Harmatz, P.R.; Scarpa, M.; Furlanetto, B.; Kampmann, C.; Loehr, J.P.; Ponder, K.P.; Roberts, W.C.; Rosenfeld, H.M.; Giugliani, R. Cardiac disease in patients with mucopolysaccharidosis: Presentation, diagnosis and management. *J. Inherit. Metab. Dis.* **2011**, *34*, 1183–1197. [CrossRef]
6. Valayannopoulos, V.; Nicely, H.; Harmatz, P.; Turbeville, S. Mucopolysaccharidosis vi. *Orphanet J. Rare Dis.* **2010**, *5*, 5. [CrossRef]
7. Berger, K.I.; Fagondes, S.C.; Giugliani, R.; Hardy, K.A.; Lee, K.S.; McArdle, C.; Scarpa, M.; Tobin, M.J.; Ward, S.A.; Rapoport, D.M. Respiratory and sleep disorders in mucopolysaccharidosis. *J. Inherit. Metab. Dis.* **2013**, *36*, 201–210. [CrossRef]
8. Muhlebach, M.S.; Wooten, W.; Muenzer, J. Respiratory manifestations in mucopolysaccharidoses. *Paediatr. Respir. Rev.* **2011**, *12*, 133–138. [CrossRef]
9. Tsara, V.; Amfilochiou, A.; Papagrigorakis, J.; Georgopoulos, D.; Liolios, E.; Kadiths, A.; Koudoumnakis, E.; Aulonitou, E.; Emporiadou, M.; Tsakanikos, M. Guidelines for diagnosing and treating sleep related breathing disorders in adults and children (Part 3: Obstructive sleep apnea in children, diagnosis and treatment). *Hippokratia* **2010**, *14*, 57.
10. Dalewski, B.; Kamińska, A.; Syrico, A.; Kałdunska, A.; Pałka, Ł.; Sobolewska, E. The Usefulness of Modified Mallampati Score and CT Upper Airway Volume Measurements in Diagnosing OSA among Patients with Breathing-Related Sleep Disorders. *Appl. Sci.* **2021**, *11*, 3764. [CrossRef]
11. Huang, H.-H.; Lee, M.-S.; Shih, Y.-L.; Chu, H.-C.; Huang, T.-Y.; Hsieh, T.-Y. Modified Mallampati classification as a clinical predictor of peroral esophagogastroduodenoscopy tolerance. *BMC Gastroenterol.* **2011**, *11*, 1–7. [CrossRef] [PubMed]
12. Thurtell, M.J.; Bruce, B.B.; Rye, D.B.; Newman, N.J.; Biousse, V. The Berlin questionnaire screens for obstructive sleep apnea in idiopathic intracranial hypertension. *J. Neuro-Ophthalmol.* **2011**, *31*, 316–319. [CrossRef] [PubMed]
13. Wraith, J.E. The first 5years of clinical experience with laronidase enzyme replacement therapy for mucopolysaccharidosis I. *Expert Opin. Pharmacother.* **2005**, *6*, 489–506. [CrossRef] [PubMed]
14. Wraith, J.E.; Beck, M.; Lane, R.; Van Der Ploeg, A.; Shapiro, E.; Xue, Y.; Kakkis, E.D.; Guffon, N. Enzyme replacement therapy in patients who have mucopolysaccharidosis I and are younger than 5 years: Results of a multinational study of recombinant human α-L-iduronidase (laronidase). *Pediatrics* **2007**, *120*, e37–e46. [CrossRef]
15. Hendriksz, C.J.; Giugliani, R.; Harmatz, P.; Mengel, E.; Guffon, N.; Valayannopoulos, V.; Parini, R.; Hughes, D.; Pastores, G.M.; Lau, H.A. Multi-domain impact of elosulfase alfa in Morquio A syndrome in the pivotal phase III trial. *Mol. Genet. Metab.* **2015**, *114*, 178–185. [CrossRef] [PubMed]
16. Hendriksz, C.J.; Burton, B.; Fleming, T.R.; Harmatz, P.; Hughes, D.; Jones, S.A.; Lin, S.-P.; Mengel, E.; Scarpa, M.; Valayannopoulos, V. Efficacy and safety of enzyme replacement therapy with BMN 110 (elosulfase alfa) for Morquio A syndrome (mucopolysaccharidosis IVA): A phase 3 randomised placebo-controlled study. *J. Inherit. Metab. Dis.* **2014**, *37*, 979–990. [CrossRef]

17. Clarke, L.A.; Wraith, J.E.; Beck, M.; Kolodny, E.H.; Pastores, G.M.; Muenzer, J.; Rapoport, D.M.; Berger, K.I.; Sidman, M.; Kakkis, E.D. Long-term efficacy and safety of laronidase in the treatment of mucopolysaccharidosis I. *Pediatrics* **2009**, *123*, 229–240. [CrossRef] [PubMed]
18. Harmatz, P.; Giugliani, R.; Schwartz, I.V.D.; Guffon, N.; Teles, E.L.; Miranda, M.C.S.; Wraith, J.E.; Beck, M.; Arash, L.; Scarpa, M. Long-term follow-up of endurance and safety outcomes during enzyme replacement therapy for mucopolysaccharidosis VI: Final results of three clinical studies of recombinant human N-acetylgalactosamine 4-sulfatase. *Mol. Genet. Metab.* **2008**, *94*, 469–475. [CrossRef]
19. Aldenhoven, M.; Wynn, R.F.; Orchard, P.J.; O'Meara, A.; Veys, P.; Fischer, A.; Valayannopoulos, V.; Neven, B.; Rovelli, A.; Prasad, V.K. Long-term outcome of Hurler syndrome patients after hematopoietic cell transplantation: An international multicenter study. *Blood J. Am. Soc. Hematol.* **2015**, *125*, 2164–2172. [CrossRef] [PubMed]
20. Arn, P.; Bruce, I.A.; Wraith, J.E.; Travers, H.; Fallet, S. Airway-related symptoms and surgeries in patients with mucopolysaccharidosis I. *Ann. Otol. Rhinol. Laryngol.* **2015**, *124*, 198–205. [CrossRef]
21. Pal, A.R.; Mercer, J.; Jones, S.A.; Bruce, I.A.; Bigger, B.W. Substrate accumulation and extracellular matrix remodelling promote persistent upper airway disease in mucopolysaccharidosis patients on enzyme replacement therapy. *PLoS ONE* **2018**, *13*, e0203216. [CrossRef]
22. Kirkpatrick, K.; Ellwood, J.; Walker, R.W. Mucopolysaccharidosis type I (Hurler syndrome) and anesthesia: The impact of bone marrow transplantation, enzyme replacement therapy, and fiberoptic intubation on airway management. *Pediatric Anesth.* **2012**, *22*, 745–751. [CrossRef]
23. Katz, J.A.; Avram, M.J. 4th National Audit Project of the Royal College of Anaesthetists and The Difficult Airway Society: Major Complications of Airway Management in the United Kingdom: Report and Findings. *J. Am. Soc. Anesthesiol.* **2012**, *116*, 496. [CrossRef]
24. Apfelbaum, J.; Hagberg, C.; Caplan, R.; Blitt, C.; Connis, R.; Nickinovich, D.; Benumof, J.; Berry, F. American Society of Anesthesiologists Task Force on Management of the Difficult Airway Practice guidelines for management of the difficult airway: An updated report by the American Society of Anesthesiologists Task Force on Management of the Difficult Airway. *Anesthesiology* **2013**, *118*, 251–270. [PubMed]
25. Roth, D.; Pace, N.; Lee, A.; Hovhannisyan, K.; Warenits, A.; Arrich, J.; Herkner, H. Bedside tests for predicting difficult airways: An abridged Cochrane diagnostic test accuracy systematic review. *Anaesthesia* **2019**, *74*, 915–928. [CrossRef] [PubMed]
26. Mallampati, S.R.; Gatt, S.P.; Gugino, L.D.; Desai, S.P.; Waraksa, B.; Freiberger, D.; Liu, P.L. A clinical sign to predict difficult tracheal intubation; a prospective study. *Can. Anaesth. Soc. J.* **1985**, *32*, 429–434. [CrossRef] [PubMed]
27. Wilson, M.; Spiegelhalter, D.; Robertson, J.; Lesser, P. Predicting difficult intubation. *BJA Br. J. Anaesth.* **1988**, *61*, 211–216. [CrossRef] [PubMed]
28. Crawley, S.; Dalton, A. Predicting the difficult airway. *BJA Educ.* **2015**, *15*, 253–257. [CrossRef]
29. Cattano, D.; Killoran, P.; Iannucci, D.; Maddukuri, V.; Altamirano, A.; Sridhar, S.; Seitan, C.; Chen, Z.; Hagberg, C. Anticipation of the difficult airway: Preoperative airway assessment, an educational and quality improvement tool. *Br. J. Anaesth.* **2013**, *111*, 276–285. [CrossRef] [PubMed]
30. Wittenborg, M.; Gyepes, M.; Crocker, D. Tracheal dynamics in infants with respiratory distress, stridor, and collapsing trachea. *Radiology* **1967**, *88*, 653–662. [CrossRef]
31. Murgu, S.D.; Colt, H.G. Description of a multidimensional classification system for patients with expiratory central airway collapse. *Respirology* **2007**, *12*, 543–550. [CrossRef]
32. Boiselle, P.M.; O'Donnell, C.R.; Bankier, A.A.; Ernst, A.; Millet, M.E.; Potemkin, A.; Loring, S.H. Tracheal collapsibility in healthy volunteers during forced expiration: Assessment with multidetector CT. *Radiology* **2009**, *252*, 255–262. [CrossRef]
33. Baroni, R.H.; Feller-Kopman, D.; Nishino, M.; Hatabu, H.; Loring, S.H.; Ernst, A.; Boiselle, P.M. Tracheobronchomalacia: Comparison between end-expiratory and dynamic expiratory CT for evaluation of central airway collapse. *Radiology* **2005**, *235*, 635–641. [CrossRef] [PubMed]
34. Murgu, S.D.; Colt, H.G. Treatment of adult tracheobronchomalacia and excessive dynamic airway collapse. *Treat. Respir. Med.* **2006**, *5*, 103–115. [CrossRef] [PubMed]
35. Svetanoff, W.J.; Jennings, R.W. Updates on surgical repair of tracheobronchomalacia. *J. Lung Health Dis.* **2018**, *2*, 17–23. [CrossRef]
36. Pizarro, C.; Davies, R.R.; Theroux, M.; Spurrier, E.A.; Averill, L.W.; Tomatsu, S. Surgical reconstruction for severe tracheal obstruction in Morquio A syndrome. *Ann. Thorac. Surg.* **2016**, *102*, e329–e331. [CrossRef] [PubMed]
37. Kenth, J.J.; Thompson, G.; Fullwood, C.; Wilkinson, S.; Jones, S.; Bruce, I. The characterisation of pulmonary function in patients with mucopolysaccharidoses IVA: A longitudinal analysis. *Mol. Genet. Metab. Rep.* **2019**, *20*, 100487. [CrossRef]
38. Taylor, M.; Khan, S.; Stapleton, M.; Wang, J.; Chen, J.; Wynn, R.; Yabe, H.; Chinen, Y.; Boelens, J.J.; Mason, R.W. Hematopoietic stem cell transplantation for mucopolysaccharidoses: Past, present, and future. *Biol. Blood Marrow Transplant.* **2019**, *25*, e226–e246. [CrossRef]
39. Concolino, D.; Deodato, F.; Parini, R. Enzyme replacement therapy: Efficacy and limitations. *Ital. J. Pediatrics* **2018**, *44*, 117–126. [CrossRef] [PubMed]

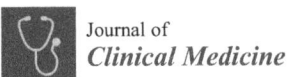

Review

A Systematic Review and Meta-Analysis of Enzyme Replacement Therapy in Late-Onset Pompe Disease

Alícia Dorneles Dornelles [1,2], Ana Paula Pedroso Junges [2,3], Tiago Veiga Pereira [4,5], Bárbara Corrêa Krug [6], Candice Beatriz Treter Gonçalves [6], Juan Clinton Llerena, Jr. [7], Priya Sunil Kishnani [8], Haliton Alves de Oliveira, Jr. [9] and Ida Vanessa Doederlein Schwartz [1,2,3,6,10,*]

1. Postgraduate Program in Medical Sciences, Faculty of Medicine, Universidade Federal do Rio Grande do Sul, Porto Alegre CEP 90035003, Brazil; alidorneles@gmail.com
2. Medical Genetics Service, Hospital de Clínicas de Porto Alegre, Porto Alegre CEP 90035903, Brazil; apjunges@hcpa.edu.br
3. Faculty of Medicine, Universidade Federal do Rio Grande do Sul, Porto Alegre CEP 90035003, Brazil
4. Applied Health Research Centre, Li Ka Shing Knowledge Institute, St Michael's Hospital, Toronto, ON M5B 1T8, Canada; tiago.pereira@metadatum.com.br
5. Department of Health Sciences, College of Medicine, University of Leicester, Leicester LE1 7RH, UK
6. Nuclimed, Clinical Research Center, Hospital de Clinicas de Porto Alegre, Porto Alegre CEP 90035903, Brazil; krugbarbara@gmail.com (B.C.K.); candicebtg@gmail.com (C.B.T.G.)
7. Instituto Fernandes Figueira, Fiocruz, Rio de Janeiro CEP 22250020, Brazil; juan.llerena@iff.fiocruz.br
8. Department of Pediatrics, Duke University Medical Center, Durham, NC 27710, USA; priya.kishnani@duke.edu
9. Health Technology Assessment Unit, Hospital Alemão Oswaldo Cruz, São Paulo CEP 01323903, Brazil; haoliveira@haoc.com.br
10. Department of Genetics, Universidade Federal do Rio Grande do Sul, Porto Alegre CEP 91501970, Brazil
* Correspondence: idadschwartz@gmail.com; Tel.: +55-51-33598011; Fax: +55-51-33598010

Citation: Dornelles, A.D.; Junges, A.P.P.; Pereira, T.V.; Krug, B.C.; Gonçalves, C.B.T.; Llerena, J.C., Jr.; Kishnani, P.S.; de Oliveira, H.A., Jr.; Schwartz, I.V.D. A Systematic Review and Meta-Analysis of Enzyme Replacement Therapy in Late-Onset Pompe Disease. *J. Clin. Med.* **2021**, *10*, 4828. https://doi.org/10.3390/jcm10214828

Academic Editors: Sylvia Lee-Huang, Karolina M. Stepien, Christian J. Hendriksz and Gregory M. Pastores

Received: 1 September 2021
Accepted: 12 October 2021
Published: 21 October 2021

Publisher's Note: MDPI stays neutral with regard to jurisdictional claims in published maps and institutional affiliations.

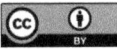

Copyright: © 2021 by the authors. Licensee MDPI, Basel, Switzerland. This article is an open access article distributed under the terms and conditions of the Creative Commons Attribution (CC BY) license (https://creativecommons.org/licenses/by/4.0/).

Abstract: Pompe disease (PD) is a glycogen storage disorder caused by deficient activity of acid alpha-glucosidase (GAA). We sought to review the latest available evidence on the safety and efficacy of recombinant human GAA enzyme replacement therapy (ERT) for late-onset PD (LOPD). Methods: We systematically searched the MEDLINE (via PubMed), Embase, and Cochrane databases for prospective clinical studies evaluating ERT for LOPD on pre-specified outcomes. A meta-analysis was also performed. Results: Of 1601 articles identified, 22 were included. Studies were heterogeneous and with very low certainty of evidence for most outcomes. The following outcomes showed improvements associated with GAA ERT, over a mean follow-up of 32.5 months: distance walked in the 6-min walking test (6MWT) (mean change 35.7 m (95% confidence interval [CI] 7.78, 63.75)), physical domain of the SF-36 quality of life (QOL) questionnaire (mean change 1.96 (95% CI 0.33, 3.59)), and time on ventilation (TOV) (mean change −2.64 h (95% CI −5.28, 0.00)). There were no differences between the pre- and post-ERT period for functional vital capacity (FVC), Walton and Gardner-Medwin Scale score, upper-limb strength, or total SF-36 QOL score. Adverse events (AEs) after ERT were mild in most cases. Conclusion: Considering the limitations imposed by the rarity of PD, our data suggest that GAA ERT improves 6MWT, physical QOL, and TOV in LOPD patients. ERT was safe in the studied population. PROSPERO register: 135102.

Keywords: glycogen storage disease type II; alpha-glucosidase; Pompe disease; enzyme replacement therapy

1. Introduction

Pompe disease (PD), or type II glycogenosis, is a rare genetic disease characterized by progressive neuromuscular involvement, often fatal in severe forms [1]. It is caused by deficient activity of acid alpha-glucosidase (also known as acid maltase), a lysosomal enzyme encoded by the *GAA* gene that breaks down glycogen into glucose [1]. This deficient activity, caused by biallelic pathogenic variants in *GAA*, leads to lysosomal glycogen accumulation in the skeletal and cardiac muscles, hindering cell function and ultimately destroying cells by hypertrophy and lysosome rupture [1–6].

Residual enzyme activity correlates positively with age at disease onset and inversely with the rate of disease progression, which allows PD to be classified according to the age of onset, cardiac involvement, and speed of progression. When clinical onset occurs before the age of 12 months and cardiomyopathy is present, it is known as infantile-onset PD (IOPD); all other forms are referred to as late-onset PD (LOPD) [1,7]. LOPD occurs on a spectrum; patients may present through the second year of life without cardiomyopathy, in childhood, adolescence, or at any point in adult life [1,7]. Although the overall severity of involvement is variable, life expectancy is generally shorter than in healthy individuals [1,2,8].

The overall incidence of PD worldwide is around 1 in 40,000 newborns (NBs). The incidence is higher in African Americans (1/12,000 NBs) and lower in Chinese (1/40,000 to 1/50,000 NBs) individuals [1–3]. After the inclusion of PD in the newborn screening programs of some countries, more reliable estimates of its incidence have emerged: 1/26,319 NBs in Illinois (USA) [9], 1/17,134 NBs in Pennsylvania (USA) [10], 1/10,152 NBs in Missouri (USA) [11], and 1/34,402 NBs in the Asian population of Japan [12].

There is no curative treatment for PD. Currently available treatment options are designed to address the mutant protein and consist of enzyme replacement therapy (ERT) with alglucosidase alfa (Myozyme™), a form of human acid alpha-glucosidase (GAA) produced by recombinant DNA technology in Chinese hamster ovary cells [2]. The recommended dosage regimen of alglucosidase alfa is 20 mg/kg body weight, administered every 2 weeks by intravenous (IV) infusion [8].

Two previous systematic reviews aimed to assess the effectiveness, safety, and appropriate dose regimen of enzyme replacement therapy (ERT) for treating LOPD; however, both have limitations in important domains. One, which included a meta-analysis, evaluated survival, vital capacity, and performance in the 6-min walking test (6MWT), reporting improvements in all outcomes [13]. The second, which did not perform a meta-analysis, showed improvement in the 6MWT but failed to include relevant prospective cohort studies [14]. Therefore, the impact of alglucosidase alfa treatment on key outcomes, such as quality of life (QOL) and time on ventilatory support (TOV), is still unclear. A further, significant knowledge gap that still remains is the ideal timing of ERT initiation. Within this context, the present systematic review with meta-analysis was designed to evaluate the effects of alglucosidase alfa ERT in LOPD.

2. Methodology

This study aimed to review the latest available evidence on the effects of alglucosidase alfa ERT in LOPD and its safety. To guide the literature search, a structured PICO question was formulated as follows: "Is the use of alglucosidase alfa as effective and safe as ERT in patients with PD?". The systematic review is reported as proposed by the PRISMA Guidelines [15] and has been registered in the PROSPERO database (123700).

2.1. Information Sources and Search Strategy

The MEDLINE (via PubMed), Embase, and Cochrane Central Register of Controlled Trials databases were searched for studies published before 30 May 2021. The search strategies are shown in Table 1; for the Cochrane Library, we used both strategies combined.

Table 1. Database search queries.

Database	Search Query
MEDLINE (via PubMed)	"Glycogen Storage Disease Type II" [Mesh] AND "alpha-Glucosidases" [Mesh] AND "humans" [MeSH]
Embase	"glycogen storage disease type 2"/exp AND "recombinant glucan 1, 4 alpha glucosidase"/exp OR "recombinant glucan 1,4 alpha glucosidase"

2.2. Eligibility Criteria and Study Selection

We planned to include only randomized clinical trials (RCT) and observational comparative studies in which ERT with alglucosidase alfa was used for the treatment of patients with LOPD. Other prospective study designs were included (open-label and non-randomized trials, controlled or otherwise, including quasi-experimental designs) if the sample size was ≥5. In vitro studies or animal models, reviews, expert opinions, and retrospective studies were excluded. Unpublished work was covered by the identification of conference abstracts containing data deemed to be of interest. The final published articles were then included when available.

Studies that did not evaluate at least one of the eight outcomes of interest, defined a priori by a team of experts, were excluded. These outcomes were QOL, functional capacity (6MWT, forced vital capacity (FVC), and Walton and Gardner-Medwin Scale (WGMS) score), survival, TOV in hours/day, muscle strength, sleep quality, swallowing, and safety. For FVC, an increase of at least 10% after the intervention was considered a clinically relevant improvement [16,17]. For 6MWT, an increase of at least 26 m was considered a clinically significant change, as recommended by Schrover et al. for muscular diseases [18]. The WGMS is a scale that evaluates functional activity on a point system ranging from 0 = normal to 10 = bedridden.

The selection stage was performed independently by two investigators (APPJ, CG), who assessed the abstracts retrieved during the search for eligibility. Decisions were compared, and articles deemed relevant were forwarded to two other investigators (ADD, BK) who, independently, using standardized data collection forms, extracted information on the characteristics of these studies (design, randomization methods, population of participants, interventions, and outcomes). The two investigators then took part in a consensus meeting. Any disagreement that remained was addressed by the intervention of a third investigator (IVDS). Finally, the references of the selected articles were hand-searched for potentially relevant studies not identified by the previous search strategies. When such information could not be retrieved, an email was sent to authors requesting non-reported data.

2.3. Data Collection

Studies with overlapping data were excluded from meta-analyses. In these cases, the study with the largest sample (or, if both studies had the same sample size, that with the longest follow-up) was retained for analysis.

2.4. Statistical Analysis

We summarized results using mean changes from baseline with 95% confidence intervals (CIs) for continuous outcomes. To incorporate follow-up time, we used incidence rates (IRs) with 95% CIs to summarize events. To facilitate interpretation, we standardized all IR estimates in events per 100 person-years. Study-specific mean changes were combined through an inverse-variance random-effects model with the restricted maximum-likelihood estimator (REML) of between-study variance ($\tau 2$) for continuous variables. Events were combined with a generalized linear mixed model (GLMM) [19], in which a random intercept logistic regression model was fitted (log transformation) with a maximum-likelihood (ML) estimator. Sparse data were naturally taken into account in the GLMM, and no continuity corrections were used. The random-effects model was used for the primary analysis, but summary estimates obtained with a fixed-effects model (inverse-variance) were presented as a sensitivity analysis.

When not directly reported, mean change from baseline and standard error estimates were approximated based on reported statistics (95% CI, *p*-values, median, and interquartile range). We imputed standard deviations for baseline changes, assuming a correlation of 0.7 between baseline and follow-up scores. When only the median and interquartile range were informed, we used an approximate Bayesian computation (ABC) model to estimate means and standard deviations [20]. We employed clinically plausible ranges for the prior [~uniform (0,100)] distributions derived from studies reporting complete information and the opinion of specialists. Statistical heterogeneity was tested with Cochran's Q test and quantified with the I^2 metric. Cochran's Q was considered statistically significant for heterogeneity if $p < 0.10$ [21]. No threshold for statistical significance was used for the evaluation of clinical variables. Analyses were performed with Stata (version 16, StataCorp, College Station, TX, USA) and R (version 3.2.3, R Core Team, The R Foundation, Vienna, Austria).

2.5. Evaluation of the Quality of Included Studies

The quality of included studies was evaluated with tools appropriate for the study designs: Risk of Bias tool (RoB) 2.0 for RCTs and Risk Of Bias In Non-randomized Studies of Interventions tool (ROBINS-I) for non-randomized studies of interventions (NRSI) [22,23]. Certainty of evidence of outcomes defined a priori was evaluated according to GRADE criteria [24–26]. Assessment of certainty of evidence for outcomes was performed independently by two investigators (ADD, HAOJ).

3. Results

The broad search strategy retrieved 1601 references (768 from MEDLINE, 833 from EMBASE, none from the Cochrane Library), of which 242 were duplicated. The titles and abstracts of 1359 references were read, and 33 publications were selected for full-text evaluation. Of these, 22 were selected for eligibility, and 11 were excluded. A flow diagram of evidence selection is shown in Figure 1. Ultimately, 22 studies were identified for LOPD, including one RCT.

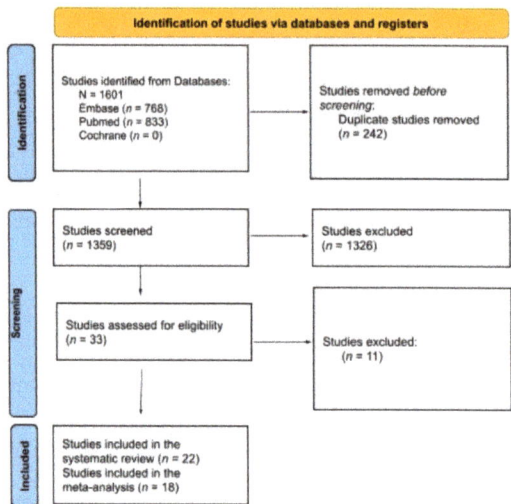

Figure 1. PRISMA flow diagram of search results.

Studies that evaluated the outcomes defined a priori are described in Table 2. Our search did not retrieve any articles evaluating sleep quality, survival, or swallowing disorder that matched the inclusion criteria; therefore, these outcomes could not be evaluated.

Table 2. Outcomes of interest defined a priori and studies that met the inclusion criteria.

Outcome	Number of Articles	References
Assessment of functional capacity:		
-FVC	15	[13,27–40]
-6MWT	14	[13,27–31,34–39,41,42]
-WGMS	6	[13,27,30,31,40,43]
Safety	14	[13,28–31,33,34,36,39,40,42–45]
Upper-limb strength	9	[13,28–30,33,34,36,39,46]
Quality of life	6	[13,28,30,36,43,47]
Time on ventilation	6	[30,31,33,40,42,43]
Survival	0	-
Sleep quality	0	-
Swallowing disorder	0	-

FVC = forced vital capacity. 6MWT = 6-min walking test. WGMS = Walton and Gardner-Medwin Scale.

3.1. Characteristics of Included Studies

All included studies and their characteristics are described in Table 3. Only one double-blind RCT was identified and included [36].

Table 3. Included studies and their characteristics.

Author	Patients (n/Male)	Design	Age at Onset of ERT—yo–μ (sd) (Range)	Follow-Up Duration	Control	Patients on Ventilation (n)
Angelini et al. (2009) [37]	11/3	Cohort	31.1 (8)	* N/A	-	1/11
Angelini et al. (2012) [31]	68/33	Cohort	43 (15.4) (7 to 72)	36 months	-	27/68
Bembi et al. (2010) [42]	24/14	NRSI	Young: 12 (3.3) Adults: 47.6 (10.7)	36 months	-	9/24
de Vries et al. (2012) [33]	49/21	Cohort	52.1 (median) (26.2 to 76.3)	23 months	-	13/49
de Vries et al. (2017) [45]	73/37	NRSI	52 (26 to 74)	36 months	-	22/73
Forsha et al. (2011) [44]	87/44	Post-hoc analysis of RCT	44 (39 to 52)	19.5 months	Placebo	N/A
Furusawa et al. (2011) [32]	5/2	Case series	47 (13.6) (32 to 66)	24 months	-	5/5
Gungor et al. (2016) [47]	174/81	Cohort	50 (median) (24 to 76)	*120 months	-	84/174
Kuperus et al. (2017) [39]	88/45	Cohort	52 (median) (24 to 76)	73.2 months (median)	-	21/88
Montagnese et al. (2015) [27]	14/N/A	Cohort	53.2 (11.1) (36 to 72)	31 months (mean)	-	N/A
Orlikowski et al. (2011) [43]	5/2	NRSI	47.8 (14.4) (28 to 62)	12 months	-	5/5
Papadimas et al. (2011) [46]	5/1	Cohort	46.8 (14.4) (40 to 73)	12 months	-	N/A
Ravaglia et al. (2010) [35]	11/6	NRSI	54.2 (11.2)	at least 24 months	-	N/A
Ravaglia et al. (2012) [41]	16/7	NRSI	54.5 (15.1)	at least 24 months	-	N/A
Regnery et al. (2012) [30]	38/18	NRSI	53.1 (27 to 73)	36 months	-	13/38
Strothotte et al. (2010) [13]	44/24	NRSI	48.9 (12.9) (21 to 69)	12 months	-	16/44
van Capelle et al. (2010) [34]	5/3	Phase II open study, followed by an extension period	11.1 (3.7) (5.9 to 15.2)	36 months	-	1/5
van der Ploeg et al. (2010) [36]	90/45	RCT (LOTS)	45.3 (12.4) (15.9 to 70)	19.5 months	Placebo	ERT = 20/60 Placebo = 11/30
van der Ploeg et al. (2012) [29]	60/34	Open study (LOTS extension)	45.3 (12.4) (15.9 to 79)	26 months	-	20/60

Table 3. *Cont.*

Author	Patients (n/Male)	Design	Age at Onset of ERT—yo-μ (sd) (Range)	Follow-Up Duration	Control	Patients on Ventilation (n)
van der Ploeg et al. (2016) [28]	16/7	NRSI	51.6 (13.7) (24.5 to 70.7)	6 months	-	0/16
Vianello et al. (2013) [40]	Group A: 8/5 Group B: 6/1	Cohort with historical control	Group A: 51.5 (12.2) (29 to 65) Group B: 43.8 (15.8) (18 to 59)	Group A = 35.8 months (mean)	Group B (Historical control without ERT) = 52.6 months (mean)	Group A=8/8 Group B=6/6
Witkowski et al. (2018) [38]	5/2	Case series	35.8 (26 to 41)	72 months	-	N/A
TOTAL	896/388	-	42.8 (7 to 72.3)	32.5 months	-	265

NRSI = non-randomized study of interventions. N/A = not available. LOTS = late-onset treatment study. All studies used alglucosidase alfa IV 20 mg/kg/biweekly, except those marked with *, in which dosage was not specified.

3.2. Assessment of Functional Capacity

3.2.1. Forced Vital Capacity

Based on data from 15 studies (participants = 348; mean follow-up = 36.8 mo; Table 2 [13,27–40]), there was no evidence of improvement in FVC during the performance of spirometry in the sitting, supine, or orthostatic positions (within-group mean change: 0.41% (95% CI: −0.3 to 1.12%)), as shown in Figure 2 and Supplementary Table S1. There was low heterogeneity between studies and very low certainty of evidence (Supplementary Table S2).

3.2.2. Six-Minute Walking Test

Performance on the 6MWT was evaluated in 14 studies before and after ERT (participants = 348; mean follow-up = 36.8 mo), as shown in Table 2 [13,27–31,34–39,41,42] and Supplementary Table S3. Van der Ploeg et al. (2010) [36] included the same population as van der Ploeg et al. (2012) [29] and was thus excluded; Kuperus et al. [39] measured the outcome as median and, therefore, was excluded from meta-analysis as well. Despite the considerable heterogeneity between studies and very low certainty of evidence (Supplementary Table S4), there was evidence of clinically significant improvement after treatment (within-group mean change: 35.7 m (95% CI: 7.78 to 63.75); Figure 3).

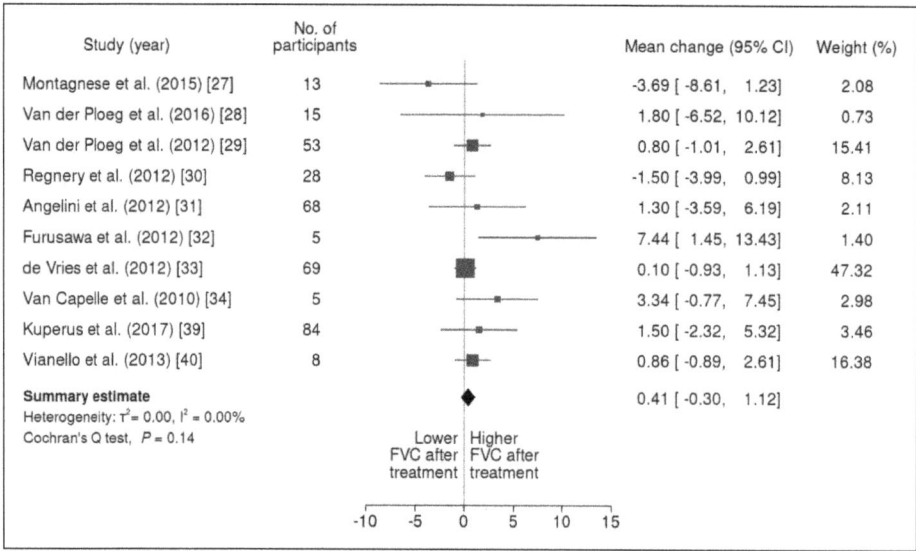

Figure 2. Evaluation of forced vital capacity (% of predicted) in upright position in patients with late-onset Pompe disease

on enzyme replacement therapy with alglucosidase alfa. Weights are inverse-variance weights and are proportional to the contribution of each study to the summary estimate. I^2 is the fraction of variance that is due to statistical heterogeneity and not chance. Tau^2 denotes the between-study variance.

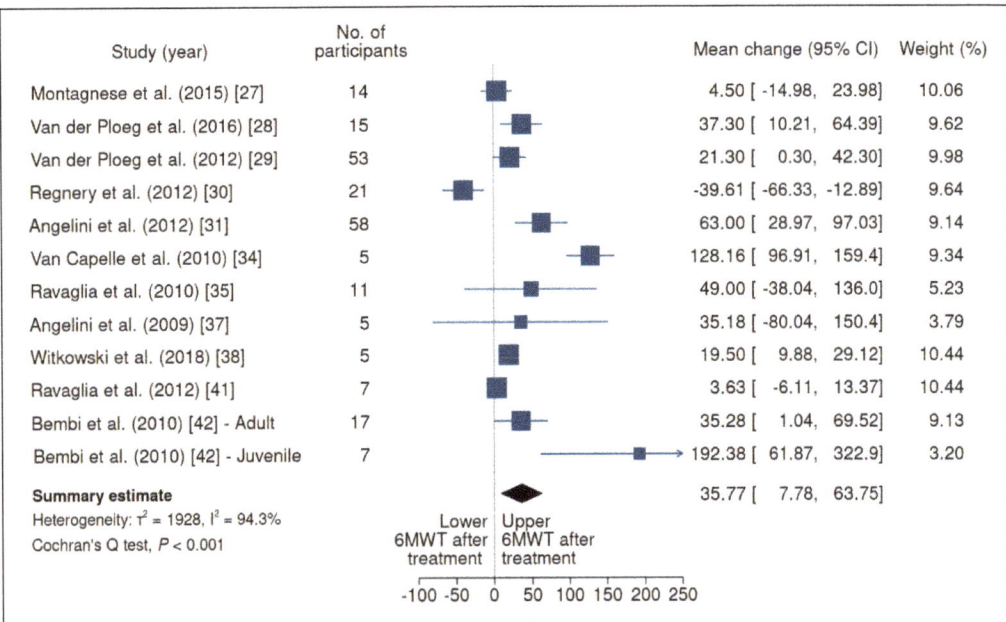

Figure 3. Evaluation of 6-min walking test performance (distance walked in meters) in patients with late-onset Pompe disease on enzyme replacement therapy with alglucosidase alfa. Weights are inverse-variance weights and are proportional to the contribution of each study to the summary estimate. I^2 is the fraction of variance that is due to statistical heterogeneity and not chance. Tau^2 denotes the between-study variance.

3.2.3. Walton and Gardner-Medwin Scale (WGMS)

Six studies evaluated WGMS scores, as shown in Table 2 [13,27,30,31,40,43] (results shown in Supplementary Table S5). The data suggest that ERT had no effect on the WGMS score in any of the included studies. Certainty of evidence was very low (Supplementary Table S6), mainly due to the imprecision of the results of the included studies.

3.3. Upper-Limb Strength

Nine studies evaluated strength in the upper limbs, but did so very heterogeneously (Supplementary Table S7). Although several studies carried out strength assessment according to the Medical Research Council (MRC) scale [13,30,33,46], they reported different methods of calculating it, evaluated different muscle groups, and some did not evaluate upper and lower limbs separately, limiting the comparability of this outcome. Thereby, muscle strength was evaluated through a meta-analysis in relation to two variables: handheld dynamometry and the Quick Motor Function Test. Handheld dynamometry was evaluated in 2 of 9 studies, without significant differences (mean change 244.05 (95% CI −151.18, 639.27)) (Figure 4), with considerable heterogeneity between studies; the Quick Motor Function Test was evaluated in 3 of 9 studies, without a significant difference (mean change 7.85 (95% CI −2.48, 18.18)) (Figure 5), with substantial heterogeneity between studies and very low certainty of evidence (Supplementary Table S8).

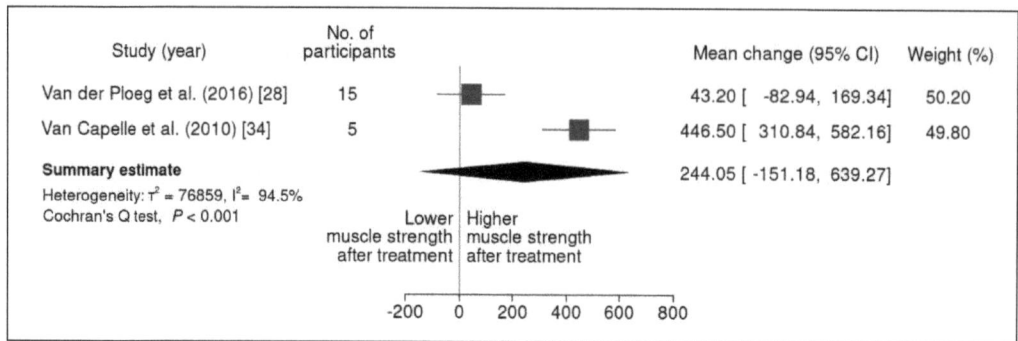

Figure 4. Evaluation of handheld dynamometry in patients with late-onset Pompe disease on enzyme replacement therapy with alglucosidase alfa. Weights are inverse-variance weights and are proportional to the contribution of each study to the summary estimate. I^2 is the fraction of variance that is due to statistical heterogeneity and not chance. Tau^2 denotes the between-study variance.

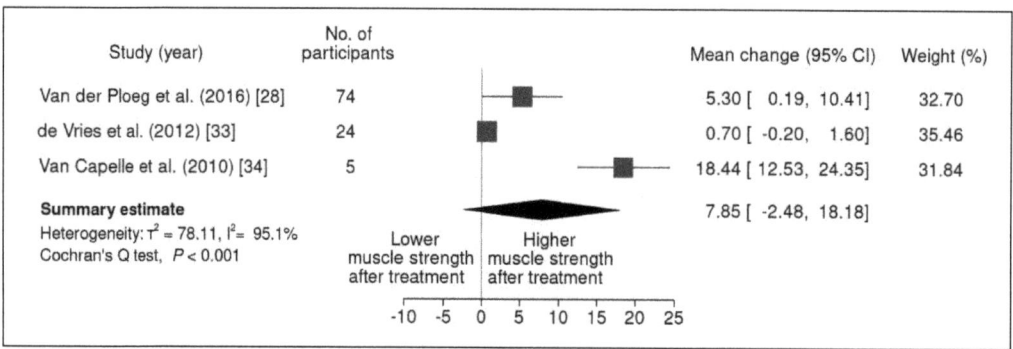

Figure 5. Evaluation of the Quick Motor Function Test in patients with late-onset Pompe disease on enzyme replacement therapy with alglucosidase alfa. Weights are inverse-variance weights and are proportional to the contribution of each study to the summary estimate. I^2 is the fraction of variance that is due to statistical heterogeneity and not chance. Tau^2 denotes the between-study variance.

3.4. Quality of Life

Six studies evaluated this outcome; the meta-analysis of their results is shown in Figure 6 and detailed in Supplementary Table S9. The instrument most commonly used to assess QOL was the Medical Outcome Study 36-item Short Form Health Survey, or SF-36 questionnaire [13,30,36,43,47]. The SF-36 is a generic instrument that has been widely used, has been translated into many languages, and has been shown to have good reliability and validity. Strothotte et al. [13] was excluded from the meta-analysis due to incomplete data available, and van der Ploeg et al. (2016) was excluded due to the use of the Pediatric Quality of Life Inventory™ (PedsQL) [28].

There were no differences in overall QOL (mean change 7.05 (95% CI −7.30, 21.41)) or in the mental component of the SF-36 (mean change 5.37 (95% CI −4.04, 14.78)), with considerable heterogeneity. However, there was a difference in the physical component (mean change 1.96 (95% CI 0.33, 3.59)) (Figure 6), with substantial heterogeneity and very low certainty of evidence (Supplementary Table S10).

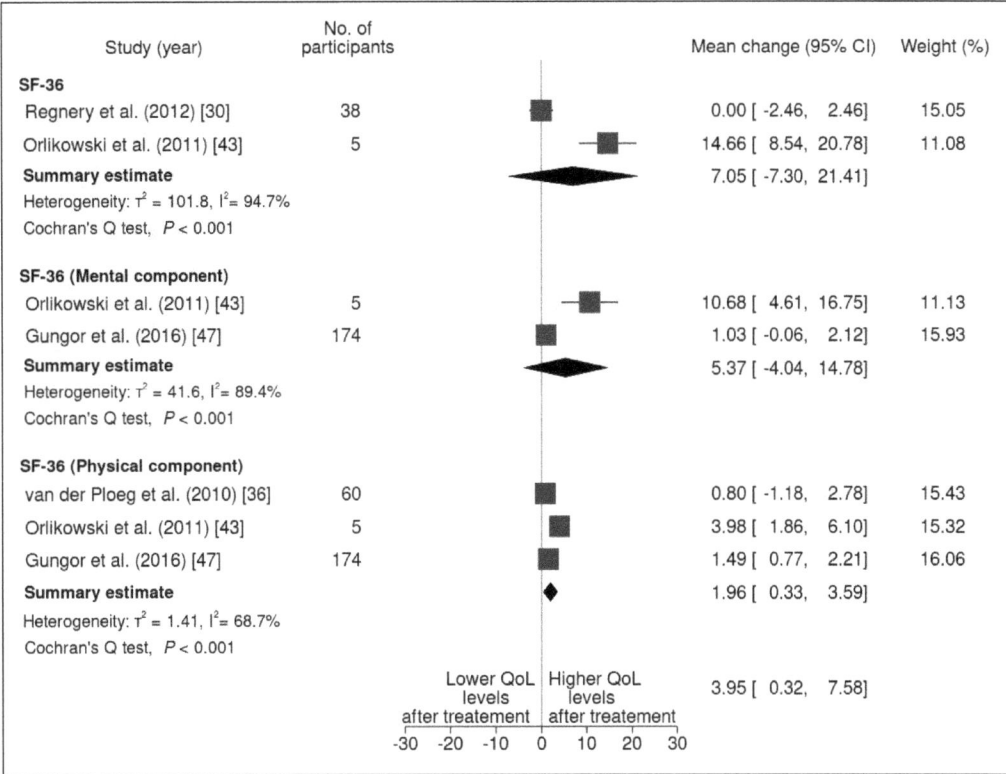

Figure 6. Evaluation of the quality of life of patients with late-onset Pompe disease on enzyme replacement therapy with alglucosidase alfa. Weights are inverse-variance weights and are proportional to the contribution of each study to the summary estimate. I^2 is the fraction of variance that is due to statistical heterogeneity and not chance. Tau^2 denotes the between-study variance.

3.5. Time on Ventilation

Six studies evaluated this outcome in LOPD; a synthesis of their results is shown in Figure 7 and Supplementary Table S11. Two studies [30,33] were not included in the meta-analysis due to a lack of data. There was weak evidence indicating that ERT, on average, is associated with a positive effect on TOV, despite substantial heterogeneity between studies and low certainty of evidence (Supplementary Table S12) (mean change −2.64 h (95% CI −5.28, 0.00)).

3.6. Safety

3.6.1. Adverse Events

Several studies have assessed the safety profile of ERT concerning the presence of adverse events (AEs) and infusion-associated reactions (IARs), as shown in Table 4 and Supplementary Table S13 [13,28–31,33,34,36,39,40,42–45]. The reported AEs are tachycardia, desaturation, malaise, chills, facial erythema, erythema at the enzyme infusion site, urticarial reactions, hyperhidrosis, chest discomfort, vomiting, systemic arterial hypertension, flu-like symptoms, pruritus, bronchospasm, and hyperthermia. Certainty of evidence is presented in Supplementary Table S14.

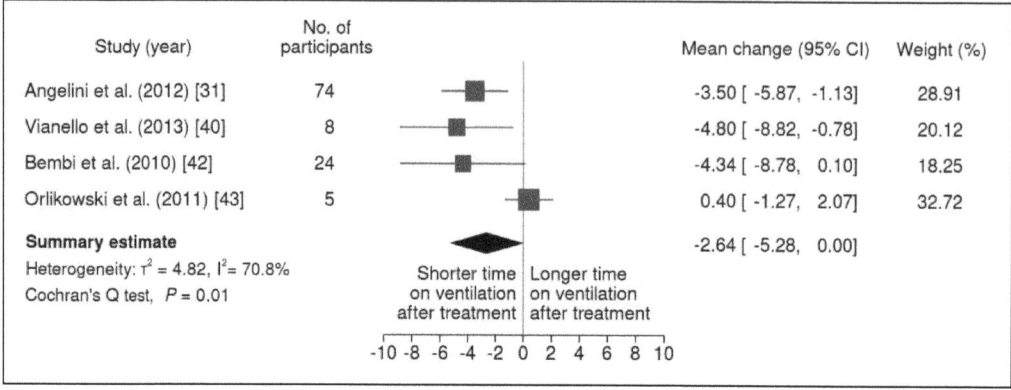

Figure 7. Evaluation of the time on ventilation (h) of patients with late-onset Pompe disease on enzyme replacement therapy with alglucosidase alfa. Weights are inverse-variance weights and are proportional to the contribution of each study to the summary estimate. I^2 is the fraction of variance that is due to statistical heterogeneity and not chance. Tau^2 denotes the between-study variance.

Table 4. Summary estimates for incidence of safety outcomes of enzyme replacement therapy for patients with late-onset Pompe disease.

Outcome	Studies	Participants	P_Q	I^2	Summary IR (95% CI) Random-Effects Model	Fixed-Effects Model
Mortality	9	675	0.66	38.9	0.44 (0.15 to 1.28)	0.56 (0.31 to 1.01)
AB+	7	323	<0.001	94.7	42.63 (24.07 to 75.49)	35.28 (31.41 to 39.62)
AE	3	139	<0.001	97.4	30.93 (2.96 to 323.51)	26.59 (21.0 to 33.67)
SAE	5	367	<0.001	89.7	4.19 (0.63 to 27.69)	2.32 (1.52 to 3.57)
IAR	4	43	<0.001	97.2	3.03 (0.03 to 305.58)	23.71 (16.26 to 34.58)
Patients with IAR	7	274	<0.001	94.1	6.58 (1.67 to 25.93)	6.69 (5.20 to 8.60)

AE = adverse event. SAE = serious adverse event. IAR = infusion-associated reaction. AB+ = presence of anti-alglucosidase alfa antibodies. P_Q denotes the p-value for Cochran's Q test. I^2 is the fraction of variance that is due to statistical heterogeneity and not chance. 95% CI = 95% confidence interval. IR = incidence rate (expressed in number of events per 100 person-years).

In the study by van der Ploeg et al. (2016) [28], there was only one severe AE (not specified), unrelated to treatment. Mild and moderate AEs occurred in 35.5% of patients, with 25% experiencing IARs. The incidence of IARs reported by de Vries et al. (2017) [45] was 18% (13/73 patients), the most common being malaise, chills, and hyperthermia. In another study by the same author [33], 12/69 patients (17%) developed an infusion reaction; however, only three patients remained symptomatic after administration of antihistamines and corticosteroids.

Angelini et al. (2012) [31] reported the following adverse reactions to ERT, occurring in 4/74 patients (6%) and considered of moderate intensity: facial erythema, erythema at the infusion site, flu-like symptoms, generalized pruritus, and bronchospasm (also described by Bembi et al. [42]). The symptoms were controlled with antihistamines. In another study by Orlikowski et al. with five patients, 58 mild to moderate AEs were described after starting treatment, including erythema and hyperthermia.

In the LOTS RCT, the ERT group and the placebo group had similar frequencies of severe AEs, treatment-related events, and infusion reactions (Supplementary Table S13). The treatment group had a higher frequency of mild to moderate AEs, which did not prevent the continuation of treatment. Urticariform reactions (also described by Bembi et al. [42]), hyperhidrosis, chest discomfort, flushing, vomiting, and increased blood pressure occurred in up to 8% of patients treated with alglucosidase alfa, and were not reported in the placebo group. These findings were corroborated by an extension study with the same population (LOTS Extension) [29]. In addition, Forsha et al. [44], using data obtained in the LOTS study, evaluated only the safety of ERT regarding cardiovascular events that occurred after the initiation of alglucosidase alfa, and found no significant difference between the treatment and placebo groups in change in ejection fraction ($p = 0.8$), PR interval ($p = 0.71$), ventricular mass ($p = 0.71$), or QRS duration ($p = 0.67$).

In the study by Kuperus et al. [39], 19 patients (22%) had at least one AE, all of which were controlled by a reduced infusion rate or premedication (antihistamines or corticosteroids). ERT was discontinued in four patients, but in only one for safety reasons (a patient with a history of autoimmune diseases and drug allergies before treatment developed multiple IARs). AEs have also been described in the study by Strothotte et al. [13], not included in meta-analysis due to incomplete data, and by Regnery et al. [30]: erythema, tachycardia, desaturation, rash, and pruritus, with no deaths occurring during the 12 and 36 months, respectively, of these studies. In the study by Vianello et al. [40], no AE has been described. In the study by van Capelle et al. [34], five patients were treated with ERT for 3 years and no AEs were observed in any of the 390 total intravenous infusions.

3.6.2. Mortality

Data on mortality were described in nine studies (Table 4 and Supplementary Table S15); however, only five described the occurrence of the event [31,33,36,39,43]. In the study conducted by Orlikowski et al. [43] with five patients, there was one death due to tracheal hemorrhage not related to treatment. In the study with the highest overall mortality rate, Kuperus et al. [39], 1/19 patients died of respiratory failure at 56 years of age, 1.1 years after discontinuing ERT for personal reasons. Another 6/19 patients on ERT died, though no deaths were considered treatment-related. The incidence rate of death (events per person-year) across all included studies was 4.4 events per 1000 person-years (95% CI 1.5 to 12.8).

3.6.3. Anti-Alglucosidase Alfa Antibodies

Data on anti-alglucosidase alfa antibody (Ab) titers for patients receiving ERT are shown in Table 5. Although most patients presented with elevated Ab titers, few showed a reduction in response to treatment or higher incidence of AEs. The most in-depth evaluation of Ab titers for patients receiving ERT was by de Vries et al. (2017) [45], and this study will therefore be described in greater detail. The patients were divided into three groups, according to their respective Ab titers: the first, of 16 patients, corresponded to high titers (>1: 31,250); the second, of 29 patients, corresponded to moderate titers (1: 1250 to <1: 31,250); the third, of 28 patients, to low titers (0 to <1: 1250). Three patterns of progression were observed concerning anti-ERT Ab titers; in the vast majority of patients (97%), titers either decreased or remained stable after 12 months of treatment, except in two patients, one of whom belonged to the group with the highest titers and the other to intermediate titers. Using the combined score of the MRC scale and the standing FVC, the authors compared treatment responses between the three Ab titer groups and found no significant differences between them, whether at baseline or after 3 years of treatment ($p = 0.35$ and $p = 0.38$, respectively). In one patient with high titers, the Ab had neutralizing effects on the enzyme, with a decline in FVC and strength. De Vries et al. (2017) [45] concluded, therefore, that there was a relationship between anti-alglucosidase alfa Ab titers and the development of AEs (statistical analysis not shown). Only 1/28 (4%) patients in the low-titer group had AEs, while 5/29 (17%) in the intermediate-titer group and 7/16 (44%) in the high-titer group experienced them.

Table 5. Antibody titers for patients with late-onset Pompe disease receiving enzyme replacement therapy, reduction in response to treatment, and incidence of AEs.

Study	N of Patients	N Ab Titer ≥ 1:250	Method of Measuring Ab	Reduced Response to Treatment	AEs Attributable to Ab Presence
Angelini et al. (2012) [31]	15	11	N/A	N/E	Yes ($n = 1$)
de Vries et al. (2017) [45]	73	46	Van Gelder et al. (2014) [48]	Yes ($n = 1$)	Yes
Kuperus et al. (2017) [39]	73	44	Van Gelder et al. (2014) [48]	Yes ($n = 1$)	N/E
Orlikowski et al. (2011) [43]	5	5	N/A	No	N/E
Regnery et al. (2012) [30]	38	38	N/A	Yes ($n = 1$)	N/E
van Capelle et al. (2010) [34]	5	5	N/A	No	N/E
Van der Ploeg et al. (2010) [36]	59	59	Kishnani et al. (2006) [49]	N/E	No
Van der Ploeg et al. (2012) [29]	59	59	Kishnani et al. (2006) [49]	Yes ($n = 2$)	No

AE = adverse event. Ab = anti-alglucosidase alfa antibodies (measured by different methods). N/A = not available. N/E = not evaluated.

3.7. Risk of Bias and Quality of Included Studies

The risk of bias of the included NRSI is shown in Figure 8. The RCT included had some concerning issues, such as an imbalance in age at baseline and possible conflict of interest of the investigators. Most included articles showed a moderate to severe risk of bias, independently of the study design; only one showed a critical risk of bias [46].

3.8. Certainty of Evidence by Outcomes

All outcomes were assessed for certainty of evidence, with low certainty only for TOV. All other outcomes had very low certainty of evidence, mainly due to the uncontrolled observational design of the included studies, with data from secondary outcomes. A full analysis is available in the Supplementary Materials.

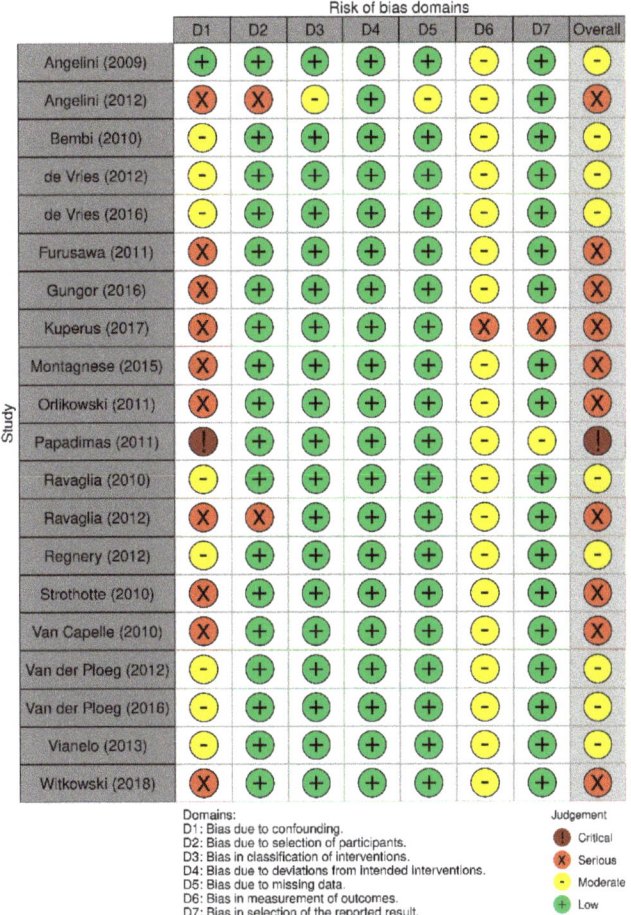

Figure 8. Risk of bias of included studies evaluated through the ROBIN-I tool.

4. Discussion

LOPD is a rare, serious disease with no specific treatment available other than ERT. Interpretation of the available evidence must always consider these facts. Given that only one double-blind RCT of GAA ERT for LOPD has been conducted [36], prospective observational trials were also evaluated in this review. The included studies all had small sample sizes (which is to be expected given the rarity of LOPD), as well as different ages (children, adolescents, and adults), stages, durations of disease burden prior to start of ERT, and phenotypic manifestations. Among the outcomes evaluated for LOPD, we showed a benefit for 6MWT, as also demonstrated in a previous meta-analysis [50]. Otherwise, this was the first meta-analysis to evaluate the effect of ERT on TOV and QOL. An improvement in functional capacity, measured through FVC, was not confirmed.

Two systematic reviews have already been published on the efficacy of alglucosidase alfa, neither of which assessed safety directly [14,50]: the first one in 2013, by Toscano et al. [14], and the second one in 2017, by Schoser et al. [50]. The latter included 22 papers (of which 10 were included in the present review), comprising case series and retrospective studies, with or without a control group, and evaluated 6MWT, FVC, and mortality by conducting a meta-analysis. The average age of patients included in the review was 46 years. [50] Toscano et al. included 21 papers (of which 14 were included in the present review), also comprising case series and retrospective studies, with or without a control group. They evaluated, among other outcomes, 6MWT, FVC, the need for ventilatory support, and QOL, with most patients aged between 40 and 59 years (44%); any improvement was considered meaningful, without defined criteria for clinical relevance [14]. Our review included 22 papers only with prospective data, excluding case series, and the mean age of the included participants was 42.8 years (range, 7 to 76.3 years), with 32.5 months of follow-up.

The systematic review carried out by Toscano et al. [14] evaluated FVC for 124 treated patients and identified an improvement in 51.6%, stable disease in 13.7%, and decline in 34.7%. There was no correlation between the duration of treatment and improvement in lung capacity, with no description of comparison with a control group. Likewise, the meta-analysis carried out by Schoser et al. [50] demonstrated a beneficial effect of ERT on FVC in groups receiving alglucosidase alfa; their conclusion was based on an analysis using a fixed-effect model, which is not considered the best method of evaluating studies with heterogeneous populations. The results showed that untreated patients had a 2.3% decline in FVC% after 12 months and 6.2% after 4 years; treated patients had an initial increase in FVC% of 1.4% after 2 months, with a return to baseline FVC% and a slight decline in follow-up, with data not detailed. The difference in efficacy between control (a historical cohort without treatment) and treated patients varied from 4.5% after 1 year to 6% at 4 years, and therefore cannot be considered clinically significant. Our data, retrieved from 348 patients, do not confirm the findings of Schoser et al., suggesting that there is little effect of ERT on FVC.

Our results confirm a previously published meta-analysis concerning the effect of ERT on 6MWT (mean change 36.6 m (95% CI 10.72, 62.48)). Schoser et al. [50] demonstrated a beneficial effect of ERT on 6MWT in the groups receiving alglucosidase alfa at 12 months, with an average improvement 43 m greater than in controls, based on data from 171 patients undergoing treatment in comparison to a historical cohort without treatment. Toscano et al. [14] also included the 6MWT among their outcomes of interest and reported data from 122 patients, of which 77.9% improved, 8.2% stabilized, and 13.9% worsened. We found an increase of 36 m in this outcome, above the 26 m cutoff considered clinically relevant, and the improvement in walking distance described in the included articles ranged from 33 to 1000 m. The inclusion of the results from Bembi et al. (2010) [42] for this outcome highlights the issue of early intervention, as the greatest benefit of intervention was seen in the young group, which is of fundamental importance for the analysis of the available evidence, since additional benefits or a greater effect size may not have been found in other studies due to the inclusion of patients with established disease and very heterogeneous age at initiation of treatment.

Our study also indicates a beneficial effect of ERT on the physical component of QOL (mean change 1.96 (95% CI 0.33, 3.59)), and this improvement in endurance has positive aspects in making patients less dependent on caregivers. However, it bears stressing that generic QOL instruments were used, as there is no specific validated instrument for assessing the QOL of patients with PD. One systematic review without meta-analysis also evaluated QOL [14], and all included studies in this systematic review with $n \geq 5$ were included in our search. In addition, 9 of the 21 included articles evaluated QOL, with 156 patients evaluated for this outcome using the SF-36 questionnaire. Qualitative synthesis of these studies showed that only 13/156 patients (8.3%) improved their QOL scores after treatment.

This is the first meta-analysis to show a trend toward a beneficial effect of ERT on TOV (mean change -2.64 h (95% CI -5.28, 0.00)), although previous systematic reviews have evaluated this outcome in different ways. In Schoser et al. [50], the percentage of patients dependent on ventilation varied between 14 and 100%, which is considered very high, due to the early age of the sample. They also reported that the number of patients requiring ventilation was maintained in patients treated with ERT, compared to a historical cohort that presented an increased proportion of patients using ventilation (data not provided by Schoser et al.)—with great heterogeneity between studies, however. Toscano et al. [14] evaluated data from 66 patients and demonstrated that ERT resulted in an improvement in the need for MV in 59.1% of patients, stabilization in 36.4% of patients, and worsening in only 4.5% of patients. Regarding the need for non-invasive ventilation, 64.1% improved, 32.1% stabilized, and 3.8% worsened (data not detailed). In our study, 265 patients were on any type of ventilatory support.

Concerning mortality, our study showed an incidence rate of 4.4/1000 events per person-year of patients with LOPD treated with ERT, which is considered very low. A previous systematic review with meta-analysis [50] was able to estimate that patients on ERT had a lower mortality rate compared to those not treated, using mortality data from included studies. It is important to note that the results of this study should be interpreted with caution, as the methodological steps followed by authors were not clearly mentioned.

Schoser et al. included six observational studies [31,32,43,46,51,52], of which only one [51] presented comparative data between a group on alglucosidase alfa ERT and untreated controls. According to this meta-analysis, the summary measure showed a 79% reduction in risk of death for those patients on alglucosidase alfa (HR = 0.21 (95% CI 0.11; 0.41)). However, it should be noted that the other studies, which were non-comparative case series, might have led to an overestimation of the effect. Although this study corrected the meta-analysis by covariables (meta-regression adjusted for age, sex, and severity of PD) and interpreted the sources of heterogeneity, the review had a serious risk of bias, according to the AMSTAR-2 tool. Gungor et al. (2013) [51] showed a 59% reduced risk of death for those patients on alglucosidase alfa compared to those who did not receive the therapy (HR = 0.41 (95% CI 0.19; 0.87)). This analysis was adjusted for age, sex, country of residence, and severity of PD. The other studies were case series, with no comparator group, reported a small number of deaths, and did not discuss whether these were related to treatment (absolute frequency in the five studies: 3 deaths among 151 patients). Gungor et al. (2013) [51] was the only study with a comparator group and cohort adjusted for potential confounders.

Although treatment-emergent or infusion-related AEs are common in ERT recipients, in most cases, these are mild and easily treatable. The development of IgG antibodies to alglucosidase alfa is also frequent; however, it does not seem to be related to the presence or absence of AEs or to the effect of treatment, although the measures used may not be sensitive enough to identify these. In IOPD, where the outcome is clearer, there is a direct correlation between patients with highly sustained and sustained intermediate Ab titers and clinical outcome. Therefore, more studies in LOPD are needed evaluating outcome measures that have the ability to capture small changes caused by ERT on them [53]. A systematic review conducted by Toscano et al. [14] described AEs as mostly mild to moderate in 303 patients undergoing treatment, with severe AEs reported in only four patients, all in studies included in the present article. They also reported the development of antibodies in 128 patients, three of whom had an anaphylactic reaction. It bears stressing that the evidence for safety is low, but although these studies have already reached a substantial length of follow-up, ERT is generally understood to be safe. No studies have demonstrated, for example, the effectiveness of physical therapy as the sole treatment strategy for these patients.

The included studies were highly heterogeneous, enrolling patients from different age groups and with different disease severities. Therefore, the findings of this review and meta-analysis should be interpreted with caution. In addition, most included studies were non-randomized studies of interventions, with low methodological quality, no comparison group, or comparison with a historical cohort. Another challenge is incompletely reported data, as publication bias was present. Usually, data from secondary outcomes were poorly reported, as studies were not designed to measure them. In most cases, however, conclusions were made without showing full data and results. Proper reporting of data is essential. One strength of the present study was that we included only prospective trials, in an attempt to avoid memory and selection bias. Prospective trials also have the advantage of collecting data accordingly with the predefined outcomes of interest, which does not happen in retrospective trials.

In conclusion, alglucosidase alfa effectively increases the distance achieved in 6MWT, improves the physical component of QOL, and may decrease TOV in treated patients. Stabilization of functional capacity, measured through FVC, was not confirmed. The treatment is safe in the studied population, with generally mild adverse events. Further studies could evaluate the impact of the duration of follow-up in the included studies, taking into consideration that the efficacy of ERT may present some secondary decline after 3 to 5 years of treatment [54]. Moreover, the age at ERT initiation is an important aspect that should be addressed in future reviews.

Supplementary Materials: The following are available online at https://www.mdpi.com/2077-0383/10/21/4828/s1, Table S1: Evaluation of the effect of enzyme replacement therapy on forced vital capacity in late-onset Pompe disease; Table S2: GRADEpro of forced vital capacity outcome; Table S3: Evaluation of the effect of enzyme replacement therapy on 6-min walking test in late-onset Pompe disease; Table S4: GRADEpro of 6-min walking test outcome; Table S5: Evaluation of the effect of enzyme replacement therapy on Walton & Gardner-Medwin scale scores in late-onset Pompe disease; Table S6: GRADEpro of Walton & Gardner-Medwin Scale outcome; Table S7: Evaluation of the effect of enzyme replacement therapy on upper limb strength in late-onset Pompe disease; Table S8: GRADEpro of upper limb strength outcome (assessed with QMFT and HHD); Table S9: Evaluation of the effect of enzyme replacement therapy on quality of life in late-onset Pompe disease; Table S10: GRADEpro of quality of life outcome (assessed with SF-36); Table S11: Evaluation of the effect of enzyme replacement therapy on time on ventilation in late-onset Pompe disease; Table S12: GRADEpro of time on ventilation; Table S13. Safety assessment of enzyme replacement therapy for patients with late-onset Pompe disease; Table S14: GRADEpro of safety outcomes; Table S15: GRADEpro of mortality.

Author Contributions: Conceptualization, A.D.D. and I.V.D.S.; Methodology, A.D.D., T.V.P., H.A.d.O.J. and I.V.D.S.; Software, T.V.P.; Formal Analysis, T.V.P.; Selection stage, A.P.P.J. and C.B.T.G.; Data extraction, A.D.D. and B.C.K.; Writing—Original Draft Preparation, A.D.D.; Writing—Review and Editing, A.P.P.J., P.S.K., J.C.L.J. and H.A.d.O.J.; Supervision, H.A.d.O.J.; Project Administration, I.V.D.S.; Funding Acquisition, I.V.D.S. All authors have read and agreed to the published version of the manuscript.

Funding: This research was funded by the Hospital de Clínicas de Porto Alegre Event Incentive Fund (FIPE/HCPA), grant number (protocol code) 2019-0495, by the Pro-BIC HCPA/CNPq Undergraduate Research Program, by Casa dos Raros, Center for Comprehensive Care and Training in Rare Diseases, and by Casa Hunter. The funding body had no role in the design of the study, in the collection, analysis, and interpretation of data, or in writing the manuscript. T.V.P. is funded by the Chevening Scholarship Programme (Foreign and Commonwealth Office, UK).

Institutional Review Board Statement: The study was conducted according to the guidelines of the Declaration of Helsinki and approved by the Institutional Review Board (or Ethics Committee) of Hospital de Clínicas de Porto Alegre (protocol code 2019-0495, date of approval 11 February 2020) and Plataforma Brasil (protocol code 20996919000005327, date of approval 11 February 2020).

Informed Consent Statement: Not applicable.

Data Availability Statement: The datasets analyzed during the current study are available from the corresponding author on reasonable request.

Conflicts of Interest: P.S.K. has received research/grant support from Sanofi Genzyme, Valerion Therapeutics, Shire Pharmaceuticals, and Amicus Therapeutics. P.S.K. has received consulting fees and honoraria from Sanofi Genzyme, Shire Pharmaceuticals, Amicus Therapeutics, Vertex Pharmaceuticals, Maze Therapeutics, JCR Pharmaceutical and Asklepios BioPharmaceuticalBiopharmaceutical, Inc. (AskBio). P.S.K. is a member of the Pompe and Gaucher Disease Registry Advisory Board for Sanofi Genzyme., Amicus Therapeutics, and Baebies. P.S.K. has equity in Asklepios Biopharmaceutical, Inc. (AskBio), which is developing gene therapy for Pompe disease and Maze Therapeutics, which is developing small molecule in Pompe disease. All other authors declare that they have no competing interests.

Abbreviations

6MWT	6 min walking test
ABC	approximate Bayesian computation model
AE	adverse event
CI	confidence interval
OPD	infantile-onset Pompe disease
ERT	enzyme replacement therapy
FVC	forced vital capacity
GAA	acid alpha-glucosidase
GLMM	generalized linear mixed model
IAR	infusion-associated reaction
IgG	immunoglobulin G
IR	incidence rate
LOPD	late-onset Pompe disease
LOTS	late-onset treatment study
ML	maximum likelihood
MRC	Medical Research Council
NB	newborn
NRSI	non-randomized studies of interventions
PD	Pompe disease
PedsQL	Pediatric Quality of Life Inventory™
PICO	patients, intervention, control, outcome
QOL	quality of life
RCT	randomized clinical trial
REML	restricted maximum-likelihood estimator
RoB	Risk of Bias tool
ROBINS-I	Risk Of Bias In Non-randomized Studies of Interventions tool
SM	Supplementary Materials
TOV	time on ventilatory support
WGMS	Walton and Gardner-Medwin Scale

References

1. Llerena, J.C.; Horovitz, D.M.; Marie, S.K.; Porta, G.; Giugliani, R.; Rojas, M.V.; Martins, A.M.; Brazilian Network for Studies in Pompe Disease (ReBrPOM). The Brazilian consensus on the management of Pompe disease. *J. Pediatr.* **2009**, *155*, S47–S56. [CrossRef]
2. Levine, J.C.; Kishnani, P.S.; Chen, Y.T.; Herlong, J.R.; Li, J.S. Cardiac remodeling after enzyme replacement therapy with acid alpha-glucosidase for infants with Pompe disease. *Pediatr. Cardiol.* **2008**, *29*, 1033–1042. [CrossRef]
3. Slonim, A.E.; Bulone, L.; Goldberg, T.; Minikes, J.; Slonim, E.; Galanko, J.; Martiniuk, F. Modification of the natural history of adult-onset acid maltase deficiency by nutrition and exercise therapy. *Muscle Nerve* **2007**, *35*, 70–77. [CrossRef]
4. Geel, T.M.; McLaughlin, P.M.; de Leij, L.F.; Ruiters, M.H.; Niezen-Koning, K.E. Pompe disease: Current state of treatment modalities and animal models. *Mol. Genet. Metab.* **2007**, *92*, 299–307. [CrossRef] [PubMed]
5. Winchester, B.; Bali, D.; Bodamer, O.A.; Caillaud, C.; Christensen, E.; Cooper, A.; Cupler, E.; Deschauer, M.; Fumić, K.; Jackson, M.; et al. Methods for a prompt and reliable laboratory diagnosis of Pompe disease: Report from an international consensus meeting. *Mol. Genet. Metab.* **2008**, *93*, 275–281. [CrossRef] [PubMed]
6. Bembi, B.; Cerini, E.; Danesino, C.; Donati, M.A.; Gasperini, S.; Morandi, L.; Musumeci, O.; Parenti, G.; Ravaglia, S.; Seidita, F.; et al. Diagnosis of glycogenosis type II. *Neurology* **2008**, *71*, S4–S11. [CrossRef] [PubMed]
7. Chen, M.; Zhang, L.; Quan, S. Enzyme replacement therapy for infantile-onset Pompe disease. *Cochrane Database Syst. Rev.* **2017**, *11*, CD011539. [CrossRef]
8. Llerena Junior, J.C.; Nascimento, O.J.; Oliveira, A.S.; Dourado Junior, M.E.; Marrone, C.D.; Siqueira, H.H.; Sobreira, C.F.; Dias-Tosta, E.; Werneck, L.C. Guidelines for the diagnosis, treatment and clinical monitoring of patients with juvenile and adult Pompe disease. *Arq Neuropsiquiatr.* **2016**, *74*, 166–176. [CrossRef]
9. Burton, B.K.; Charrow, J.; Hoganson, G.E.; Fleischer, J.; Grange, D.K.; Braddock, S.R.; Hitchins, L.; Hickey, R.; Christensen, K.M.; Groepper, D.; et al. Newborn Screening for Pompe Disease in Illinois: Experience with 684,290 Infants. *Int. J. Neonatal Screen.* **2020**, *6*, 4. [CrossRef]

10. Ficicioglu, C.; Ahrens-Nicklas, R.C.; Barch, J.; Cuddapah, S.R.; DiBoscio, B.S.; DiPerna, J.C.; Gordon, P.L.; Henderson, N.; Menello, C.; Luongo, N.; et al. Newborn Screening for Pompe Disease: Pennsylvania Experience. *Int. J. Neonatal Screen.* **2020**, *6*, 89. [CrossRef]
11. Klug, T.L.; Swartz, L.B.; Washburn, J.; Brannen, C.; Kiesling, J.L. Lessons Learned from Pompe Disease Newborn Screening and Follow-up. *Int. J. Neonatal Screen.* **2020**, *6*, 11. [CrossRef]
12. Momosaki, K.; Kido, J.; Yoshida, S.; Sugawara, K.; Miyamoto, T.; Inoue, T.; Okumiya, T.; Matsumoto, S.; Endo, F.; Hirose, S.; et al. Newborn screening for Pompe disease in Japan: Report and literature review of mutations in the GAA gene in Japanese and Asian patients. *J. Hum. Genet.* **2019**, *64*, 741–755. [CrossRef]
13. Strothotte, S.; Strigl-Pill, N.; Grunert, B.; Kornblum, C.; Eger, K.; Wessig, C.; Deschauer, M.; Breunig, F.; Glocker, F.X.; Vielhaber, S.; et al. Enzyme replacement therapy with alglucosidase alfa in 44 patients with late-onset glycogen storage disease type 2: 12-month results of an observational clinical trial. *J. Neurol.* **2010**, *257*, 91–97. [CrossRef] [PubMed]
14. Toscano, A.; Schoser, B. Enzyme replacement therapy in late-onset Pompe disease: A systematic literature review. *J. Neurol.* **2013**, *260*, 951–959. [CrossRef] [PubMed]
15. Page, M.J.; McKenzie, J.E.; Bossuyt, P.M.; Boutron, I.; Hoffmann, T.C.; Mulrow, C.D.; Shamseer, L.; Tetzlaff, J.M.; Akl, E.A.; Brennan, S.E.; et al. The PRISMA 2020 statement: An updated guideline for reporting systematic reviews. *Int. J. Surg.* **2021**, *88*, 105906. [CrossRef] [PubMed]
16. Plotkin, S.R.; Davis, S.D.; Robertson, K.A.; Akshintala, S.; Allen, J.; Fisher, M.J.; Blakeley, J.O.; Widemann, B.C.; Ferner, R.E.; Marcus, C.L.; et al. Sleep and pulmonary outcomes for clinical trials of airway plexiform neurofibromas in NF1. *Neurology* **2016**, *87*, S13–S20. [CrossRef] [PubMed]
17. Rozov, T.; Silva, F.A.; Santana, M.A.; Adde, F.V.; Mendes, R.H.; Group, B.C.F.M.S. A first-year dornase alfa treatment impact on clinical parameters of patients with cystic fibrosis: The Brazilian cystic fibrosis multicenter study. *Rev. Paul Pediatr.* **2013**, *31*, 420–430. [CrossRef]
18. Schrover, R.; Evans, K.; Giugliani, R.; Noble, I.; Bhattacharya, K. Minimal clinically important difference for the 6-min walk test: Literature review and application to Morquio A syndrome. *Orphanet J. Rare Dis.* **2017**, *12*, 78. [CrossRef]
19. Schwarzer, G.; Chemaitelly, H.; Abu-Raddad, L.J.; Rücker, G. Seriously misleading results using inverse of Freeman-Tukey double arcsine transformation in meta-analysis of single proportions. *Res. Synth. Methods* **2019**, *10*, 476–483. [CrossRef]
20. Kwon, D.; Reis, I.M. Simulation-based estimation of mean and standard deviation for meta-analysis via Approximate Bayesian Computation (ABC). *BMC Med. Res. Methodol.* **2015**, *15*, 61. [CrossRef]
21. Pereira, T.V.; Patsopoulos, N.A.; Salanti, G.; Ioannidis, J.P. Critical interpretation of Cochran's Q test depends on power and prior assumptions about heterogeneity. *Res. Synth. Methods* **2010**, *1*, 149–161. [CrossRef] [PubMed]
22. Sterne, J.A.C.; Savović, J.; Page, M.J.; Elbers, R.G.; Blencowe, N.S.; Boutron, I.; Cates, C.J.; Cheng, H.Y.; Corbett, M.S.; Eldridge, S.M.; et al. RoB 2: A revised tool for assessing risk of bias in randomised trials. *BMJ* **2019**, *366*, l4898. [CrossRef] [PubMed]
23. Sterne, J.A.; Hernán, M.A.; Reeves, B.C.; Savović, J.; Berkman, N.D.; Viswanathan, M.; Henry, D.; Altman, D.G.; Ansari, M.T.; Boutron, I.; et al. ROBINS-I: A tool for assessing risk of bias in non-randomised studies of interventions. *BMJ* **2016**, *355*, i4919. [CrossRef] [PubMed]
24. Balshem, H.; Helfand, M.; Schünemann, H.J.; Oxman, A.D.; Kunz, R.; Brozek, J.; Vist, G.E.; Falck-Ytter, Y.; Meerpohl, J.; Norris, S.; et al. GRADE guidelines: 3. Rating the quality of evidence. *J. Clin. Epidemiol.* **2011**, *64*, 401–406. [CrossRef] [PubMed]
25. Guyatt, G.H.; Oxman, A.D.; Vist, G.E.; Kunz, R.; Falck-Ytter, Y.; Alonso-Coello, P.; Schünemann, H.J.; Group, G.W. GRADE: An emerging consensus on rating quality of evidence and strength of recommendations. *BMJ* **2008**, *336*, 924–926. [CrossRef]
26. Guyatt, G.H.; Oxman, A.D.; Schünemann, H.J.; Tugwell, P.; Knottnerus, A. GRADE guidelines: A new series of articles in the Journal of Clinical Epidemiology. *J. Clin. Epidemiol.* **2011**, *64*, 380–382. [CrossRef]
27. Montagnese, F.; Barca, E.; Musumeci, O.; Mondello, S.; Migliorato, A.; Ciranni, A.; Rodolico, C.; De Filippi, P.; Danesino, C.; Toscano, A. Clinical and molecular aspects of 30 patients with late-onset Pompe disease (LOPD): Unusual features and response to treatment. *J. Neurol.* **2015**, *262*, 968–978. [CrossRef]
28. van der Ploeg, A.; Carlier, P.G.; Carlier, R.Y.; Kissel, J.T.; Schoser, B.; Wenninger, S.; Pestronk, A.; Barohn, R.J.; Dimachkie, M.M.; Goker-Alpan, O.; et al. Prospective exploratory muscle biopsy, imaging, and functional assessment in patients with late-onset Pompe disease treated with alglucosidase alfa: The EMBASSY Study. *Mol. Genet. Metab.* **2016**, *119*, 115–123. [CrossRef]
29. van der Ploeg, A.T.; Barohn, R.; Carlson, L.; Charrow, J.; Clemens, P.R.; Hopkin, R.J.; Kishnani, P.S.; Laforêt, P.; Morgan, C.; Nations, S.; et al. Open-label extension study following the Late-Onset Treatment Study (LOTS) of alglucosidase alfa. *Mol. Genet. Metab.* **2012**, *107*, 456–461. [CrossRef]
30. Regnery, C.; Kornblum, C.; Hanisch, F.; Vielhaber, S.; Strigl-Pill, N.; Grunert, B.; Müller-Felber, W.; Glocker, F.X.; Spranger, M.; Deschauer, M.; et al. 36 months observational clinical study of 38 adult Pompe disease patients under alglucosidase alfa enzyme replacement therapy. *J. Inherit. Metab. Dis.* **2012**, *35*, 837–845. [CrossRef] [PubMed]
31. Angelini, C.; Semplicini, C.; Ravaglia, S.; Bembi, B.; Servidei, S.; Pegoraro, E.; Moggio, M.; Filosto, M.; Sette, E.; Crescimanno, G.; et al. Observational clinical study in juvenile-adult glycogenosis type 2 patients undergoing enzyme replacement therapy for up to 4 years. *J. Neurol.* **2012**, *259*, 952–958. [CrossRef]
32. Furusawa, Y.; Mori-Yoshimura, M.; Yamamoto, T.; Sakamoto, C.; Wakita, M.; Kobayashi, Y.; Fukumoto, Y.; Oya, Y.; Fukuda, T.; Sugie, H.; et al. Effects of enzyme replacement therapy on five patients with advanced late-onset glycogen storage disease type II: A 2-year follow-up study. *J. Inherit. Metab. Dis.* **2012**, *35*, 301–310. [CrossRef]

33. de Vries, J.M.; van der Beek, N.A.; Hop, W.C.; Karstens, F.P.; Wokke, J.H.; de Visser, M.; van Engelen, B.G.; Kuks, J.B.; van der Kooi, A.J.; Notermans, N.C.; et al. Effect of enzyme therapy and prognostic factors in 69 adults with Pompe disease: An open-label single-center study. *Orphanet J. Rare Dis.* **2012**, *7*, 73. [CrossRef]
34. van Capelle, C.I.; van der Beek, N.A.; Hagemans, M.L.; Arts, W.F.; Hop, W.C.; Lee, P.; Jaeken, J.; Frohn-Mulder, I.M.; Merkus, P.J.; Corzo, D.; et al. Effect of enzyme therapy in juvenile patients with Pompe disease: A three-year open-label study. *Neuromuscul. Disord.* **2010**, *20*, 775–782. [CrossRef] [PubMed]
35. Ravaglia, S.; Pichiecchio, A.; Ponzio, M.; Danesino, C.; Saeidi Garaghani, K.; Poloni, G.U.; Toscano, A.; Moglia, A.; Carlucci, A.; Bini, P.; et al. Changes in skeletal muscle qualities during enzyme replacement therapy in late-onset type II glycogenosis: Temporal and spatial pattern of mass vs. strength response. *J. Inherit. Metab. Dis.* **2010**, *33*, 737–745. [CrossRef] [PubMed]
36. van der Ploeg, A.T.; Clemens, P.R.; Corzo, D.; Escolar, D.M.; Florence, J.; Groeneveld, G.J.; Herson, S.; Kishnani, P.S.; Laforet, P.; Lake, S.L.; et al. A randomized study of alglucosidase alfa in late-onset Pompe's disease. *N. Engl. J. Med.* **2010**, *362*, 1396–1406. [CrossRef]
37. Angelini, C.; Semplicini, C.; Tonin, P.; Filosto, M.; Pegoraro, E.; Sorarù, G.; Fanin, M. Progress in Enzyme Replacement Therapy in Glycogen Storage Disease Type II. *Ther. Adv. Neurol. Disord.* **2009**, *2*, 143–153. [CrossRef] [PubMed]
38. Witkowski, G.; Konopko, M.; Rola, R.; Ługowska, A.; Ryglewicz, D.; Sienkiewicz-Jarosz, H. Enzymatic replacement therapy in patients with late-onset Pompe disease—6-Year follow up. *Neurol. Neurochir. Pol.* **2018**, *52*, 465–469. [CrossRef]
39. Kuperus, E.; Kruijshaar, M.E.; Wens, S.C.A.; de Vries, J.M.; Favejee, M.M.; van der Meijden, J.C.; Rizopoulos, D.; Brusse, E.; van Doorn, P.A.; van der Ploeg, A.T.; et al. Long-term benefit of enzyme replacement therapy in Pompe disease: A 5-year prospective study. *Neurology* **2017**, *89*, 2365–2373. [CrossRef]
40. Vianello, A.; Semplicini, C.; Paladini, L.; Concas, A.; Ravaglia, S.; Servidei, S.; Toscano, A.; Mongini, T.; Angelini, C.; Pegoraro, E. Enzyme replacement therapy improves respiratory outcomes in patients with late-onset type II glycogenosis and high ventilator dependency. *Lung* **2013**, *191*, 537–544. [CrossRef]
41. Ravaglia, S.; De Filippi, P.; Pichiecchio, A.; Ponzio, M.; Saeidi Garaghani, K.; Poloni, G.U.; Bini, P.; Danesino, C. Can genes influencing muscle function affect the therapeutic response to enzyme replacement therapy (ERT) in late-onset type II glycogenosis? *Mol. Genet. Metab.* **2012**, *107*, 104–110. [CrossRef] [PubMed]
42. Bembi, B.; Pisa, F.E.; Confalonieri, M.; Ciana, G.; Fiumara, A.; Parini, R.; Rigoldi, M.; Moglia, A.; Costa, A.; Carlucci, A.; et al. Long-term observational, non-randomized study of enzyme replacement therapy in late-onset glycogenosis type II. *J. Inherit. Metab. Dis.* **2010**, *33*, 727–735. [CrossRef] [PubMed]
43. Orlikowski, D.; Pellegrini, N.; Prigent, H.; Laforêt, P.; Carlier, R.; Carlier, P.; Eymard, B.; Lofaso, F.; Annane, D. Recombinant human acid alpha-glucosidase (rhGAA) in adult patients with severe respiratory failure due to Pompe disease. *Neuromuscul. Disord.* **2011**, *21*, 477–482. [CrossRef] [PubMed]
44. Forsha, D.; Li, J.S.; Smith, P.B.; van der Ploeg, A.T.; Kishnani, P.; Pasquali, S.K.; Investigators, L.-O.T.S. Cardiovascular abnormalities in late-onset Pompe disease and response to enzyme replacement therapy. *Genet. Med.* **2011**, *13*, 625–631. [CrossRef]
45. de Vries, J.M.; Kuperus, E.; Hoogeveen-Westerveld, M.; Kroos, M.A.; Wens, S.C.; Stok, M.; van der Beek, N.A.; Kruijshaar, M.E.; Rizopoulos, D.; van Doorn, P.A.; et al. Pompe disease in adulthood: Effects of antibody formation on enzyme replacement therapy. *Genet. Med.* **2017**, *19*, 90–97. [CrossRef]
46. Papadimas, G.K.; Spengos, K.; Konstantinopoulou, A.; Vassilopoulou, S.; Vontzalidis, A.; Papadopoulos, C.; Michelakakis, H.; Manta, P. Adult Pompe disease: Clinical manifestations and outcome of the first Greek patients receiving enzyme replacement therapy. *Clin. Neurol. Neurosurg.* **2011**, *113*, 303–307. [CrossRef]
47. Güngör, D.; Kruijshaar, M.E.; Plug, I.; Rizopoulos, D.; Kanters, T.A.; Wens, S.C.; Reuser, A.J.; van Doorn, P.A.; van der Ploeg, A.T. Quality of life and participation in daily life of adults with Pompe disease receiving enzyme replacement therapy: 10 years of international follow-up. *J. Inherit. Metab. Dis.* **2016**, *39*, 253–260. [CrossRef]
48. van Gelder, C.M.; Hoogeveen-Westerveld, M.; Kroos, M.A.; Plug, I.; van der Ploeg, A.T.; Reuser, A.J. Enzyme therapy and immune response in relation to CRIM status: The Dutch experience in classic infantile Pompe disease. *J. Inherit. Metab. Dis.* **2015**, *38*, 305–314. [CrossRef]
49. Kishnani, P.S.; Nicolino, M.; Voit, T.; Rogers, R.C.; Tsai, A.C.; Waterson, J.; Herman, G.E.; Amalfitano, A.; Thurberg, B.L.; Richards, S.; et al. Chinese hamster ovary cell-derived recombinant human acid alpha-glucosidase in infantile-onset Pompe disease. *J. Pediatr.* **2006**, *149*, 89–97. [CrossRef]
50. Schoser, B.; Stewart, A.; Kanters, S.; Hamed, A.; Jansen, J.; Chan, K.; Karamouzian, M.; Toscano, A. Survival and long-term outcomes in late-onset Pompe disease following alglucosidase alfa treatment: A systematic review and meta-analysis. *J. Neurol.* **2017**, *264*, 621–630. [CrossRef] [PubMed]
51. Güngör, D.; Kruijshaar, M.E.; Plug, I.; D'Agostino, R.B.; Hagemans, M.L.; van Doorn, P.A.; Reuser, A.J.; van der Ploeg, A.T. Impact of enzyme replacement therapy on survival in adults with Pompe disease: Results from a prospective international observational study. *Orphanet J. Rare Dis.* **2013**, *8*, 49. [CrossRef]
52. Anderson, L.J.; Henley, W.; Wyatt, K.M.; Nikolaou, V.; Waldek, S.; Hughes, D.A.; Lachmann, R.H.; Logan, S. Effectiveness of enzyme replacement therapy in adults with late-onset Pompe disease: Results from the NCS-LSD cohort study. *J. Inherit. Metab. Dis.* **2014**, *37*, 945–952. [CrossRef]
53. Herbert, M.; Kazi, Z.B.; Richards, S.; Rosenberg, A.S.; Kishnani, P.S. Response to de Vries et al. *Genet. Med.* **2017**, *19*, 1281–1282. [CrossRef]

54. Harlaar, L.; Hogrel, J.Y.; Perniconi, B.; Kruijshaar, M.E.; Rizopoulos, D.; Taouagh, N.; Canal, A.; Brusse, E.; van Doorn, P.A.; van der Ploeg, A.T.; et al. Large variation in effects during 10 years of enzyme therapy in adults with Pompe disease. *Neurology* **2019**, *93*, e1756–e1767. [CrossRef]

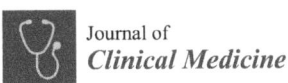

Article

Impact of Intravenous Trehalose Administration in Patients with Niemann–Pick Disease Types A and B

Moein Mobini [1], Shabnam Radbakhsh [2,3], Francyne Kubaski [4,5,6], Peyman Eshraghi [7], Saba Vakili [8], Rahim Vakili [8], Manijeh Khalili [9], Majid Varesvazirian [10], Tannaz Jamialahmadi [11], Seyed Ali Alamdaran [12], Seyed Javad Sayedi [13], Omid Rajabi [14], Seyed Ahmad Emami [15], Željko Reiner [16] and Amirhossein Sahebkar [17,18,19,*]

1. Faculty of Medicine, Mashhad University of Medical Sciences, Mashhad 9177948564, Iran; Mobinim891@gmail.com
2. Student Research Committee, Mashhad University of Medical Sciences, Mashhad 9177948564, Iran; Radbakhshs971@mums.ac.ir
3. Department of Medical Biotechnology and Nanotechnology, Mashhad University of Medical Sciences, Mashhad 9177948564, Iran
4. Department of Genetics, UFRGS, Porto Alegre 91501970, Brazil; fkubaski@udel.edu
5. Medical Genetics Service, HCPA, Porto Alegre 90035903, Brazil
6. Biodiscovery Lab, HCPA, Porto Alegre 90035903, Brazil
7. Department of Pediatric Diseases, Akbar Hospital, Faculty of Medicine, Mashhad University of Medical Sciences, Mashhad 9177897157, Iran; Eshraghip2@mums.ac.ir
8. Medical Genetic Research Center, Mashhad University of Medical Sciences, Mashhad 9177948564, Iran; Vakilis@mums.ac.ir (S.V.); Vakilir@mums.ac.ir (R.V.)
9. Children and Adolescents Health Research Center, Research Institute of cellular and Molecular Science in Infectious Diseases, Zahedan University of Medical Science, Zahedan 9816743463, Iran; dr_khalili2000@yahoo.com
10. Shafa Hospital, Kerman University of Medical Sciences, Kerman 7618751151, Iran; dr.vazirian@gmail.com
11. Department of Nutrition, Faculty of Medicine, Mashhad University of Medical Sciences, Mashhad 9177948564, Iran; jamiat931@gmail.com
12. Pediatric Radiology Department, Faculty of Medicine, Mashhad University of Medical Sciences, Mashhad 9177948564, Iran; Alamdarana@mums.ac.ir
13. Department of Pediatrics, Mashhad University of Medical Sciences, Mashhad 9177948564, Iran; Sayedij@mums.ac.ir
14. Department of Pharmaceutical and Food Control, School of Pharmacy, Mashhad University of Medical Sciences, Mashhad 9177948954, Iran; Rajabio@mums.ac.ir
15. Department of Traditional Pharmacy, School of Pharmacy, Mashhad University of Medical Sciences, Mashhad 9177948954, Iran; Emamia@mums.ac.ir
16. Department of Internal Medicine, University Hospital Center Zagreb, University of Zagreb, Kišpatićeva 12, 1000 Zagreb, Croatia; zreiner@kbc-zagreb.hr
17. Applied Biomedical Research Center, Mashhad University of Medical Sciences, Mashhad 9177948564, Iran
18. Biotechnology Research Center, Pharmaceutical Technology Institute, Mashhad University of Medical Sciences, Mashhad 9177948954, Iran
19. Department of Biotechnology, School of Pharmacy, Mashhad University of Medical Sciences, Mashhad 9177948954, Iran
* Correspondence: amir_saheb2000@yahoo.com

Abstract: Background and Aims: Niemann–Pick disease (NPD) types A (NPA) and B (NPB) are caused by deficiency of the acid sphingomyelinase enzyme, which is encoded by the *SMPD1* gene, resulting in progressive pathogenic accumulation of lipids in tissues. Trehalose has been suggested as an autophagy inducer with therapeutic neuroprotective effects. We performed a single-arm, open-label pilot study to assess the potential efficacy of trehalose treatment in patients with NPA and NPB patients. Methods: Five patients with NPD type A and B were enrolled in an open-label, single-arm clinical trial. Trehalose was administrated intravenously (IV) (15 g/week) for three months. The efficacy of trehalose in the management of clinical symptoms was evaluated in patients by assessing the quality of life, serum biomarkers, and high-resolution computed tomography (HRCT) of the lungs at the baseline and end of the interventional trial (day 0 and week 12). Results: The mean of TNO-AZL Preschool children Quality of Life (TAPQOL) scores increased in all patients after intervention at W12 compared to the baseline W0, although the difference was not statistically significant. The serum levels of lyso-SM-509 and lyso-SM were decreased in three and four patients out of five, respectively, compared with baseline. Elevated ALT and AST levels were decreased in all patients after 12 weeks of treatment; however, changes were not statistically significant. Pro-oxidant antioxidant balance (PAB) was also decreased and glutathione peroxidase (GPX) activity was increased in serum of patients at the end of the study. Imaging studies of spleen and lung HRCT showed improvement of symptoms in two patients. Conclusions: Positive trends in health-related quality of life (HRQoL), serum biomarkers, and organomegaly were observed after 3 months of treatment with trehalose in patients with NPA and NPB. Although not statistically significant, due to the small number of patients enrolled, these results are encouraging and should be further explored.

Keywords: lysosomal storage disease (LSD); Niemann–Pick type A; Niemann–Pick type B; acid sphingomyelinase; sphingolipid deposition; Trehalose

1. Introduction

Niemann–Pick disease (NPD) is a lysosomal storage disorder (LSDs) caused by the deficiency of acid sphingomyelinase activity (ASM) NP type A and B or cholesterol transporter function (NP type C) leading to lipid accumulation in different tissues and organs [1]. The estimated prevalence of NPA and NPB is 0.4–0.6 in 100,000 individuals [2]. Hepatosplenomegaly, pulmonary insufficiency, and profound central nervous system (CNS) involvement can lead to death in untreated patients within the first few years of life in NPA [3]. In contrast, NPB is the non-neuropathic form of the disorder with milder symptoms and clinical manifestations starting at later ages, with most patients reaching adulthood [4]. Low levels or total deficiency of ASM is the main cause of sphingomyelin accumulation and lipid abnormalities as well as downstream cell signaling pathways that affect ceramide generation as an important secondary pathway [1]. A common histopathological occurrence in NP patients is lipid-laden macrophages, also called foam cells, in the liver, spleen, lung airways, bone marrow, and cerebral cortex that lead to progressive destruction of target tissues [5]. Early diagnosis and treatment are required to attenuate outcome and to improve the quality of life in NP patients; however, bone marrow transplantation (BMT), enzyme replacement therapy (ERT), and other therapeutic approaches are still in stages of research and have not been adequately effective [6–8].

Trehalose is a natural non reducing (1–1 α-linkage) disaccharide in various organisms, from bacteria to animals, that exerts cell-protective effects under tensions, such as temperature, drought, and oxidative stress [9]. Trehalose has been recognized as a safe additive by the Joint WHO/FOA Expert Committee on Food Additive (JECFA) and U.S. Food and Drug Administration (FDA) in 2000, and was approved for use in food in Europe in 2001 [10]. Apart from basic and experimental evidence [11–16], several clinical trials were performed to evaluate the safety and efficacy of trehalose in healthy subjects or patients with different diseases, both orally and intravenously [17,18]. At doses up to 50 g, trehalose is safe for humans, and no adverse effect has been reported in most subjects; however, gastrointestinal side effects may occur in trehalose-deficient individuals [19].

In addition, trehalose has also been reported to prevent neuronal damage and attenuate neurodegenerative disorders caused by LSDs [19,20]. Antiaggregant, anti-inflammatory, and antioxidant properties, along with autophagy inducer, might be proposed as potential mechanisms of neuroprotective activities of trehalose in both cell cultures and in-vivo animal models [21,22]. Several lines of evidence suggest the chaperone-like activity of trehalose to prevent protein misfolding or aggregation and to contribute to clearance of accumulated proteins through promoting autophagy in neurodegenerative diseases (NDs) [21]. As such, trehalose is emerging as a novel therapeutic alternative to repressing oxidative stress and inflammation by decreasing the production of reactive oxygen species (ROS) and proinflammatory cytokines, such as interleukin 1 beta (IL-1β) and tumor necrosis factor-alpha (TNF-α), respectively [23]. Deposition of sphingomyelin and other lipids [24], neuroinflammation [25], and oxidative stress [26] have been considered as leading causes of NP. Therefore, trehalose might be effective at attenuating the negative outcomes in NP patients by reducing lipid accumulation, inflammation, and oxidative damage [9,27]. Trehalose can be used by either oral or intravenous (IV) administration; however, its absorption is decreased to 0.5% in the oral route due to enzymatic metabolization with Trehalase exhibiting in the intestinal brush border, and (IV) trehalose administration is more efficient for clinical trials [10,28]. Nevertheless, oral administration of trehalose in both preclinical and clinical studies of oculopharyngeal muscular dystrophy (OPMD) and Machado–Joseph disease (MJD) can stabilize neurological impairment and improve the severity of clinical disease scores [17,18].

This study reports clinical research aimed to investigate the efficacy of intravenous trehalose infusion (15 g/week) for a period of 12 weeks in five NPA and NPB patients.

2. Patients and Methods

2.1. Study Design and Participants

A single-arm, open-label pilot study was performed to assess trehalose therapeutic potential in NPA and NPB patients. All patients received IV trehalose infusions once a week (15 gr) for 90 min during three months of treatment. Follow-up visits were also conducted weekly during the study period. This clinical research was approved by the Ethics Committee of the Mashhad University of Medical Sciences, registered in the Iranian Registry of Clinical Trials (Code: IRCT20130829014521N16). Five patients aged 2–12 years old who had been diagnosed with NPA and NPB (confirmation by genotype and clinical examination) were considered for enrollment in the present study. The parents or legal guardians of the children signed the informed consent forms before any procedures were performed.

2.2. Test Substances

For our research, the pharmaceutical grade of trehalose has been used as a form of aqueous 15% solution in 100 mL sterile sealed vials manufactured by Dr. Rajabi Pharmaceutical Company, Khorasan Razavi, Iran.

2.3. Endpoints and Assessments

The main objective was to determine the therapeutic efficacy of trehalose in patients with NPA and NPB. Primary endpoints included quality of life assessment and reduction in serum biomarker levels (lysosphingomyelin-lysoSM, and lysosphingomyelin-509 (lysoSM-509)). The secondary endpoints of the study were to assess the condition of the liver, spleen, and lung, and measurement of the aminotransferases enzymes (AST and ALT levels), as well as oxidative stress status at the baseline and end of the interventional trial (day 0 and week 12).

2.3.1. Primary Endpoints

Quality of life assessment: TAPQOL (TNO-AZL Preschool children Quality of Life) index was used during this research to evaluate the physical, social, emotional, and cognitive function of patients. TAPQOL is a multidimensional questionnaire-parent form with 43 items comprising 12 scales, which was developed to measure health-related quality of life (HRQoL) in preschool children (aged 2–48 months) [29].

Sample preparation and lyso-SM and lyso-SM-509 quantification: Blood samples were obtained from all patients before and after treatment. Samples were collected in tubes containing serum gel separator and were centrifuged at $750 \times g$ for 20 min to obtain serum. Serum samples were aliquoted and were stored at $-80\ °C$ until required for measurements. Changes in serum lyso-SM and lyso-SM-509 levels were measured by ultra-performance liquid chromatography tandem mass spectrometry (UPLC–MS/MS) in a Xevo TQ-S micro (Waters Technology, Milford, MA, USA) at baseline (day 0) and the end of the study (week 12). The method used for the quantification of lyso-SM and lyso-SM-509 was adapted from Polo et al., 2019 [30].

2.3.2. Secondary Endpoints

Liver, spleen, and lung scans: Serum levels of alanine aminotransferase (ALT) and aspartate transaminase (AST) were measured by the kinetic method using a colorimetric assay kit to assess liver function at baseline and the end of the trehalose treatment period. Moreover, the spleen and liver size were measured using ultrasonography, and volumetric analyses were performed at the baseline and end of the study. Chest high-resolution computed tomography (HRCT) was also performed to compare the lung condition of patients between the W0 and W12.

Oxidative stress status: To evaluate whether trehalose could improve the antioxidant status, investigation of (anti)oxidant parameters pre- and post-treatment were performed by commercial kits (Kiazist; Iran). In this study, PAB (pro-oxidant antioxidant balance) was measured to evaluate the total oxidants and antioxidants in a single measurement simultaneously according to the previously described method [31], which is based on the oxidation of the chromogen 3,3′,5,5′-tetramethylbenzidine (TMB) to a color cation by pro-oxidants in an enzymatic reaction and reduction of the TMB cation to a colorless compound in a chemical reaction. The antioxidant enzyme activity of the glutathione peroxidase (GPx) was also assayed based on the reduction of hydrogen peroxide to water accompanied by the oxidation of glutathione.

2.3.3. Statistical Analysis

Statistical analysis was performed with GraphPad Prism version 8 software and Microsoft Excel (2019) The results were analyzed using paired t-test to evaluate the significance of differences before and after the treatment period. Results with $p < 0.05$ were considered statistically significant.

3. Results

3.1. Clinical Characteristics of Patients

Five male patients with a mean age of 4.4 years (range = 2–12 years of age) were enrolled who were diagnosed clinically and genetically with Niemann–Pick (NP) type A and B, genotype analysis results were homozygous. All children were born from consanguineous families. No subjects discontinued from the study, and all patients received all 12 of their scheduled doses.

3.2. Quality of Life Assessment

TAPQOL Test: To determine whether trehalose treatment could improve the health status in patients, we compared the TAPQOL score, which was used to assess the patients' health-related quality of life between the W12 and W0. The TAPQOL index score can vary from 0–100, and higher scores indicate better quality of life. The TAPQOL score was elevated in all patients, and the mean score for quality of life was increased after intervention at W12 compared to the baseline (difference between means ± standard error mean (SEM): 6/000 ± 2/449), although the difference was not statistically significant. The results suggested an improvement in health-related quality of life after 12 weeks of trehalose treatment (Figure 1) in patients 2–5.

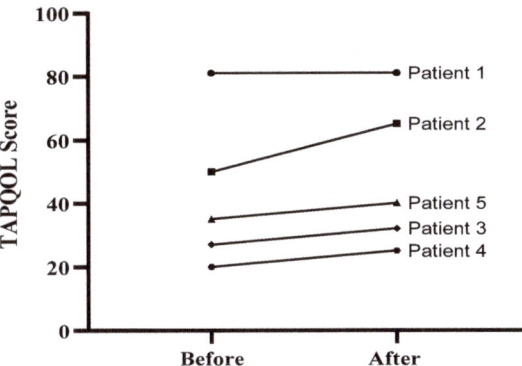

Figure 1. TAPQOL score of five patients at baseline (week 0) and at the end of treatment (week 12).

3.3. Serum Lysosphingomyelin Levels (lyso-SM and lyso-SM509)

The levels of serum lysosphingomyelin are shown at baseline and week 12 (Figure 2). The average of lyso-SM-509 at the baseline was 30.511 (nmoL/L), while the average post-treatment is 25.051 (nmoL/L); the average of lyso-SM at the baseline was 72 (nmoL/L) while the average post-treatment was 12 (nmoL/L). Overall, out of five patients there was a reduction in the levels of lyso-SM-509 in three patients, and a reduction in levels of lyso-SM in four patients (Figure 2). However, the changes were not statistically significant.

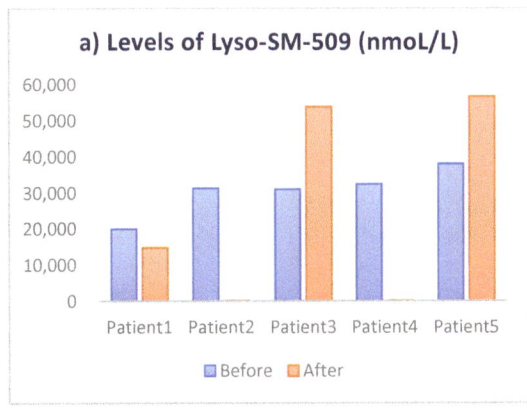
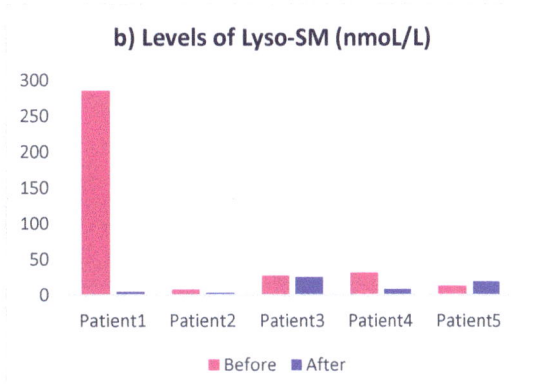

Figure 2. Levels of serum lysosphingomyelin (**a**) lyso-SM509 and (**b**) lyso-SM in patients before and after 3 months treatment with trehalose.

3.4. Serum ALT and AST Levels

The average of ALT at the baseline was 94.40 (IU/L), while the average post-treatment was 14.40 (IU/L); the average of AST at the baseline was 94.20 (IU/L), while the average post-treatment was 21.80 (IU/L). Overall, there was a reduction in the levels of ALT and AST post-treatment (Figure 3). Although changes were not statistically significant, improved results (reduction in ALT and AST levels) showed improvement in liver function after trehalose treatment.

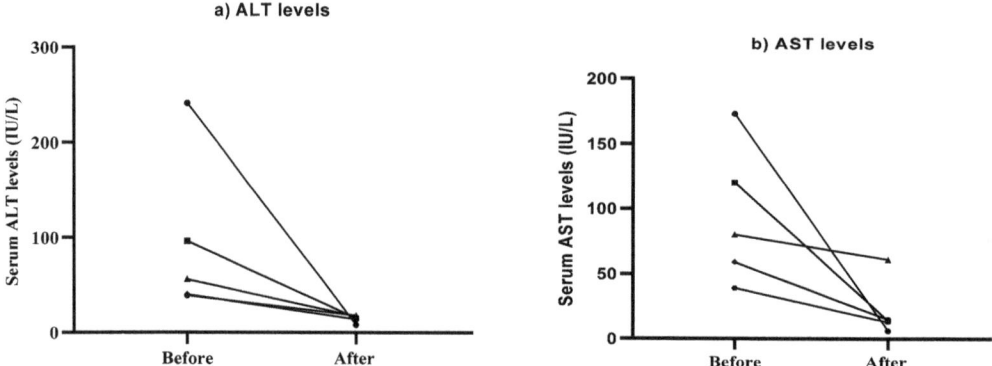

Figure 3. Alterations in serum ALT (**a**) and AST (**b**) levels in patients following 12 weeks of treatment with trehalose.

3.5. Oxidative Stress Index (OSI)

The mean of pro-oxidant-antioxidant balance (PAB) before treatment was 10.734 (HK unit), while post-treatment was 11.018 (HK unit) (Figure 4b). The level of GPX activity before treatment was 7.93 (mU/mL), while post-treatment was 9.09 (mU/mL) (Figure 4a). Although, differences were not statistically significant neither in PAB values nor in GPX activity.

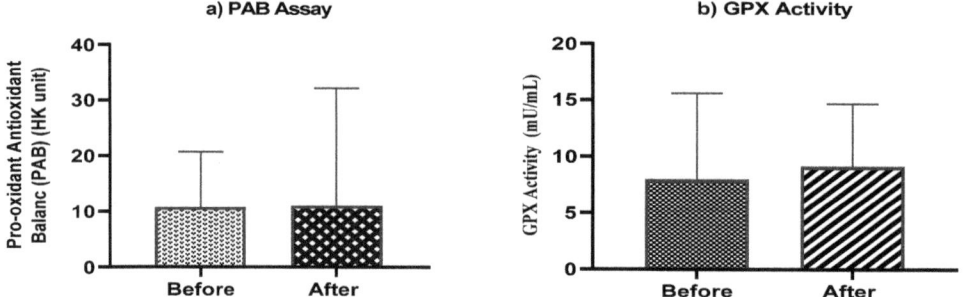

Figure 4. (**a**) Mean serum pro-oxidant antioxidant balance (PAB) and (**b**) mean serum activities of GPX (mU/mL) at baseline and end of the study.

3.6. Sonographic Liver and Spleen Dimensions

Table 1 includes the alteration of spleen and liver size in patients pre-and post-treatment with trehalose. Although spleen size was found to have decreased in two patients (patients 2 and 4) compared with baseline, a progressive increase in the mean splenic length and the average liver volume was observed at the end of the study. It is worth mentioning that the liver diameter was reported by measuring the liver span below the costal margin in the midclavicular line by using the ultrasound scan because it could assist clinicians to confirm these changes in practice.

Table 1. Spleen and liver diameter changes pre-and post-treatment with trehalose.

Patient ID	Spleen cranio-Caudal Diameter (mm)		Liver Diameter Changes, Measuring the Liver Span below the Costa Margin by Ultrasound Scan (mm)	
	Before	After	Before	After
01	204	224	30	30
02	125	122	10	30
03	120	138	30	10
04	150	145	10	30
05	115	115	30	30

3.7. Lung HRCT

Follow-up HRCT chest was carried out in all patients. Improvement of symptoms in HRCT chest findings were observed in two patients out of five after 3 months treatment with trehalose (Figure 5).

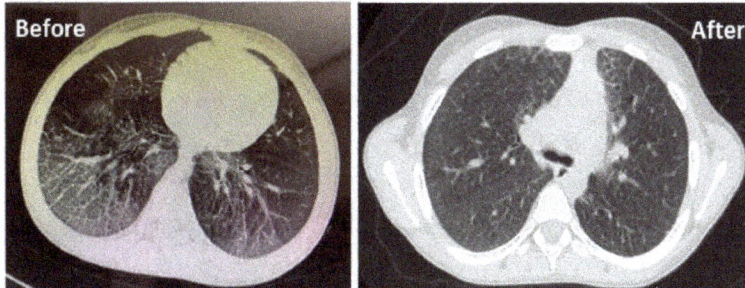

Figure 5. HRCT scan of the chest showing ground–glass changes in both lung fields before and after 3 months of treatment with trehalose in a patient.

4. Discussion

ASMD (acid sphingomyelinase deficiency), also known as Niemann–Pick disease, is a rare autosomal recessive LSD that includes two subtypes (A and B) associated with lipid metabolism abnormalities and intracellular deposition of glycosphingolipids [32]. Abnormal lipid accumulation due to a deficiency of specific lysosomal enzymes has been shown to impact morphologic alterations in different tissues, leading to multi-organ failure and early death in children with NPA and NPB [3]. Currently, no effective treatment is available for NPA/NPB patients [33]. A considerable body of evidence suggests the role of impaired autophagy in the pathophysiology and progression of lipid storage disorders [34–36]. Therefore, the possible use of the autophagy-inducing compounds in decreasing lipid accumulation has been proposed to attenuate severe LSDs manifestations [37]. In recent years, trehalose has been described as a natural non-reducing disaccharide that promotes the autophagy process in both in vitro and in vivo models by activating transcription factor EB (TFEB) and enhancing target genes such as *GLA*, *LAMP2A*, *MCOLN1*, *CTSB*. Furthermore, it can also induce the autophagy process via the mTOR-independent pathway in cells of the nervous system [38–41]. This study aimed to evaluate the potential efficacy of IV trehalose (at a dose of 15 mg/week) in NPA and NPB patients. The dose of 15 mg/week was selected based on recent evidence and a previous similar clinical study showing the safety and efficacy of 15 mg IV trehalose in patients with Machado–Joseph disease (MJD) [18]. We hypothesized that trehalose could slow disease progression and improve neuropathologic features by decreasing sphingolipid deposition post three months of treatment. Disruption of sphingolipid homeostasis leads to several pathological consequences, and the accumulation of these metabolites can trigger a high level of apoptosis by activating proapoptotic genes and proteins [42,43]. Elevated levels of lysosphingolipids (lyso-SM and lyso-SM-509) have been identified as specific and reliable biomarkers for the diagnosis of NP and early assessment of drug effects during the treatment process in all types of NP (A/B and C), which might be detected via different methods in plasma, serum, or dried blood spots of patients [30,44]. The results of this study might suggest that treatment with trehalose could potentially lead to a decrease in the levels of both lyso-SM and lyso-SM-509; however, additional studies are required to further elucidate the efficacy of trehalose treatment and to confirm if the mechanism is associated with the autophagy-inducing effect of this small molecule that contributes to the clearance of accumulated lysosomal lipid substrates.

In addition, as important signaling mediators involved in the control of cell survival, sphingolipids also have an essential role in regulating proinflammatory cytokines and inflammation processes. Sphingosine-1-phosphate can induce interleukin 8 (IL-8) expression and activated protein 1 (AP-1) inflammatory transcriptional action via activating ERK and p38 MAPK pathways, which are involved in many inflammatory responses, particularly in lung inflammation and progressive respiratory failure [45,46]. Pulmonary involvement is considered one of the main causes of morbidity and mortality in NPA and NPB patients [47]. It has been shown that trehalose can attenuate inflammation in different animal models by reducing the production of inflammatory cytokines, such as TNF-α, MCP-1 (monocyte chemotactic protein-1) and PAI-1 (plasminogen activator inhibitor-1) [23]. Our lung function tests and high-resolution computed tomography (HRCT) findings showed improved lung function in two patients during three months of trehalose treatment that might be due to anti-inflammatory effects of trehalose and modulation of pro-inflammatory cytokines. Furthermore, recent studies have uncovered the link between sphingolipid deposition and cellular stress responses, such as ER and oxidative stress [48,49]. The accumulation of complex sphingolipid inositol phosphorylceramide (IPC) can increase ROS generation in mitochondria, which in turn decreases mitochondrial mass by activating Ras and affecting Snf1/AMPK pathways [49]. It has also been suggested that trehalose might exhibit a protective effect against oxidative stress by either upregulation of antioxidant enzymes such as superoxide dismutase (SOD), glutathione peroxidase (GPX) [50,51], or scavenging ROS [52]. In line with this, we investigated pro-oxidant antioxidant balance and GPX activity after treatment to evaluate if trehalose has antioxidant effects. A decrease in levels of PAB and increased GPX activity could be due to the antioxidant activity of trehalose in the serum of NPA and NPB patients.

Besides anti-inflammatory and antioxidant properties, neuroprotective effects of trehalose to ameliorate neurological pathologies have been established in several experimental models of neurodegenerative diseases (NDs) [19]. Significant improvement has been observed on multiple behavioral tasks along with a marked increase in synaptophysin, doublecortin, and progranulin in the hippocampus and cortex of mice treated with oral administration of 2% trehalose for one month [53–55]. Moreover, a clinical study showed the effect of trehalose in patients with MJD with the optimal dose of 15 mg/week to improve disease severity and clinical symptoms [18]. Neurological involvement in NP varies in frequency and severity of disease, loss of mental abilities, and cognitive impairment more prominent in NPA, while type B patients tend to have milder symptoms with later-onset [56]. Our data confirmed previous similar reports in the literature and demonstrated significant improvement in health-related quality of life assessment through increased TAPQOL scores in four out of five patients after three months of treatment.

Hepatosplenomegaly accompanied by liver failure is another typical sign in NP patients [56]. Two clinical studies indicated liver dysfunction and elevated transaminase levels (ALT and AST) in 51% to 75% of NP patients [57,58]. Our results showed improvements in liver transaminase levels, and a reduction in the levels of both ALT and AST were observed in all patients treated with trehalose. Furthermore, a slight decrease in the spleen dimensions were found in two patients.

Our study has several limitations, including it being an open-label pilot research with limited sample size. Larger controlled, blind studies are required to demonstrate whether trehalose is effective in NPA and NPB patients. The length of treatment in our research is also not long enough to evaluate trehalose's effects on behavioral problems. Finally, future dose-ranging studies are needed to indicate the optimal therapeutic dose of trehalose.

In conclusion, the treatment of NPA and NPB in patients with 15 mg/week of trehalose may be effective to reduce serum levels of sphingomyelins and possibly improving disease symptoms caused by lipid accumulation, although large-scale randomized trials with longer follow-up are needed to confirm whether trehalose has clinical efficacy in patients with LSDs.

Author Contributions: Conceptualization, M.M., M.K. and A.S.; data curation, F.K. and M.V.; investigation, R.V.; methodology, S.V. and S.J.S.; project administration, S.A.A.; validation, S.A.E.; writing–original draft, S.R., P.E., T.J. and O.R.; writing–review and editing, Ž.R. All authors have read and agreed to the published version of the manuscript.

Funding: This study was financially supported by the Mashhad University of Medical Sciences (grant no. 981217) and the Iran National Science Foundation (grant no. 99014887).

Institutional Review Board Statement: This study was approved by the Ethics Committee of the Mashhad University of Medical Sciences (Ethics ID: IR.MUMS.REC.1398.257). Trial registration: IRCT20130829014521N16.

Informed Consent Statement: The parents or legal guardians of the children signed the informed consent forms before any procedures were performed.

Data Availability Statement: Data are available from the corresponding author upon a reasonable request.

Conflicts of Interest: The authors declare no conflict of interest.

References

1. Schuchman, E.H.; Desnick, R.J. Types A and B niemann-pick disease. *Mol. Genet. Metab.* **2017**, *120*, 27–33. [CrossRef] [PubMed]
2. Cerón-Rodríguez, M.; Vázquez-Martínez, E.R.; García-Delgado, C.; Ortega-Vázquez, A.; Valencia-Mayoral, P.; Ramírez-Devars, L.; Arias-Villegas, C.; Monroy-Muñoz, I.E.; López, M.; Cervantes, A.; et al. Niemann-Pick disease A or B in four pediatric patients and SMPD1 mutation carrier frequency in the Mexican population. *Ann. Hepatol.* **2019**, *18*, 613–619. [CrossRef] [PubMed]
3. Schuchman, E.H.; Wasserstein, M.P. Types A and B niemann-pick disease. *Best Pract. Res. Clin. Endocrinol. Metab.* **2015**, *29*, 237–247. [CrossRef]
4. Ordieres-Ortega, L.; Galeano-Valle, F.; Mallén-Pérez, M.; Muñoz-Delgado, C.; Apaza-Chavez, J.E.; Menárguez-Palanca, F.J.; Alvarez-Sala Walther, L.A.; Demelo-Rodríguez, P. Niemann-Pick disease type-B: A unique case report with compound heterozygosity and complicated lipid management. *BMC Med. Genet.* **2020**, *21*, 94. [CrossRef] [PubMed]
5. Pick, L., II. Niemann-Pick's disease and other forms of so-called xanthomatosis. *Am. J. Med. Sci.* **1933**, *185*, 615–616. [CrossRef]
6. McGovern, M.M.; Wasserstein, M.P.; Kirmse, B.; Duvall, W.L.; Schiano, T.; Thurberg, B.L.; Richards, S.; Cox, G.F. Novel first-dose adverse drug reactions during a phase I trial of olipudase alfa (recombinant human acid sphingomyelinase) in adults with Niemann-Pick disease type B (acid sphingomyelinase deficiency). *Genet. Med. Off. J. Am. Coll. Med. Genet.* **2016**, *18*, 34–40. [CrossRef]
7. Coelho, G.R.; Praciano, A.M.; Rodrigues, J.P.; Viana, C.F.; Brandão, K.P.; Valenca, J.T., Jr.; Garcia, J.H. Liver transplantation in patients with niemann-pick disease–single-center experience. *Transplant. Proc.* **2015**, *47*, 2929–2931. [CrossRef]
8. Victor, S.; Coulter, J.; Besley, G.; Ellis, I.; Desnick, R.; Schuchman, E.; Vellodi, A. Niemann–Pick disease: Sixteen-year follow-up of allogeneic bone marrow transplantation in a type B variant. *J. Inherit. Metab. Dis.* **2003**, *26*, 775–785. [CrossRef]
9. Tang, Q.; Zheng, G.; Feng, Z.; Chen, Y.; Lou, Y.; Wang, C.; Zhang, X.; Zhang, Y.; Xu, H.; Shang, P.; et al. Trehalose ameliorates oxidative stress-mediated mitochondrial dysfunction and ER stress via selective autophagy stimulation and autophagic flux restoration in osteoarthritis development. *Cell Death Dis.* **2017**, *8*, e3081. [CrossRef]
10. Richards, A.B.; Krakowka, S.; Dexter, L.B.; Schmid, H.; Wolterbeek, A.P.; Waalkens-Berendsen, D.H.; Shigoyuki, A.; Kurimoto, M. Trehalose: A review of properties, history of use and human tolerance, and results of multiple safety studies. *Food Chem. Toxicol.* **2002**, *40*, 871–898. [CrossRef]
11. DeBosch, B.J.; Heitmeier, M.R.; Mayer, A.L.; Higgins, C.B.; Crowley, J.R.; Kraft, T.E.; Chi, M.; Newberry, E.P.; Chen, Z.; Finck, B.N.; et al. Trehalose inhibits solute carrier 2A (SLC2A) proteins to induce autophagy and prevent hepatic steatosis. *Sci. Signal.* **2016**, *9*, ra21. [CrossRef]
12. Nazari-Robati, M.; Akbari, M.; Khaksari, M.; Mirzaee, M. Trehalose attenuates spinal cord injury through the regulation of oxidative stress, inflammation and GFAP expression in rats. *J. Spinal Cord Med.* **2019**, *42*, 387–394. [CrossRef] [PubMed]
13. Hosseinpour-Moghaddam, K.; Caraglia, M.; Sahebkar, A. Autophagy induction by trehalose: Molecular mechanisms and therapeutic impacts. *J. Cell. Physiol.* **2018**, *233*, 6524–6543. [CrossRef] [PubMed]
14. Khalifeh, M.; Barreto, G.E.; Sahebkar, A. Trehalose as a promising therapeutic candidate for the treatment of Parkinson's disease. *Br. J. Pharmacol.* **2019**, *176*, 1173–1189. [CrossRef] [PubMed]

15. Khalifeh, M.; Read, M.I.; Barreto, G.E.; Sahebkar, A. Trehalose against Alzheimer's disease: Insights into a potential therapy. *BioEssays* **2020**, *42*, 1900195. [CrossRef]
16. Sahebkar, A.; Hatamipour, M.; Tabatabaei, S.A. Trehalose administration attenuates atherosclerosis in rabbits fed a high-fat diet. *J. Cell. Biochem.* **2019**, *120*, 9455–9459. [CrossRef] [PubMed]
17. Davies, J.E.; Sarkar, S.; Rubinsztein, D.C. Trehalose reduces aggregate formation and delays pathology in a transgenic mouse model of oculopharyngeal muscular dystrophy. *Hum. Mol. Genet.* **2005**, *15*, 23–31. [CrossRef]
18. Zaltzman, R.; Elyoseph, Z.; Lev, N.; Gordon, C.R. Trehalose in machado-joseph disease: Safety, tolerability, and efficacy. *Cerebellum* **2020**, *19*, 672–679. [CrossRef]
19. Khalifeh, M.; Barreto, G.E.; Sahebkar, A. Therapeutic potential of trehalose in neurodegenerative diseases: The knowns and unknowns. *Neural Regen. Res.* **2021**, *16*, 2026–2027. [CrossRef]
20. Lotfi, P.; Tse, D.Y.; Di Ronza, A.; Seymour, M.L.; Martano, G.; Cooper, J.D.; Pereira, F.A.; Passafaro, M.; Wu, S.M.; Sardiello, M. Trehalose reduces retinal degeneration, neuroinflammation and storage burden caused by a lysosomal hydrolase deficiency. *Autophagy* **2018**, *14*, 1419–1434. [CrossRef]
21. Emanuele, E. Can trehalose prevent neurodegeneration? Insights from experimental studies. *Curr. Drug Targets* **2014**, *15*, 551–557. [CrossRef] [PubMed]
22. Assoni, G.; Frapporti, G.; Colombo, E.; Gornati, D.; Perez-Carrion, M.D.; Polito, L.; Seneci, P.; Piccoli, G.; Arosio, D. Trehalose-based neuroprotective autophagy inducers. *Bioorg. Med. Chem. Lett.* **2021**, *40*, 127929. [CrossRef]
23. Taya, K.; Hirose, K.; Hamada, S. Trehalose inhibits inflammatory cytokine production by protecting IkappaB-alpha reduction in mouse peritoneal macrophages. *Arch. Oral Biol.* **2009**, *54*, 749–756. [CrossRef] [PubMed]
24. Gabandé-Rodríguez, E.; Boya, P.; Labrador, V.; Dotti, C.G.; Ledesma, M.D. High sphingomyelin levels induce lysosomal damage and autophagy dysfunction in Niemann Pick disease type A. *Cell Death Differ.* **2014**, *21*, 864–875. [CrossRef] [PubMed]
25. Cologna, S.M.; Cluzeau, C.V.; Yanjanin, N.M.; Blank, P.S.; Dail, M.K.; Siebel, S.; Toth, C.L.; Wassif, C.A.; Lieberman, A.P.; Porter, F.D. Human and mouse neuroinflammation markers in Niemann-Pick disease, type C1. *J. Inherit. Metab. Dis.* **2014**, *37*, 83–92. [CrossRef] [PubMed]
26. Pérez-Cañamás, A.; Benvegnù, S.; Rueda, C.B.; Rábano, A.; Satrústegui, J.; Ledesma, M.D. Sphingomyelin-induced inhibition of the plasma membrane calcium ATPase causes neurodegeneration in type A Niemann-Pick disease. *Mol. Psychiatry* **2017**, *22*, 711–723. [CrossRef] [PubMed]
27. Yaribeygi, H.; Yaribeygi, A.; Sathyapalan, T.; Sahebkar, A. Molecular mechanisms of trehalose in modulating glucose homeostasis in diabetes. *Diabetes Metab. Syndr.* **2019**, *13*, 2214–2218. [CrossRef]
28. Ohtake, S.; Wang, Y.J. Trehalose: Current use and future applications. *J. Pharm. Sci.* **2011**, *100*, 2020–2053. [CrossRef]
29. Bunge, E.; Essink-Bot, M.-L.; Kobussen, M.; van Suijlekom-Smit, L.; Moll, H.; Raat, H. Reliability and validity of health status measurement by the TAPQOL. *Arch. Dis. Child.* **2005**, *90*, 351–358. [CrossRef]
30. Polo, G.; Burlina, A.P.; Ranieri, E.; Colucci, F.; Rubert, L.; Pascarella, A.; Duro, G.; Tummolo, A.; Padoan, A.; Plebani, M.; et al. Plasma and dried blood spot lysosphingolipids for the diagnosis of different sphingolipidoses: A comparative study. *Clin. Chem. Lab. Med.* **2019**, *57*, 1863–1874. [CrossRef]
31. Ghayour-Mobarhan, M.; Alamdari, D.H.; Moohebati, M.; Sahebkar, A.; Nematy, M.; Safarian, M.; Azimi-Nezhad, M.; Parizadeh, S.M.; Tavallaie, S.; Koliakos, G.; et al. Determination of prooxidant—Antioxidant balance after acute coronary syndrome using a rapid assay: A pilot study. *Angiology* **2009**, *60*, 657–662. [CrossRef]
32. Von Ranke, F.M.; Pereira Freitas, H.M.; Mançano, A.D.; Rodrigues, R.S.; Hochhegger, B.; Escuissato, D.; Araujo Neto, C.A.; da Silva, T.K.; Marchiori, E. Pulmonary involvement in Niemann-Pick disease: A state-of-the-art review. *Lung* **2016**, *194*, 511–518. [CrossRef]
33. Santos-Lozano, A.; Villamandos García, D.; Sanchis-Gomar, F.; Fiuza-Luces, C.; Pareja-Galeano, H.; Garatachea, N.; Nogales Gadea, G.; Lucia, A. Niemann-Pick disease treatment: A systematic review of clinical trials. *Ann. Transl. Med.* **2015**, *3*, 360. [CrossRef]
34. Myerowitz, R.; Puertollano, R.; Raben, N. Impaired autophagy: The collateral damage of lysosomal storage disorders. *EBioMedicine* **2021**, *63*, 103166. [CrossRef]
35. Pacheco, C.D.; Lieberman, A.P. The pathogenesis of Niemann–Pick type C disease: A role for autophagy? *Expert Rev. Mol. Med.* **2008**, *10*, e26. [CrossRef] [PubMed]
36. Canonico, B.; Cesarini, E.; Salucci, S.; Luchetti, F.; Falcieri, E.; Di Sario, G.; Palma, F.; Papa, S. Defective autophagy, mitochondrial clearance and lipophagy in Niemann-Pick type B lymphocytes. *PLoS ONE* **2016**, *11*, e0165780. [CrossRef] [PubMed]
37. Rusmini, P.; Cortese, K.; Crippa, V.; Cristofani, R.; Cicardi, M.E.; Ferrari, V.; Vezzoli, G.; Tedesco, B.; Meroni, M.; Messi, E.; et al. Trehalose induces autophagy via lysosomal-mediated TFEB activation in models of motoneuron degeneration. *Autophagy* **2019**, *15*, 631–651. [CrossRef]
38. Chen, X.; Li, M.; Li, L.; Xu, S.; Huang, D.; Ju, M.; Huang, J.; Chen, K.; Gu, H. Trehalose, sucrose and raffinose are novel activators of autophagy in human keratinocytes through an mTOR-independent pathway. *Sci. Rep.* **2016**, *6*, 28423. [CrossRef] [PubMed]
39. Zhang, Y.; Higgins, C.B.; Mayer, A.L.; Mysorekar, I.U.; Razani, B.; Graham, M.J.; Hruz, P.W.; DeBosch, B.J. TFEB-dependent induction of thermogenesis by the hepatocyte SLC2A inhibitor trehalose. *Autophagy* **2018**, *14*, 1959–1975. [CrossRef] [PubMed]
40. Wang, Q.; Ren, J. mTOR-Independent autophagy inducer trehalose rescues against insulin resistance-induced myocardial contractile anomalies: Role of p38 MAPK and Foxo1. *Pharmacol. Res.* **2016**, *111*, 357–373. [CrossRef]
41. Evans, T.D.; Jeong, S.-J.; Zhang, X.; Sergin, I.; Razani, B. TFEB and trehalose drive the macrophage autophagy-lysosome system to protect against atherosclerosis. *Autophagy* **2018**, *14*, 724–726. [CrossRef] [PubMed]

42. Phan, V.H.; Herr, D.R.; Panton, D.; Fyrst, H.; Saba, J.D.; Harris, G.L. Disruption of sphingolipid metabolism elicits apoptosis-associated reproductive defects in Drosophila. *Dev. Biol.* **2007**, *309*, 329–341. [CrossRef] [PubMed]
43. Mignard, V.; Dubois, N.; Lanoé, D.; Joalland, M.P.; Oliver, L.; Pecqueur, C.; Heymann, D.; Paris, F.; Vallette, F.M.; Lalier, L. Sphingolipid distribution at mitochondria-associated membranes (MAMs) upon induction of apoptosis. *J. Lipid Res.* **2020**, *61*, 1025–1037. [CrossRef] [PubMed]
44. Maekawa, M.; Jinnoh, I.; Matsumoto, Y.; Narita, A.; Mashima, R.; Takahashi, H.; Iwahori, A.; Saigusa, D.; Fujii, K.; Abe, A.; et al. Structural determination of lysosphingomyelin-509 and discovery of novel class lipids from patients with Niemann–Pick disease type C. *Int. J. Mol. Sci.* **2019**, *20*, 5018. [CrossRef]
45. Ghidoni, R.; Caretti, A.; Signorelli, P. Role of sphingolipids in the pathobiology of lung inflammation. *Mediat. Inflamm.* **2015**, *2015*, 487508. [CrossRef]
46. Chandru, H.; Boggaram, V. The role of sphingosine 1-phosphate in the TNF-alpha induction of IL-8 gene expression in lung epithelial cells. *Gene* **2007**, *391*, 150–160. [CrossRef]
47. Uyan, Z.S.; Karadağ, B.; Ersu, R.; Kiyan, G.; Kotiloğlu, E.; Sirvanci, S.; Ercan, F.; Dağli, T.; Karakoç, F.; Dağli, E. Early pulmonary involvement in Niemann-Pick type B disease: Lung lavage is not useful. *Pediatric Pulmonol.* **2005**, *40*, 169–172. [CrossRef]
48. Park, W.J.; Park, J.W. The role of sphingolipids in endoplasmic reticulum stress. *FEBS Lett.* **2020**, *594*, 3632–3651. [CrossRef] [PubMed]
49. Knupp, J.; Martinez-Montañés, F.; Van Den Bergh, F.; Cottier, S.; Schneiter, R.; Beard, D.; Chang, A. Sphingolipid accumulation causes mitochondrial dysregulation and cell death. *Cell Death Differ.* **2017**, *24*, 2044–2053. [CrossRef] [PubMed]
50. Mizunoe, Y.; Kobayashi, M.; Sudo, Y.; Watanabe, S.; Yasukawa, H.; Natori, D.; Hoshino, A.; Negishi, A.; Okita, N.; Komatsu, M.; et al. Trehalose protects against oxidative stress by regulating the Keap1-Nrf2 and autophagy pathways. *Redox Biol.* **2018**, *15*, 115–124. [CrossRef]
51. Sun, L.; Zhao, Q.; Xiao, Y.; Liu, X.; Li, Y.; Zhang, J.; Pan, J.; Zhang, Z. Trehalose targets Nrf2 signal to alleviate d-galactose induced aging and improve behavioral ability. *Biochem. Biophys. Res. Commun.* **2020**, *521*, 113–119. [CrossRef] [PubMed]
52. Lin, C.F.; Kuo, Y.T.; Chen, T.Y.; Chien, C.T. Quercetin-rich guava (*Psidium guajava*) juice in combination with trehalose reduces autophagy, apoptosis and pyroptosis formation in the kidney and pancreas of type II diabetic rats. *Molecules* **2016**, *21*, 334. [CrossRef] [PubMed]
53. Portbury, S.D.; Hare, D.J.; Sgambelloni, C.; Perronnes, K.; Portbury, A.J.; Finkelstein, D.I.; Adlard, P.A. Trehalose improves cognition in the transgenic Tg2576 mouse model of Alzheimer's disease. *J. Alzheimer's Dis.* **2017**, *60*, 549–560. [CrossRef]
54. Portbury, S.D.; Hare, D.J.; Finkelstein, D.I.; Adlard, P.A. Trehalose improves traumatic brain injury-induced cognitive impairment. *PLoS ONE* **2017**, *12*, e0183683. [CrossRef] [PubMed]
55. Berry, A.; Marconi, M.; Musillo, C.; Chiarotti, F.; Bellisario, V.; Matarrese, P.; Gambardella, L.; Vona, R.; Lombardi, M.; Foglieni, C.; et al. Trehalose administration in C57BL/6N old mice affects healthspan improving motor learning and brain anti-oxidant defences in a sex-dependent fashion: A pilot study. *Exp. Gerontol.* **2020**, *129*, 110755. [CrossRef]
56. McGovern, M.M.; Avetisyan, R.; Sanson, B.-J.; Lidove, O. Disease manifestations and burden of illness in patients with acid sphingomyelinase deficiency (ASMD). *Orphanet J. Rare Dis.* **2017**, *12*, 41. [CrossRef]
57. McGovern, M.M.; Wasserstein, M.P.; Giugliani, R.; Bembi, B.; Vanier, M.T.; Mengel, E.; Brodie, S.E.; Mendelson, D.; Skloot, G.; Desnick, R.J.; et al. A prospective, cross-sectional survey study of the natural history of Niemann-Pick disease type B. *Pediatrics* **2008**, *122*, e341–e349. [CrossRef] [PubMed]
58. Wasserstein, M.P.; Desnick, R.J.; Schuchman, E.H.; Hossain, S.; Wallenstein, S.; Lamm, C.; McGovern, M.M. The natural history of type B Niemann-Pick disease: Results from a 10-year longitudinal study. *Pediatrics* **2004**, *114*, e672–e677. [CrossRef]

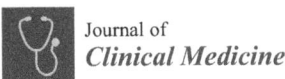

Article

New Insights into Gastrointestinal Involvement in Late-Onset Pompe Disease: Lessons Learned from Bench and Bedside

Aditi Korlimarla [1,*], Jeong-A Lim [1], Paul McIntosh [2], Kanecia Zimmerman [3], Baodong D. Sun [1] and Priya S. Kishnani [1,*]

[1] Division of Medical Genetics, Department of Pediatrics, Duke University Medical Center, Durham, NC 27710, USA; jeonga.lim@duke.edu (J.-A.L.); baodong.sun@duke.edu (B.D.S.)
[2] Department of Neurology, Duke University Medical Center, Durham, NC 27710, USA; paul_mcintosh@duke.edu
[3] Duke Clinical Research Institute, Durham, NC 27710, USA; kanecia.zimmerman@duke.edu
* Correspondence: aditi.korlimarla@duke.edu (A.K.); priya.kishnani@duke.edu (P.S.K.)

Abstract: Background: There are new emerging phenotypes in Pompe disease, and studies on smooth muscle pathology are limited. Gastrointestinal (GI) manifestations are poorly understood and underreported in Pompe disease. Methods: To understand the extent and the effects of enzyme replacement therapy (ERT; alglucosidase alfa) in Pompe disease, we studied the histopathology (entire GI tract) in Pompe mice (GAAKO $6^{neo}/6^{neo}$). To determine the disease burden in patients with late-onset Pompe disease (LOPD), we used Patient-Reported Outcomes Measurements Information System (PROMIS)-GI symptom scales and a GI-focused medical history. Results: Pompe mice showed early, extensive, and progressive glycogen accumulation throughout the GI tract. Long-term ERT (6 months) was more effective to clear the glycogen accumulation than short-term ERT (5 weeks). GI manifestations were highly prevalent and severe, presented early in life, and were not fully amenable to ERT in patients with LOPD (n = 58; age range: 18–79 years, median age: 51.55 years; 35 females; 53 on ERT). Conclusion: GI manifestations cause a significant disease burden on adults with LOPD, and should be evaluated during routine clinical visits, using quantitative tools (PROMIS-GI measures). The study also highlights the need for next generation therapies for Pompe disease that target the smooth muscles.

Keywords: late-onset Pompe disease; gastrointestinal; smooth muscles; PROMIS–GI symptom scales; GAAKO mice; glycogen storage disorder; translational research; patient-reported outcomes measures

1. Introduction

Pompe disease (glycogen storage disease type II, OMIM ID: 232300) is an autosomal recessive disorder caused by deficiency of the enzyme acid α-glucosidase (GAA) [1]. This deficiency leads to an abnormal accumulation of glycogen in the cardiac, skeletal and smooth muscles, and the nervous system. Pompe disease is broadly classified as infantile-onset (IPD) or late-onset Pompe disease (LOPD) [2]. Patients with IPD have little or no GAA enzyme activity, resulting in cardiomyopathy in the first year of life, and if untreated, die from cardiorespiratory complications before two years of age [2]. Patients with LOPD have residual GAA activity, and present with a slowly progressive myopathy and respiratory failure, with symptom onset ranging from the first year of life to the sixth decade [2,3]. Enzyme replacement therapy (ERT; alglucosidase alfa) is the standard of care for IPD and LOPD. Prior to its advent in 2006, LOPD was considered a proximal limb girdle muscle dystrophy with pulmonary involvement [4]. Over time, there has been a growing evidence of smooth muscle involvement in individuals with Pompe disease with reports of life-threatening basilar artery and ascending aorta aneurysms, difficulties in swallowing and speech, and the involvement of eyes, genitourinary tract, and gastrointestinal (GI) tract [3,5–9].

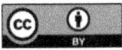

GI manifestations are poorly understood, often underreported, or misdiagnosed as a separate entity [10–12]. GI manifestations in LOPD include abdominal pain, feeding and swallowing difficulties, gastroesophageal reflux, postprandial bloating, early satiety, abdominal discomfort, chronic diarrhea, constipation, poor weight gain, and decreased gag reflex [7,13–15]. Patients with LOPD were found to have significantly more stool urgency, incontinence, and diarrhea, when compared to age- and gender-matched controls [7,13,16,17]. There are a few case reports and small case series describing improvement in GI symptoms with ERT therapy [11,14,15]. However, objective evidence of glycogen clearance within the GI tract is lacking. This could be attributable to the inefficient delivery of ERT to the target tissues (skeletal and smooth muscles). Therefore, many patients on long-term ERT still encounter a multitude of clinical symptoms, such as skeletal muscle weakness, respiratory failure, sleep disturbances, gastro-intestinal (GI), and genitourinary problems.

Autopsy data from patients with Pompe disease show a mild to moderate accumulation of glycogen in the tongue (skeletal muscles) and proximal third of esophagus (striated muscles) contributing to dysphagia, and in the smooth muscles of the distal esophagus and small intestines causing gastrointestinal symptoms [18–20]. Severe fibrosis, dilatation, increased vacuolization of myocytes, and autophagic buildup were noted in the esophagus in two adult patients with LOPD [18,21]. Although three available Pompe disease knockout (GAAKO) mice are extensively used in preclinical studies, the entire GI tract and its response to ERT have not been studied. Data from two of three mouse models show extensive glycogen accumulation in the stomach, small intestine, and colon (including the nervous supply or plexus) in a 15-month-old $\Delta 13/\Delta 13$ model, generated by the targeted disruption of exon 13; and glycogen accumulation in the esophagus in a 6-month-old $6^{neo}/6^{neo}$ model, generated by the targeted disruption of exon 6 [6,22–24].

Therefore, there are unmet needs to systematically understand the spectrum of GI involvement, the histopathology of the entire GI tract, and the impact of the available treatment (ERT) on Pompe disease. The aims of this study were (a) to better understand the wide range of GI symptoms, including their frequency and severity, as well as the disease burden in adult patients with LOPD using patient-reported outcomes, and (b) to assess the distribution of glycogen accumulation within the entire GI tract, and study the effects of ERT using the $6^{neo}/6^{neo}$ GAAKO mouse model.

2. Materials and Methods

The study design included the use of patient-reported outcome measures to understand the prevalence and severity of GI disorders (Section 2.1), and the use of a mouse model to understand the histopathology of the entire GI tract (Section 2.2).

2.1. Participants

All participants were enrolled in a long-term follow up study of Pompe disease (Pro00010830) at the Duke University Medical Center. The study protocol was approved by the Duke University Institutional Review Board (Pro00010830). Eligible participants were adults (ages $\geq$ 18 years) with a confirmed diagnosis of LOPD (n = 58), who were evaluated at Duke between April 2017 and July 2018. Written informed consent was obtained from each participant prior to all assessments.

The GI health of all the participants was prospectively evaluated during their routine clinical visits to Duke University. For participants who were evaluated more than once during the study period, their baseline data were used in the cross-sectional analysis, and the follow-up data were used in the longitudinal analysis of the study. Participants completed a GI questionnaire (Patient-Reported Outcomes Measurements Information System—Gastrointestinal (PROMIS-GI) symptom scales) and/or a GI-focused medical history was obtained by one medical geneticist (P.S.K.) during the same clinical visit, depending on the time available during clinic.

2.1.1. PROMIS-GI Symptom Scales

The PROMIS-GI symptom scales v1.0 are validated, person-centered questionnaires designed to assess patient-reported quality of life due to GI dysfunction, available on the HealthMeasures website (http://www.healthmeasures.net/explore-measurement-systems/promis, accessed on 15 February 2021), which is funded by the National Institutes of Health (NIH) [25–28]. There are eight PROMIS-GI scales available as 'fixed-length, short forms' for adult participants, with a designated unique name and number/letter—Gastrointestinal Disrupted Swallowing 7a, Gastroesophageal Reflux 13a, Gastrointestinal Gas and Bloating 13a, Gastrointestinal Belly Pain 5a, Gastrointestinal nausea and vomiting 4a, Gastrointestinal Bowel Incontinence 4a, Gastrointestinal Diarrhea 6a, and Gastrointestinal Constipation 9a. The current study used all eight available GI scales. These eight GI scales comprise a total of 54 items. Each item has a five-point categorical response (for example: 1 = never, 2 = rarely, 3 = sometimes, 4 = often, and 5 = always to evaluate severity, and frequency scales to evaluate frequency). Based on these categorical responses, a free, automated scoring system (HealthMeasures Scoring Service) and a manual scoring guide (https://www.healthmeasures.net/images/PROMIS/manuals/PROMIS_Gastrointestinal_Symptoms_Scoring_Manual.pdf; last accessed on 3 June 2020) were used to calculate statistical scores (raw and T-scores) [27,28]. In addition, HealthMeasures provides two reference populations to evaluate the PROMIS-GI measures—General population (GP; n = 1177 persons from the 2010 United States (US) census, who reported at least 1 GI symptom) and GI clinical sample (n = 865 patients with GI conditions) [27,28].

Raw scores: Raw scores were used to measure the prevalence of GI symptoms in this patient population. Based on the five-point categorical response, each item was rated 1 to 5, where 1 meant that the GI symptom was absent and a higher score (2–5) meant that a symptom was present with increasing severity and/or frequency. The item scores on each GI symptom scale were then summed to obtain a raw score. Therefore, each patient received one raw score for each GI scale. The scoring manual was then used to obtain a cut-off raw score for each GI scale, which indicated that a patient was symptom-free on a certain GI scale if they were at the cut-off value, or had GI problems if they scored above the cut-off value (depending on how many items were answered or skipped). Based on this, a 'yes'/'no' analysis was conducted for each GI scale. If a patient reported having a problem within one GI scale, it was considered a 'yes' response; if the patient was symptom-free, a 'no' response was recorded. For instance, PROMIS-GI Bowel Incontinence scale includes four items. If a patient responds to all four items, and has no problems related to bowel incontinence, the summed raw score for GI Bowel Incontinence scale would be 4 (the cut-off value). Therefore, a raw score of 4 would be a 'no' response to the GI Bowel Incontinence domain. Any score over 4 would indicate that there was some problem in the domain, and therefore, reflective of a 'yes' response.

T-scores: T-scores were used to understand the severity and prevalence of the GI symptoms. The mean T-score for the control group (US GP) was 50 with one standard deviation (SD) of 10 [27,28]. The T-scores from patients with LOPD were compared to T-scores of the reference populations (US general population and GI clinical sample) [25–28]. T-scores ranging between 55 and 59 were considered mildly symptomatic, 60–69 were moderate, and over 70 were severe, based on the available scoring guides.

To understand the impact of the GI symptoms on patients over time, baseline (first clinic visit) and follow-up (subsequent visits) T-scores were compared. The differences between the baseline and follow-up T-scores and minimally important differences (MIDs) were computed based on PROMIS databases [27]. These MIDs are estimates for the magnitude of change that corresponds to meaningful changes for patients with a specific GI symptom [29]. The estimated reference values for MIDs for each GI scale are provided on the HealthMeasures website. A change of 5–6 points (T-score) between two time points (for gas and bloating, belly pain, diarrhea, and constipation scales) would be indicative of significant clinical change in the specific GI symptom. For instance, a participant with a baseline T-score of 60 on belly pain and a follow-up T-score of ≥66 for the same scale (belly pain) would indicate clinically significant worsening. However, if the participant had a follow up T-score of ≤54, it would indicate improvement for belly pain. These are available on the HealthMeasures website.

2.1.2. GI-Focused Medical History

The GI-focused medical history was pre-designed for the current prospective study to assess the GI health of adult patients with Pompe disease. It included 16 questions, which PSK asked the participants during their clinic visits (Supplementary Table S1). The questions provided details of GI symptoms (if present), their associations with meals, diurnal variations, medications taken for GI discomfort, whether the onset of GI symptoms was before or after the diagnosis of LOPD, any changes in GI symptoms in ERT-treated patients, and whether the participants considered their GI symptoms to be one of the top three reasons to cause a reduced quality of life. It also included history of tongue weakness, chewing problems, and temporomandibular joint issues made by other medical professionals.

Medical records were reviewed to include ERT doses, age at ERT initiation, and the duration of treatment with ERT, and most recent values of creatine phosphokinase (CPK), 6-min walk test distance (6-MWT), FVC % predicted (upright), FVC % predicted (supine), and urinary hex4 (a breakdown product of glycogen, which is a biomarker of disease progression), which were available during the study period.

2.1.3. Statistical Analyses

Descriptive statistics were used to summarize the distribution of categorical variables using counts (percentages) and medians (25th and 75th percentiles) to analyze the GI-focused medical history and the responses on individual items within the PROMIS-GI questionnaire. Where appropriate, a one-sample test was used to compare T-scores to the reference T-score = 50. Pearson's chi-squared test was used to compare GI symptoms in patients who were on ERT to those who were not on ERT during the study period. A p-value of ≤0.05 was considered statistically significant for the t-test and chi-squared analyses. For all other analyses, we used Bonferroni correction for comparisons to identify a significant p-value of <0.006.

To understand the role of ERT on GI symptoms in LOPD, participants who completed the PROMIS-GI questionnaires were divided into two groups. Group I consisted of patients treated with ERT < 6 months + untreated. Patients with less than 6 months ERT were included in this group to account for the time it takes for ERT to show clinical benefits. Group II included patients who were treated ≥ 6 months with ERT. Using the two-sample Wilcoxon rank-sum (Mann–Whitney) test, we compared the T-scores/raw scores on each of the eight GI symptom scales between the two groups. The Wilcoxon rank-sum (Mann–Whitney) test was also used to explore statistical relationships between each of the eight GI T-scores/raw scores (for each group) with patient's age, sex, age at diagnosis, age at ERT start, and most recent values of CPK, 6-MWT, FVC % predicted (upright), FVC % predicted (supine), and urinary hex4.

2.2. GAAKO Mouse Model ($6^{neo}/6^{neo}$)

Animal care and experiments were conducted in accordance with Duke University Institutional Animal Care and Use Committee-approved guidelines. To study the extent of GI pathology, 3-month-old male GAAKO ($6^{neo}/6^{neo}$) mice were used. Age- and gender-matched wild type (WT) mice were used as a control. To understand the short-term effects of ERT on GI smooth muscles, a 3-month-old GAAKO mice received 20 mg/kg ERT (hGAA, alglucosidase alfa, Myozyme) through the tail vein every week for 5 weeks. Phosphate-buffered saline (PBS)-injected GAAKO mice were used as control (ERT-naïve or placebo group). To understand the long-term effects of ERT on GI smooth muscles, a 2-month-old GAAKO mouse model received 20 mg/kg ERT through the tail vein, biweekly for 6 months.

Histopathology

The following anatomical regions of the GI system were analyzed in the mice: tongue, upper 1/3rd of the esophagus, lower 1/3rd of the esophagus, stomach, gastro-esophageal (GE) junction, duodenum, small intestine (jejunum, ileum, cecum, and ileo-cecal junction), colon, and rectum.

GI tissues were fixed in 10% neutral-buffered formalin (NBF) for 48 h. After primary immersion fixation, the samples were post-fixed with 1% periodic acid in 10% NBF for 48 h at 4 °C. The samples were then washed with PBS, dehydrated with ascending grades of alcohol, cleared with xylene, and infiltrated with paraffin. Sections of paraffin-embedded tissues were stained using a Periodic acid-Schiff (PAS) stain as described [30]. Briefly, the sectioned slides were deparaffinized, re-hydrated, and oxidized with freshly made 0.5% Periodic acid for 5 min. The slides were then stained with Schiff reagent for 15 min and washed with tap water for 10 min. The tissues were counterstained with hematoxylin, dehydrated, and mounted. Paraffin-embedded sections were also processed and stained using Masson's trichrome staining kit (Sigma-Aldrich Co., St. Louis, MO, USA) following the manufacturer's protocol. The images were taken on a BZX710 microscope (Keyence America, Itasca, IL, USA).

The PAS was used to detect glycogen content within the cells of the tissues. The cells with an accumulation of glycogen stain dark pink/purple and the cell nuclei stain blue. The Masson's trichrome staining was used to explore the presence and extent of tissue fibrosis, which stains blue. Muscle fibers and cytoplasm stain red, and the cell nuclei stain dark brown.

3. Results

3.1. Participants

Patient demographics are shown in Table 1. Whenever possible, each patient completed the PROMIS-GI questionnaires, and the clinician could obtain the GI-focused medical history during the routine clinical visits. However, due to time constraints, certain patients either only completed the PROMIS-GI questionnaire or the GI-focused history was obtained. Data analysis based on the PROMIS-GI scales are shown in Section 3.1.1 (prevalence and severity using raw scores) and Section 3.1.2 (comparisons to reference population and longitudinal analysis mainly using T-scores).

3.1.1. PROMIS-GI Symptom Scales

Raw Scores

Using the 'yes/no' analysis on the raw scores, the prevalence of each GI symptom in adult patients with Pompe disease were calculated and compared to the reference populations. Details are shown in Figure 1 and Table 2.

T-Scores

Severity was computed for each GI scale. Figure 1 demonstrates the prevalence of patients with moderate to severe grades (T-scores > 60 or ≥ 1 SD compared to the reference population) for each GI scale. The prevalence of moderate-severe GI symptoms ranged from 4 to 28% (Figure 1). The mean T-scores (SD) for each GI scale at baseline were calculated and compared to the reference populations (Table 2). The mean T-scores ranged from 46.34 (belly pain) to 54.57 (gas and bloating) in the cross-sectional analyses. Though these values were not significantly different from the reference populations, the longitudinal analyses (MID) yielded meaningful, clinically significant results in a subset of patients (Table 2). These calculated MIDs indicated a clinically significant change in the GI symptoms over the study period, where some patients showed improvement, worsening, or no change in their symptoms.

Table 1. Patient demographics for the GI study in adult patients with LOPD.

Study duration	1 year, 3 months	
Total number of patients (n)	58	
(a) PROMIS-GI symptom scales	n = 52	
(b) GI-focused medical history	n = 38 (32/52 who also completed the PROMIS-GI + additional 6 patients who only had GI-focused medical history in their medical records)	
	Median age = 51.5 ± 15.5 years (age range: 18–79 years) 35 females, 23 males	
	Patients on ERT (treated group)	Patients not on ERT (untreated group)
Demographics	• n = 53 • Median age at start of ERT = 45.5 years (range: 11–77 years) • Median ERT duration = 5.5 years (range: 2 months–13 years) • n = 1/53 was included in the untreated group for statistical analysis since the duration of ERT was <6 months *	• n = 4 ERT-naïve • n = 1 discontinued ERT since 2–3 years, after being on ERT for 3 years (medical records indicated that patient had adverse effects of flushing, difficulty breathing, and GI symptoms of severe cramping, nausea, and diarrhea starting 2–3 days after each ERT infusion.
For longitudinal analysis of PROMIS-GI scales	n = 18 (1 baseline and 1 follow-up) n = 1 (1 baseline and 2 follow-ups)	

* to account for the time it takes for ERT to show clinical benefits. PROMIS-GI Patient-Reported Outcomes Measurements Information System—Gastrointestinal. ERT—Enzyme replacement therapy.

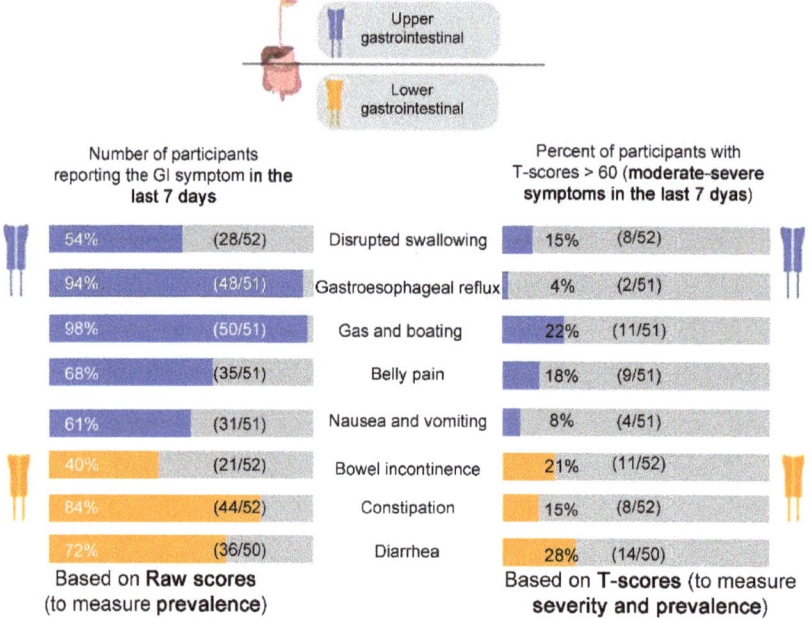

Figure 1. The prevalence and severity of gastrointestinal symptoms in adult patients with late-onset Pompe disease using PROMIS-GI symptom scales (This figure was created using BioRender.com; accessed on 5 January 2021).

Table 2. GI problems in adult patients with late-onset Pompe disease using PROMIS-GI scales, when compared to the reference populations, and a measure of meaningful change in the T-scores of patients with Pompe disease on longitudinal analysis.

PROMIS-GI Symptom Domain		Prevalence (Using Raw Scores)			Prevalence/Severity [Using Mean T-Scores (SD)]			Minimally Important Differences (MIDs) in T-Scores (n = 19) ***			
		Study Population Patients with Pompe Disease n = 52	Reference Population [29] GP n = 1177	Reference Population [29] GI Clinical Sample n = 865	Study Population Patients with Pompe Disease	Reference Population [28] GP	Reference Population [28] GI Clinical Sample	Estimated Reference Values for MIDs [29]	n with Improvement	n with Worsening	n with No MID in T-Scores
Upper GI	disrupted swallowing	54%	5.8%	u	49.15 (9.60)	50 (10)	51 (10)	u	N/A		
	gastroesophageal reflux *	94%	16–30.9%	33%	46.76 (8.06)	50 (10)	51 (10)	+5 points for improvement, −1 point for worsening	4	6	9
	gas/bloating	98%	20.6%	u	54.57 (7.68)	50 (10)	57 (10)	±6 points	4	4	10
	belly pain	68%	24.8%	u	46.34 (12.06)	50 (10)	57 (11)	±6 points	4	5	9
	nausea/vomiting	61%	9.5–19%	24%	47.07 (7.35)	50 (10)	53 (10)	u	N/A	N/A	N/A
	constipation *	84%	19.7–47%	39% total	50.05 (8.54)	50 (10)	54 (10)	±5–6 points	2	4	12
Lower GI	diarrhea	72%	6.6–20%	u	52.18 (10.38)	50 (10)	56 (11)	±5–6 points	3	2	13
	incontinence	40%	8.3%	u	48.67 (9.25)	50 (10)	53 (11)	u	N/A	N/A	N/A
Other GI condition [28]	IBS *	N/A	11%	40%	N/A				N/A		
	IBD *		4%	28%							
	systemic sclerosis *		1%	18%							
	others		47%	39% **							

GP—general population, GI—gastrointestinal, MID—minimally important differences as per the PROMIS scales, u—Unavailable, N/A—not applicable to Pompe disease (added to complete the list of GI related issues in the reference populations and to compare the characteristics between the two reference populations); * p-value was < 0.05 comparing GP versus GI clinical samples [28]. ** The most common were intestinal surgery (N = 72), symptomatic diverticular disease (N = 63), dyspepsia (N = 52), fecal incontinence (N = 44), pancreatitis (N = 25), celiac disease (N = 15), peptic ulcer (N = 15), and gastroparesis (N = 11). *** MIDs between baseline and follow-up T-scores were calculated to assess meaningful change in GI symptoms in patients with Pompe disease, over time. Note that patients within the GI-sample and LOPD groups were allowed to endorse more than one GI symptom during reporting (in our study and the other published articles). The published articles which describe the mean T-scores for the two control groups (GP and GI) [28] and the MIDs for longitudinal analyses [29] were last accessed on 3 June 2020. + is used to indicate an increase in the T-scores from baseline values, − is used to indicate a decrease in the T-scores from baseline values, and ± indicates either an increase or decrease from the baseline values.

3.1.2. GI-Focused Medical History

The 16 clinical questions (Supplementary Table S1) revealed details about the GI-symptoms, aggravating or relieving factors (diurnal variations, diet, and medications), and overall subjective perception of quality of life due to GI problems in individuals with LOPD. In the current study, 29/38 (76%) patients reported at least one GI problem, and 23 of those 29 patients (82%) reported that there were no changes in their GI symptoms after initiation of ERT. Five patients reported some changes in their GI symptoms; two felt better with additional GI medications (CoQ10 and probiotics for diarrhea, laxatives for constipation), one felt that the symptoms were reduced after an increase in the dose of ERT (from 20 to 40 mg/kg), and two had worsening symptoms with increased diarrhea and GE reflux while on ERT.

Over half of the patients with LOPD, 21/38 (55%), were on additional medications to manage their GI symptoms. The medications included antacids, anti-diarrheal, anti-spasmodic, CoQ10, probiotics (which improved diarrhea in one patient), tincture of opium, and bulking agents, such as psyllium, methylcellulose, and polyethylene glycol, stool softeners such as docusate sodium, and linactolide to treat constipation. Eleven patients reported that the GI symptoms worsened with meals.

When asked 'Did your GI symptoms start bothering you before or after your diagnosis of Pompe disease?', 16/38 (42%) patients indicated before and 14/38 (37%) indicated after the LOPD diagnosis. The rest of the patients (8/38; 21%) either could not recollect the onset of their GI manifestations or did not have a GI problem. Of the 16 patients who reported that GI symptoms presented before the LOPD diagnosis, 6 recollected that they were in their 20s at onset, one was in their 40s, and three patients had the GI symptoms since their childhood years; all 6 of these patients reported that they had no improvements in GI symptoms with ERT. Though patients could not recall the exact age at onset of GI symptoms, their responses indicated that age at onset of GI symptoms ranged from childhood to the seventies in the cohort. In addition, when asked 'Do you consider your GI symptoms to be one of your top three symptoms that affects your quality of life?', 15/38 (40%) patients replied 'yes.'

Six patients reported that they had worsening GI symptoms within 48 h of ERT infusion. All six patients reported that these were isolated (one-time) episodes, and only four of them were able to recollect the details (one patient had vomiting, two had diarrhea, and another had an upset stomach). None of these episodes reoccurred in any of the six patients.

3.1.3. Statistical Analyses

Gas and bloating was the only GI symptom scale (of the eight) to yield a significant p-value (0.0014) when the T-scores were compared to the US general population. Using Bonferroni correction for comparisons (significant p-value of <0.006) between the untreated ($n = 6$) and the treated group ($n = 46$), there were no statistically significant differences on the eight GI scales. The only exception to this was the relationship between the GI symptom scale of swallowing (higher raw scores) and FVC % predicted (low values), which yielded a p-value of 0.0036score. Other important relationships, albeit not statistically significant, are listed in Supplementary Table S2.

3.2. GAAKO Mouse Model ($6^{neo}/6^{neo}$)

Histopathology

The PAS staining showed that there was glycogen accumulation through the entire length of the GI tract (from the tongue to the rectum) in the GAAKO mouse model (Figure 2). Glycogen accumulation was seen in the smooth muscles of the esophagus, gastroesophageal junction, small intestine, rectum, duodenum, cecum, and colon. The smooth muscle layers of the submucosa and muscularis externa were the most affected (Figure 2).

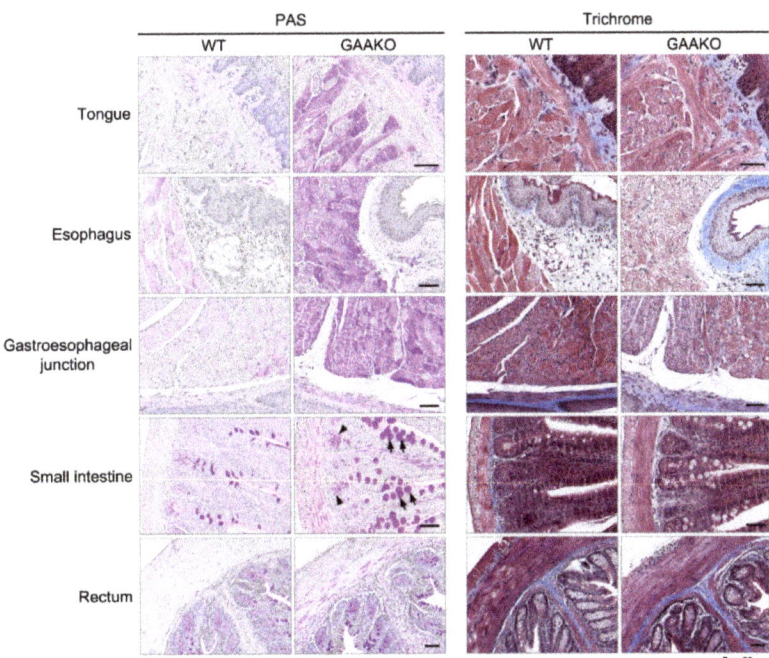

Figure 2. Periodic acid-Schiff (PAS) and Trichrome staining of the gastrointestinal tissues in Pompe mice (GAAKO), using wild type (WT) mice as controls. Extensive glycogen accumulation in the GAAKO mice, when compared to the WT mice (purple-stained skeletal muscles of the tongue and esophagus, and the smooth muscles in the esophagus, gastroesophageal junction, small intestine, and rectum). The intestinal villi (small intestine) showing hypertrophic and mild hyperplastic goblet cells (arrows) and intestinal glands (arrowheads) can be seen.

The WT mice did not have any glycogen accumulation. The glandular portions of the stomach and small intestine showed disintegrated ganglion cell structures (Aurbach's plexus) in the GAAKO mice (visualized in Figure 3).

The small intestine of the GAAKO mouse model showed hypertrophic goblet cells with hyperplasia. Duodenal sections showed hypertrophic villi in addition to the glycogen accumulation. The cecum of the GAAKO mouse model showed a mild disruption of the brush border of the epithelial lining and vacuolated nuclei of the enterocytes. The rectal section of the GAAKO mice showed some neutrophilic accumulation in the lamina propria. There was no significant sign of fibrosis in the GI tract in the GAAKO mice when compared to WT.

The effects of ERT (alglucosidase alfa) on the GI tissue in GAAKO mice were also evaluated. The short-term (5 weeks) treated mice showed clearance of the glycogen accumulation in tongue, stomach, and rectum (Figure 3). However, the smooth muscle in the esophagus, gastroesophageal junction, and small intestine still showed glycogen accumulation. The glycogen accumulation in Aurbach's plexus in the small intestine was cleared by the short-term ERT. There was no sign of fibrosis on trichrome staining in the GAAKO mice.

With long-term ERT (6 months), there was a reduction of glycogen accumulation in the entire GI tract (Figure 3). Fibrosis was seen in the old mice in the esophagus, smooth muscles of the GEJ, and submucosal region of the stomach. Fibrosis was also observed in the WT mice. The inner circular muscular layer of the stomach looked distorted, and had less muscle density (hypotrophic). Though structurally organized, the Aurbach's plexus in the esophagus had some mild fibrosis.

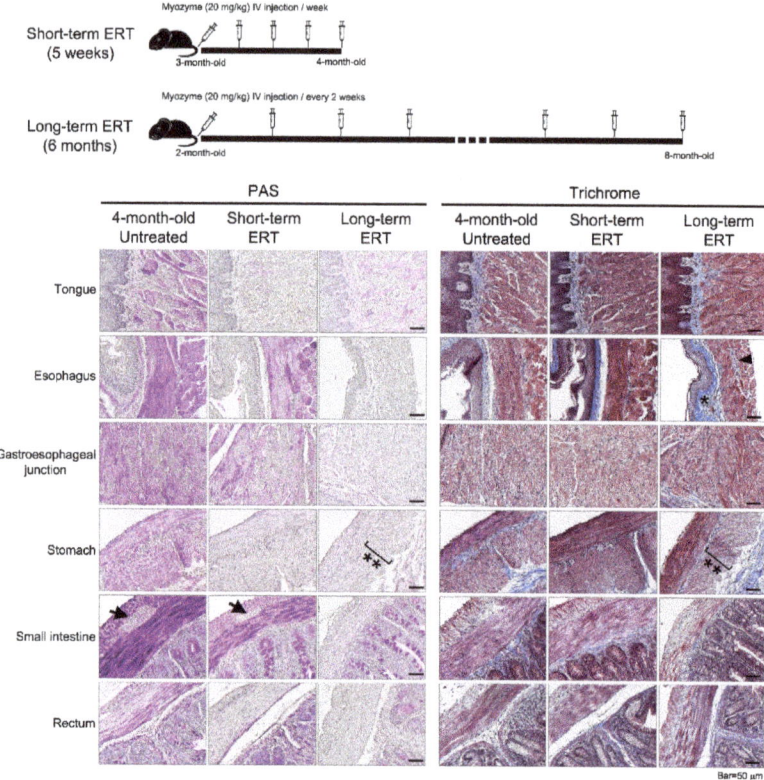

Figure 3. Short-term and long-term effects of ERT (alglucosidase alfa) on Pompe mice (GAAKO). ** Distorted muscularis externa layer in the stomach. * Fibrosis was noted in the 8-month-old mice; however, this was also seen in the wild type mice. Aurbach's plexus was seen in between the inner circular and outer longitudinal layers of the small intestine (arrows) and in the esophagus (arrowheads).

4. Discussion

LOPD is a chronic, multi-systemic disorder, with a substantial burden on health and quality of life of the patients and their caregivers [31,32]. A large number of patients with LOPD complain about GI symptoms in the clinics [7,9,11,13,14,32]. However, there still exists a knowledge gap about the impact of the GI system on LOPD, the extent of gut involvement, severity, prevalence, and treatment response to standard dose of ERT with alglucosidase alfa. There can be several factors that may influence the presence and severity of GI symptoms in LOPD, such as genotype-phenotype correlations, patient's age, age at ERT start, and overall disease burden, which can be evaluated through pulmonary function testing or muscle weakness. Patients with LOPD exhibit variable rates of progression of myopathy and pulmonary compromise, and early ERT initiation has been shown to have better outcomes compared to the untreated patients [33]. Similarly, with variable presentations of GI manifestations in LOPD, more research is needed to understand if early treatment would impact the outcomes. With an aim to bridge these knowledge gaps, the current study used Pompe mice and patient-reported outcomes measures (PROMIS-GI scales and GI-focused history).

The PROMIS-GI scales provide patient-reported information about the physical, mental, and social health related to a spectrum of GI manifestations, and therefore, by definition, provided preliminary data on quality of life [27,28,34]. The raw and T-scores from these PROMIS-GI scales indicated that the GI manifestations in LOPD were highly prevalent and severe (Figure 1, Table 2). The GI-focused medical history showed that 40% patients with LOPD (15/38) considered their GI symptoms to be one of the top three reasons affecting quality of life, and that 55% patients (21/38) were on additional medications to treat their GI symptoms, despite being on ERT. Overall, the current study showed that GI manifestations remarkably reduced quality of life in adults with LOPD.

Interestingly, the study showed that GI manifestations preceded the LOPD diagnosis in 42% (16/38), and the age of onset of GI symptoms ranged from childhood to their 40s in 6/16 patients. The GI symptoms may be an early manifestation of the disease, and their presence could be used as an adjunct to monitor disease progression, and to consider a diagnosis of Pompe disease. More than ever, monitoring disease manifestations and progression is important in LOPD with its inclusion in newborn screening programs, and with improved diagnostic criteria [35]. The use of the PROMIS-GI measures in routine follow-ups could provide useful information about clinical progression of the disease and the effectiveness of emerging therapies [36]. In addition, as GI symptoms are often under-reported by patients, awareness and focused history taking can alert clinicians to refer patients to GI specialists, when required.

Using the PROMIS-GI scales, the current study used two reference populations—the US general population and a GI sample (Figure 1, Table 2). In the US general population, there was notably a high population prevalence of GI symptoms [28,29]. The current study showed that patients with LOPD had a much higher prevalence in comparison to both reference populations—gas and bloating (98%), gastroesophageal reflux (94%), constipation (84%), diarrhea (72%), belly pain (68%), nausea and vomiting (61%), disrupted swallowing (54%), and bowel incontinence (40%) (Figure 1). This was based on raw scores. Based on T-scores, there was no significant difference in the prevalence when compared to the reference populations (Table 2). Therefore, at the population level, there was no significant difference in prevalence of GI symptoms comparing the LOPD and two reference groups. However, at the individual level (each patient with LOPD, and each GI scale as a unique symptom), the prevalence of a GI symptom requires close attention (Figure 1). Therefore, to better understand the impact and severity of each GI symptom on patients with LOPD, it is important to evaluate each patient on a case-by-case basis (individual) as well as a group (population/cohort). For instance, gastroesophageal reflux was highly prevalent (94%) in the LOPD group; of these, 4% of the patients had moderate to severe symptoms. On the other hand, while diarrhea was prevalent in 72% patients, 28% of those patients suffered from moderate to severe diarrhea. This shows that diarrhea as a presenting symptom may require early and prompt medical attention to avoid progression to severe diarrhea. Therefore, using these quantitative screening tools (PROMIS-GI and GI-focused history), all patients with LOPD should be routinely screened for GI problems during the first clinical visit and in subsequent follow-ups.

Longitudinal analyses in the current study (n = 19) showed that over time, a majority of patients had no meaningful changes (computed MIDs) in the GI scales. When the MID was identified, worsening or improvement was reported by patients in roughly equal numbers (Table 2). However, when 'worsening' and 'no change' MIDs were taken together, it indicated that ERT and the additional GI medications (over the counter) may be inefficient to treat the GI symptoms in patients with LOPD. This was further substantiated with the data from the GI-focused medical review, which suggested that 21/29 patients with at least 1 GI symptom (82%) reported no changes in their GI symptoms over time, even after the initiation of ERT (median duration of ERT = 5.5 years; range = 2 months–13 years).

Six patients reported that they had worsening GI symptoms within 48 h of ERT infusion, as per the GI-focused medical review. To understand if this could be related to GI-related adverse reactions from the ERT infusions, we checked the package insert of ERT (Lumizyme, US Food and Drug Administration). The Lumizyme package insert of ERT defines 'infusion reactions' as adverse reactions that occurred during or within 2 h of ERT infusion, and 'delayed-onset infusion reactions' occurred within 48 h [37]. As per the findings from their controlled study, GI-related infusion reactions in the LOPD group ($n = 60$) included constipation ($n = 6$), dyspepsia ($n = 5$), and vomiting ($n = 13$). There were no GI-related 'delayed onset' infusion reactions. Thus, combining the clinical data from the controlled study in the Lumizyme package insert and the current study, certain GI symptoms may be temporally associated with ERT infusions. However, this temporal association can be made only for isolated adverse events such as the ones that were reported by the six patients in the current study.

Findings from patients with other inborn errors of metabolism, such as Fabry disease and Gaucher disease, suggest that 6–7 months of treatment with agalsidase beta and ceredase ERT, respectively, led to a marked improvement in the GI symptoms [38,39]. When compared to Fabry and Gaucher-type I diseases, patients with LOPD seem to be less responsive to ERT. The high prevalence of GI symptoms from treated patients ($n = 46$) and longitudinal data from 19 patients showed that despite being on ERT, GI involvement causes a huge disease burden on adults with LOPD. All these data are contrary to the data from previous small case series, which reported that patients with LOPD ($n = 9$) had a substantial improvement in their GI symptoms following the initiation of ERT for 3–12 months [7,11,14,15]. The current study highlights that the current doses of ERT (20 mg/kg biweekly) may be insufficient to target GI symptoms effectively, as shown by no clinical change or worsening in several patients. This response to ERT could be due to a number of factors, such as low density of mannose-6-phosphate receptors in skeletal and smooth muscles as compared to cardiac muscle [40,41], using lower than recommended dose of ERT, impaired autophagy [42,43], defective mitophagy leading to abnormalities in the cellular energy metabolism [44,45], an acidic shift in the cellular pH after lysosomal rupture [44,45], and reduced uptake due to scar tissue (or residual fibrosis) in the muscles. There is also a variable response to treatment due to muscle fiber type, angiotensin-converting enzyme insertion/deletion polymorphism, and polymorphisms in the ACTN3 gene (R577X). In addition, we analyzed important factors that may influence the severity and prevalence of GI symptoms in LOPD, namely, patient's age, sex, age at diagnosis, age at ERT start, and most recent biomarkers of disease progression (CPK, 6-MWT, pulmonary function and urinary hex4). We did not identify any statistically significant relationships between these variables, potentially due to the small sample size (Supplementary Table S2).

Using the $6^{neo}/6^{neo}$ GAAKO mouse model, the current study showed that the GI tract is involved in its entirety, from the tongue and esophagus to the rectum (Figure 2). Tissue injury in the mouse model included glycogen accumulation throughout the GI tract, with vacuolization, autophagy (shown in the stomach), and fibrosis. There was hypertrophy in the intestinal villi and hyperplasia of Goblet cells, which could be a sign of compensation for the loss of functioning. In addition, there was an involvement of Aurbach's plexus (the nervous supply of the smooth muscles of the GI tissue) in the glandular portion of the stomach and small intestine. This further substantiates the need for alternate or adjuvant therapies with ERT which can target the smooth muscles and the nervous components. In the current study, short-term ERT (20 mg/kg per week for 5 weeks) could effectively clear the glycogen accumulation from the tongue, stomach, small intestine, and rectum (Figure 3). The short course of ERT also corrected the disintegrated cellular architecture in the Aurbach's plexus of the stomach and small intestine. However, it was ineffective in clearing the glycogen accumulation in the other parts of the GI tract. This shows that ERT may be inefficient for clearing glycogen accumulation in GI smooth muscle when initiated at later stage of disease, even with a 2-fold increase in dosing (from standard dose). The long-term therapy with ERT (20 mg/kg biweekly for 6 months) was more effective in clearing the glycogen accumulation throughout the gut. The age at initiation of ERT was 2 months. This showed that during early stages of disease, if ERT is started and continued for a longer duration, ERT may be effective. These mouse data will help in translational studies in children with LOPD and IPD in the advent of the newborn screening era. More research is needed at this time to follow up older mice to understand the effectiveness of ERT on the gut when it is initiated at a later stage of the disease. This will provide a better understanding about age at ERT initiation in patients with LOPD. This is important because autopsy data from three adult patients with LOPD (ages 31 years, 53 years, and 62 years) showed mild–moderate glycogen accumulation in the esophagus and ileum and vacuolation and degeneration of tongue, upper and lower esophagus, ileum, and media of arterioles [18,20,21]. The skeletal portion of the upper esophagus showed glycogen accumulation, lipofuscin, neural lipid droplets, and autophagic debris as seen on electron microscopy from a 62-year-old female patient with LOPD [20]. These data suggest that there is a need for effective therapies that minimize the gut pathologies in LOPD, even if treatment is initiated when patients are in their 30s or 40s.

Limitations: The current study has its limitations. Though subjective (patient-reported) measures were used in the study, the inclusion of objective GI tests (such as endoscopy or manometry) was beyond the scope of the current study. Future studies with objective GI testing on patients with LOPD may substantiate the findings of cellular architecture (or histopathology) in the mouse model of the current study. In addition, nutrition and dietary habits cause significant changes in the GI health; however, these causative factors could not be evaluated at this time. The study raises a question about the effectiveness of ERT on patients with LOPD. However, due to the small sample size of patients with untreated group ($n = 6$), the study could not compare the untreated with the treated group for statistical analysis. Another limitation was that PROMIS database provide estimated MIDs only for only five GI symptom scales; the clinical significance and interpretation of changes in T-scores for three other symptom scales were still unknown during the study period. Moreover, since the PROMIS-GI scales are self-reports, missed or skipped items often cause biases in data analysis. However, the automated and the manual scoring guides, provided by HealthMeasures, are built in such a way that the biases caused by missed/skipped items in self-reports are eliminated [27,28,46]. The responses in each GI symptom scale are based on the patients experience in the previous seven days, rather than longer periods in time, to reduce recall biases. Keeping in mind the varied response options and literacy demands, the items are concise and simple worded [27,28,46]. Lastly, GAAKO mouse models may not be a true representative of LOPD (mimics the IPD phenotypes more). Moreover, the long-term therapy of 6 months in the mouse model is approximately 20–30 years of therapy in humans. The 20–30 years of ERT in humans may not be feasible in patients with LOPD. However, the $6^{neo}/6^{neo}$ mouse model provided useful information about the cellular architecture in Pompe disease, and the impact of ERT on the GI tissue.

5. Conclusions

In conclusion, despite the limitations, the current study showed that about half the patients with LOPD had reduced quality of life due to GI symptoms, and these patients were on additional GI medications to treat these symptoms. However, most patients did not report any change or had worsening symptoms over time while being on ERT. Presumably, an earlier initiation of ERT may mitigate the development and progression of GI symptoms; however, this could not be concluded from the current study. Moreover, there is ineffective delivery of ERT to smooth muscles in the GI system [40–44], and the involvement of the neurological component of the gut (as seen by Aurbach plexus involvement in the current study). Recently, neurogenic dysfunction was shown in the urinary bladder of seven patients with LOPD, with probable causes of glycogen accumulation in the peripheral or central nervous system [16]. Due to a growing evidence of central nervous system involvement in Pompe disease, the neurological involvement in the GI system requires a closer evaluation [47]. In addition, the current study showed that the current recommended doses of ERT seem futile for maintaining GI health. Therefore, alternative therapies or second-generation drugs using gene therapy may be better ways to tackle the moderate to severe GI problems in patients with LOPD. In addition, since GI symptoms develop early in life, many times even before the diagnosis of LOPD, simple tools used in the current study (PROMIS-GI measures and GI-focused medical review) should be used to screen patients with clinical suspicion, and to observe progress of GI health in patients with LOPD as well as IOPD.

Supplementary Materials: The following supplementary materials will be available online at https://www.mdpi.com/2077-0383/10/15/3395/s1, Table S1: GI-focused medical history to assess the GI health of adult patients with Pompe disease, Table S2: Relationship between raw scores on PROMIS-GI symptom scales and clinical variables in patients with late-onset Pompe disease.

Author Contributions: As per the CRediT taxonomy guidelines, the individual contributions by all the authors of this manuscript are as follows—Conceptualization: A.K., P.M. and P.S.K.; Methodology: A.K., J.-A.L., K.Z., B.D.S. and P.S.K.; Validation: A.K., J.-A.L., K.Z., B.D.S. and P.S.K.; Formal analysis: A.K. and K.Z.; Investigation: A.K. and J.-A.L.; Resources: A.K., J.-A.L. and K.Z.; Data curation: A.K., J.-A.L. and K.Z.; Writing—original draft preparation: A.K.; writing—review and editing: A.K., J.-A.L., P.M., K.Z., B.D.S. and P.S.K.; Visualization and project administration: A.K. All authors have read and agreed to the published version of the manuscript.

Funding: This research received philanthropic funding from Allen Boger and family, and The Emerson and Barbara Kampen Foundation.

Institutional Review Board Statement: All participants were enrolled in a long-term follow up study of Pompe disease (Pro00010830) during the study period at the Duke University Medical Center. The study was conducted according to the guidelines of the Declaration of Helsinki, and approved by the Institutional Review Board of Duke University.

Informed Consent Statement: Written informed consent was obtained from each participant prior to all assessments in the study.

Data Availability Statement: The data presented in this study are available on request from the corresponding author.

Acknowledgments: The authors would like to thank Justin Chan, who helped with data entry during the initial phases of the study.

Conflicts of Interest: P.S.K. has received research/grant support from Sanofi Genzyme, Valerion Therapeutics, and Amicus Therapeutics and consulting fees and honoraria from Sanofi Genzyme, Amicus Therapeutics, Maze Therapeutics, JCR Pharmaceutical, and Asklepios Biopharmaceutical, Inc. (AskBio). P.S.K. is member of the Pompe and Gaucher Disease Registry Advisory Board for Sanofi Genzyme, Amicus Therapeutics, and Baebies. P.S.K. has equity in Asklepios Biopharmaceutical, Inc. (AskBio), which is developing gene therapy for Pompe disease and Maze Therapeutics, which is developing small molecule in Pompe disease. K.Z. receives support from the NIH (National Institute of Child Health and Human Development) (K23 HD091398, HHSN275201000003I), the Duke Clinical and Translational Science Award (KL2TR001115), and the industry for drug development in children. A.K., J.-A.L., P.M. and B.D.S. declare no conflict of interest. The funders had no role in the study design, data collection and analysis, decision to publish, or preparation of the manuscript.

References

1. Hers, H.G. Alpha-Glucosidase deficiency in generalized glycogenstorage disease (Pompe's disease). *Biochem. J.* **1963**, *86*, 11–16. [CrossRef] [PubMed]
2. Kishnani, P.S.; Steiner, R.; Bali, D.; Berger, K.; Byrne, B.J.; Case, L.; Crowley, J.F.; Downs, S.; Howell, R.R.; Kravitz, R.M.; et al. Pompe disease diagnosis and management guideline. *Genet. Med.* **2006**, *8*, 267–288. [CrossRef]
3. Chan, J.; Desai, A.K.; Kazi, Z.; Corey, K.; Austin, S.; Hobson-Webb, L.D.; Case, L.E.; Jones, H.N.; Kishnani, P.S. The emerging phenotype of late-onset Pompe disease: A systematic literature review. *Mol. Genet. Metab.* **2017**, *120*, 163–172. [CrossRef]
4. Kishnani, P.S.; Corzo, D.; Nicolino, M.; Byrne, B.; Mandel, H.; Hwu, W.-L.; Leslie, N.; Levine, J.; Spencer, C.; McDonald, M.; et al. Recombinant human acid -glucosidase: Major clinical benefits in infantile-onset Pompe disease. *Neurology* **2006**, *68*, 99–109. [CrossRef]
5. Montagnese, F.; Granata, F.; Musumeci, O.; Rodolico, C.; Mondello, S.; Barca, E.; Cucinotta, M.; Ciranni, A.; Longo, M.; Toscano, A. Intracranial arterial abnormalities in patients with late onset Pompe disease (LOPD). *J. Inherit. Metab. Dis.* **2016**, *39*, 391–398. [CrossRef]
6. McCall, A.L.; Salemi, J.; Bhanap, P.; Strickland, L.M.; Elmallah, M.K. The impact of Pompe disease on smooth muscle: A review. *J. Smooth Muscle Res.* **2018**, *54*, 100–118. [CrossRef]
7. Remiche, G.; Herbaut, A.-G.; Ronchi, D.; Lamperti, C.; Magri, F.; Moggio, M.; Bresolin, N.; Comi, G.P. Incontinence in Late-Onset Pompe Disease: An Underdiagnosed Treatable Condition. *Eur. Neurol.* **2012**, *68*, 75–78. [CrossRef] [PubMed]

8. El-Gharbawy, A.H.; Bhat, G.; Murillo, J.E.; Thurberg, B.L.; Kampmann, C.; Mengel, K.-E.; Kishnani, P.S. Expanding the clinical spectrum of late-onset Pompe disease: Dilated arteriopathy involving the thoracic aorta, a novel vascular phenotype uncovered. *Mol. Genet. Metab.* **2011**, *103*, 362–366. [CrossRef] [PubMed]
9. Hobson-Webb, L.D.; Jones, H.N.; Kishnani, P.S. Oropharyngeal dysphagia may occur in late-onset Pompe disease, implicating bulbar muscle involvement. *Neuromuscul. Disord.* **2013**, *23*, 319–323. [CrossRef]
10. Kishnani, P.S.; Amartino, H.M.; Lindberg, C.; Miller, T.M.; Wilson, A.; Keutzer, J. Methods of diagnosis of patients with Pompe disease: Data from the Pompe Registry. *Mol. Genet. Metab.* **2014**, *113*, 84–91. [CrossRef] [PubMed]
11. Pardo, J.; Garcia-Sobrino, T.; López-Ferreiro, A. Gastrointestinal symptoms in late-onset Pompe disease: Early response to enzyme replacement therapy. *J. Neurol. Sci.* **2015**, *353*, 181–182. [CrossRef]
12. Gesquière-Dando, A.; Attarian, S.; De Paula, A.M.; Pouget, J.; Salort-Campana, E. Fibromyalgia-like symptoms associated with irritable bowel syndrome: A challenging diagnosis of late-onset Pompe disease. *Muscle Nerve* **2015**, *52*, 300–304. [CrossRef]
13. Karabul, N.; Skudlarek, A.; Berndt, J.; Kornblum, C.; Kley, R.A.; Wenninger, S.; Tiling, N.; Mengel, E.; Plöckinger, U.; Vorgerd, M.; et al. Urge Incontinence and Gastrointestinal Symptoms in Adult Patients with Pompe Disease: A Cross-Sectional Survey. *JIMD Rep.* **2014**, *17*, 53–61. [CrossRef] [PubMed]
14. Bernstein, D.L.; Bialer, M.G.; Mehta, L.; Desnick, R.J. Pompe disease: Dramatic improvement in gastrointestinal function following enzyme replacement therapy. A report of three later-onset patients. *Mol. Genet. Metab.* **2010**, *101*, 130–133. [CrossRef] [PubMed]
15. Sacconi, S. Abnormalities of cerebral arteries are frequent in patients with late-onset Pompe disease. *J. Neurol.* **2010**, *257*, 1730–1733. [CrossRef] [PubMed]
16. Kuchenbecker, K.S.; Kirschner-Hermanns, R.; Kornblum, C.; Jaekel, A.; Anding, R.; Kohler, A. Urodynamic and clinical studies in patients with late-onset Pompe disease and lower urinary tract symptoms. *Neurourol. Urodyn.* **2020**, *39*, 1437–1446. [CrossRef] [PubMed]
17. McNamara, E.R.; Austin, S.; Case, L.; Wiener, J.S.; Peterson, A.C.; Kishnani, P.S.; Zschocke, J. Expanding Our Understanding of Lower Urinary Tract Symptoms and Incontinence in Adults with Pompe Disease. *JIMD Rep.* **2014**, *20*, 5–10. [CrossRef]
18. Walt, J.D. The pattern of involvement of adult-onset acid maltase deficiency at autopsy. *Muscle Nerve* **1987**, *10*, 272–281. [CrossRef]
19. Pena, L.D.M.; Proia, A.D.; Kishnani, P.S. Postmortem Findings and Clinical Correlates in Individuals with Infantile-Onset Pompe Disease. *JIMD Rep.* **2015**, *23*, 45–54. [CrossRef]
20. Hobson-Webb, L.D.; Proia, A.D.; Thurberg, B.L.; Banugaria, S.; Prater, S.N.; Kishnani, P.S. Autopsy findings in late-onset Pompe disease: A case report and systematic review of the literature. *Mol. Genet. Metab.* **2012**, *106*, 462–469. [CrossRef]
21. Kobayashi, H.; Shimada, Y.; Ikegami, M.; Kawai, T.; Sakurai, K.; Urashima, T.; Ijima, M.; Fujiwara, M.; Kaneshiro, E.; Ohashi, T.; et al. Prognostic factors for the late onset Pompe disease with enzyme replacement therapy: From our experience of 4 cases including an autopsy case. *Mol. Genet. Metab.* **2010**, *100*, 14–19. [CrossRef]
22. Bijvoet, A.G.; Van De Kamp, E.H.; Kroos, M.A.; Ding, J.-H.; Yang, B.Z.; Visser, P.; Bakker, C.E.; Verbeet, M.P.; Oostra, B.A.; Reuser, A.J.; et al. Generalized glycogen storage and cardiomegaly in a knockout mouse model of Pompe disease. *Hum. Mol. Genet.* **1998**, *7*, 53–62. [CrossRef]
23. Raben, N.; Nagaraju, K.; Lee, E.; Kessler, P.; Byrne, B.; Lee, L.; LaMarca, M.; King, C.; Ward, J.; Sauer, B.; et al. Targeted Disruption of the Acid α-Glucosidase Gene in Mice Causes an Illness with Critical Features of Both Infantile and Adult Human Glycogen Storage Disease Type II. *J. Biol. Chem.* **1998**, *273*, 19086–19092. [CrossRef]
24. Bijvoet, A.G.A. Recombinant Human Acid α-Glucosidase: High Level Production in Mouse Milk, Biochemical Characteristics, Correction of Enzyme Deficiency in GSDII KO Mice. *Hum. Mol. Genet.* **1998**, *7*, 1815–1824. [CrossRef]
25. Cella, D.; Riley, W.; Stone, A.; Rothrock, N.; Reeve, B.; Yount, S.; Amtmann, D.; Bode, R.; Buysse, D.; Choi, S.; et al. The Patient-Reported Outcomes Measurement Information System (PROMIS) developed and tested its first wave of adult self-reported health outcome item banks: 2005–2008. *J. Clin. Epidemiol.* **2010**, *63*, 1179–1194. [CrossRef]
26. Rothrock, N.E.; Hays, R.D.; Spritzer, K.; Yount, S.E.; Riley, W.; Cella, D. Relative to the general US population, chronic diseases are associated with poorer health-related quality of life as measured by the Patient-Reported Outcomes Measurement Information System (PROMIS). *J. Clin. Epidemiol.* **2010**, *63*, 1195–1204. [CrossRef] [PubMed]
27. Khanna, D.; Hays, R.D.; Shreiner, A.B.; Melmed, G.Y.; Chang, L.; Khanna, P.P.; Bolus, R.; Whitman, C.; Paz, S.H.; Hays, T.; et al. Responsiveness to Change and Minimally Important Differences of the Patient-Reported Outcomes Measurement Information System Gastrointestinal Symptoms Scales. *Dig. Dis. Sci.* **2017**, *62*, 1186–1192. [CrossRef] [PubMed]
28. Spiegel, B.M.R.; Hays, R.D.; Bolus, R.; Melmed, G.Y.; Chang, L.; Whitman, C.; Khanna, P.P.; Paz, S.H.; Hays, T.; Reise, S.; et al. Development of the NIH Patient-Reported Outcomes Measurement Information System (PROMIS) Gastrointestinal Symptom Scales. *Am. J. Gastroenterol.* **2014**, *109*, 1804–1814. [CrossRef] [PubMed]
29. Almario, C.V.; Ballal, M.L.; Chey, W.D.; Nordstrom, C.; Khanna, D.; Spiegel, B.M.R. Burden of Gastrointestinal Symptoms in the United States: Results of a Nationally Representative Survey of Over 71,000 Americans. *Am. J. Gastroenterol.* **2018**, *113*, 1701–1710. [CrossRef]
30. Lim, J.-A.; Yi, H.; Gao, F.; Raben, N.; Kishnani, P.S.; Sun, B. Intravenous Injection of an AAV-PHP.B Vector Encoding Human Acid α-Glucosidase Rescues Both Muscle and CNS Defects in Murine Pompe Disease. *Mol. Ther. Methods Clin. Dev.* **2019**, *12*, 233–245. [CrossRef]
31. Schoser, B.; Bilder, D.A.; Dimmock, D.; Gupta, D.; James, E.S.; Prasad, S. The humanistic burden of Pompe disease: Are there still unmet needs? A systematic review. *BMC Neurol.* **2017**, *17*, 202. [CrossRef]

32. Ajay, D.; McNamara, E.R.; Austin, S.; Wiener, J.S.; Kishnani, P. Lower Urinary Tract Symptoms and Incontinence in Children with Pompe Disease. *JIMD Rep.* **2015**, *28*, 59–67. [CrossRef]
33. Schoser, B.; Stewart, A.; Kanters, S.; Hamed, A.; Jansen, J.; Chan, K.; Karamouzian, M.; Toscano, A. Survival and long-term outcomes in late-onset Pompe disease following alglucosidase alfa treatment: A systematic review and meta-analysis. *J. Neurol.* **2017**, *264*, 621–630. [CrossRef] [PubMed]
34. Post, M. Definitions of Quality of Life: What Has Happened and How to Move On. *Top. Spinal Cord Inj. Rehabil.* **2014**, *20*, 167–180. [CrossRef] [PubMed]
35. Bodamer, O.A.; Scott, C.R.; Giugliani, R. Pompe Disease Newborn Screening Working Group; on behalf of the Pompe Disease Newborn Screening Working Group Newborn Screening for Pompe Disease. *Pediatrics* **2017**, *140*, S4–S13. [CrossRef] [PubMed]
36. Harfouche, M.; Kishnani, P.S.; Krusinska, E.; Gault, J.; Sitaraman, S.; Sowinski, A.; Katz, I.; Austin, S.; Goldstein, M.; Mulberg, A.E. Use of the patient-reported outcomes measurement information system (PROMIS®) to assess late-onset Pompe disease severity. *J. Patient-Reported Outcomes* **2020**, *4*, 1–11. [CrossRef]
37. Genzyme Corporation. Cambridge, MA. Lumizyme® (Alglucosidase Alfa) [Packet Insert] [Most Recent Major Changes in 02/2020]. Available online: https://www.accessdata.fda.gov/drugsatfda_docs/label/2010/125291lbl.pdf (accessed on 15 March 2021).
38. Banikazemi, M.; Ullman, T.; Desnick, R.J. Gastrointestinal manifestations of Fabry disease: Clinical response to enzyme replacement therapy. *Mol. Genet. Metab.* **2005**, *85*, 255–259. [CrossRef]
39. Verderese, C.L. Gaucher's disease: A pilot study of the symptomatic responses to enzyme replacement therapy. *J. Neurosci. Nurs.* **1993**, *25*, 296–301. [CrossRef] [PubMed]
40. Funk, B. Expression of the insulin-like growth factor-II/mannose-6-phosphate receptor in multiple human tissues during fetal life and early infancy. *J. Clin. Endocrinol. Metab.* **1992**, *75*, 424–431. [PubMed]
41. Cardone, M.; Porto, C.; Tarallo, A.; Vicinanza, M.; Rossi, B.; Polishchuk, E.; Donaudy, F.; Andria, G.; De Matteis, M.A.; Parenti, G. Abnormal mannose-6-phosphate receptor trafficking impairs recombinant alpha-glucosidase uptake in Pompe disease fibroblasts. *Pathogenetics* **2008**, *1*, 6. [CrossRef]
42. Shea, L.; Raben, N. Autophagy in skeletal muscle: Implications for Pompe disease. *Int. J. Clin. Pharmacol. Ther.* **2009**, *47*, S42–S47. [CrossRef] [PubMed]
43. Margeta, M. Autophagy Defects in Skeletal Myopathies. *Annu. Rev. Pathol. Mech. Dis.* **2020**, *15*, 261–285. [CrossRef] [PubMed]
44. Schoser, B. Pompe disease: What are we missing? *Ann. Transl. Med.* **2019**, *7*, 292. [CrossRef] [PubMed]
45. Meinke, P.; Limmer, S.; Hintze, S.; Schoser, B. Assessing metabolic profiles in human myoblasts from patients with late-onset Pompe disease. *Ann. Transl. Med.* **2019**, *7*, 277. [CrossRef] [PubMed]
46. PROMIS. Available online: http://www.healthmeasures.net/explore-measurement-systems/promis (accessed on 15 February 2021).
47. Korlimarla, A.; Lim, J.-A.; Kishnani, P.S.; Sun, B. An emerging phenotype of central nervous system involvement in Pompe disease: From bench to bedside and beyond. *Ann. Transl. Med.* **2019**, *7*, 289. [CrossRef] [PubMed]

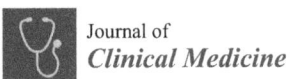

Article

COVID-19 Pandemic and Patients with Rare Inherited Metabolic Disorders and Rare Autoinflammatory Diseases—Organizational Challenges from the Point of View of Healthcare Providers

Ewa Tobór-Świętek [1,2], Jolanta Sykut-Cegielska [3], Mirosław Bik-Multanowski [4], Mieczysław Walczak [5], Dariusz Rokicki [6], Łukasz Kałużny [7], Joanna Wierzba [8], Małgorzata Pac [9], Karina Jahnz-Różyk [10], Ewa Więsik-Szewczyk [10] and Beata Kieć-Wilk [11,*]

1. Department of Metabolic Diseases, Jagiellonian University Medical College, 31-008 Cracow, Poland; ewa.tobor@doctoral.uj.edu.pl
2. Department of Metabolic Diseases, University Hospital, Jakubowskiego 2 Street, 30-688 Cracow, Poland
3. Department of Inborn Errors of Metabolism and Paediatrics, Institute of Mother and Child, Kasprzaka 17a Street, 01-211 Warsaw, Poland; jolanta.cegielska@imid.med.pl
4. Department of Medical Genetics, Medical College, Jagiellonian University, Wielicka 265 Street, 30-633 Cracow, Poland; miroslaw.bik-multanowski@uj.edu.pl
5. Department of Pediatrics, Endocrinology, Diabetology, Metabolic Diseases and Cardiology of the Developmental Age, Pomeranian Medical University, Unii Lubelskiej 1 Street, 71-242 Szczecin, Poland; ghmwal@pum.edu.pl
6. Department of Paediatrics, Nutrition and Metabolic Diseases, Institute "Children's Memorial Health Institute", al. Dzieci Polskich 20, 04-730 Warsaw, Poland; d.rokicki@ipczd.pl
7. Department of Pediatric Gastroenterology and Metabolic Diseases, Poznan University of Medical Sciences, Szpitalna 27/33 Street, 60-572 Poznan, Poland; lukasz@jerozolima.poznan.pl
8. Department of Paediatrics, Hematology and Oncology Medical University of Gdansk, Debniki 7, 80-752 Gdansk, Poland; jolanta.wierzba@gumed.edu.pl
9. Department of Immunology, Institute "Children's Memorial Health Institute", al. Dzieci Polskich 20, 04-730 Warsaw, Poland; m.pac@ipczd.pl
10. Department of Internal Diseases, Pneumology, Allergology and Clinical Immunology, Military Medical Institute, Szaserów 128 Street, 04-141 Warsaw, Poland; kjrozyk@wim.mil.pl (K.J.-R.); ewa.w.szewczyk@gmail.com (E.W.-S.)
11. Unit of Rare Metabolic Diseases, Department of Metabolic Diseases Jagiellonian University, Medical College, University Hospital, Jakubowskiego 2 Street, 30-688 Cracow, Poland
* Correspondence: mbkiec@gmail.com; Tel.: +48-12-400-29-50

Citation: Tobór-Świętek, E.; Sykut-Cegielska, J.; Bik-Multanowski, M.; Walczak, M.; Rokicki, D.; Kałużny, Ł.; Wierzba, J.; Pac, M.; Jahnz-Różyk, K.; Więsik-Szewczyk, E.; et al. COVID-19 Pandemic and Patients with Rare Inherited Metabolic Disorders and Rare Autoinflammatory Diseases—Organizational Challenges from the Point of View of Healthcare Providers. *J. Clin. Med.* **2021**, *10*, 4862. https://doi.org/10.3390/jcm10214862

Academic Editors: Karolina M. Stepien, Christian J. Hendriksz and Gregory M. Pastores

Received: 8 September 2021
Accepted: 19 October 2021
Published: 22 October 2021

Publisher's Note: MDPI stays neutral with regard to jurisdictional claims in published maps and institutional affiliations.

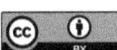

Copyright: © 2021 by the authors. Licensee MDPI, Basel, Switzerland. This article is an open access article distributed under the terms and conditions of the Creative Commons Attribution (CC BY) license (https://creativecommons.org/licenses/by/4.0/).

Abstract: COVID-19 pandemic is an organisational challenge for both healthcare providers and patients. People with rare inherited metabolic disorders (IMD) and rare autoinflammatory diseases (AD) are vulnerable patients whose well-being is deeply connected with regular follow-ups. This study aimed to assess how e one year of coronavirus pandemic has impacted the treatment of patients with IMD and AD in Poland. Surveys were distributed to all healthcare providers that coordinate the treatment of IMD and AD patients. Thirty-two responders (55%) answered the survey. They provide care to 1726 patients with IMD/AD, including 246 patients on dedicated treatment. In 35% of units, the regular appointments were disrupted, primarily because of patient infection. In 18 hospitals, remote visits were implemented, but only 66.6% of patients used this form of consultation. In 14/32 hospitals, administration of the therapy was delayed (median: 17.4 days). Forty-four patients suffered from SARS-COV-2 infection, in majority with mild symptoms. However, four adult patients developed complications, and one died following a SARS-COV-2 infection. Although most hospitals managed to maintain regular visits during the pandemic, more comprehensive implementation of telemedicine and switch to oral therapy or home infusions would be a reasonable solution for the current epidemic situation.

Keywords: COVID-19; inherited metabolic disorders; rare autoinflammatory diseases; health care providers

1. Introduction

Rare inherited metabolic disorders (IMD) and rare autoinflammatory diseases (AD) are a group of chronic and multisystem disorders with onset from the foetal period to adulthood. IMD is a heterogeneous group of c.a. 700 genetic disorders with a prevalence of around 1 in 800 live births. AD is a group of disorders characterized by recurrent, unprovoked inflammation without the typical features of autoimmune diseases (high titer autoantibodies) and the prevalence ranging from 1/10,000 to <1/1,000,000 live births. The low prevalence of the diseases and the variety of symptoms and disabilities result in high healthcare requirements and require multidisciplinary care. A large-scale survey conducted by EURORDIS in 2017 on 3450 patients with rare diseases in Europe demonstrated that 65% of patients had to frequently visit various health, social and local support services in a short time, and 51% of them found it hard to manage [1].

In 2020 healthcare coordination became even more challenging. In December 2019, several cases of pneumonia caused by novel coronavirus were detected in Wuhan, China [2]. By March 2020, severe acute respiratory syndrome coronavirus 2 (SARS-CoV-2) spread worldwide, and the World Health Organization (WHO) classified the outbreak as a pandemic [3]. The coronavirus disease (COVID-19) placed big pressure on the healthcare system and has changed the organisation of almost every hospital all over the world. Emergency departments and intensive care units were overwhelmed by COVID-19 patients, which caused that even patients with acute disorders like stroke [3] or heart attack [4] had problems getting proper help.

Decreased healthcare availability and fear of SARS-CoV-2 infection caused a series of new challenges for people with rare metabolic diseases. Reports from organizations of rare disease patients worldwide [5–14], and rare disease healthcare providers [5,15] showed the scale of disturbances: from cancelled appointments, postponed i.v. treatments and hospitalisations to shortage of medical supply and impact on mental health. EURODIS [13] and MetaBERN [5] studies involved Polish patients and health care providers, but the general report about the impact of the pandemic on patients with rare metabolic diseases in Poland is missing.

This study aimed to assess how outpatient clinics and hospitals, which provide care to patients with rare metabolic diseases, functioned and reorganised during one year of the COVID-19 pandemic in Poland and how the pandemic impacted rare metabolic disease patients.

2. Materials and Methods

It is a retrospective observational study coordinated by the Coordinating Team for Treatment of Ultra Rare Diseases in Poland. The team consists of specialists responsible for the qualification and monitoring of the treatment of patients with IMD and AD in Poland. The medical procedures in all patients are performed according to disease-specific therapeutic protocols. The study was carried out from 02 March to 30 May 2021 and assessed the first year of the COVID-19 pandemic.

The authors distributed two surveys via email (available as Supplementary Materials) with 30 questions to all 58 health care providers (HCP) taking care of adults or children patients with IMD and AD in Poland. The responders were coordinating physicians responsible for treating the patients (Figure 1).

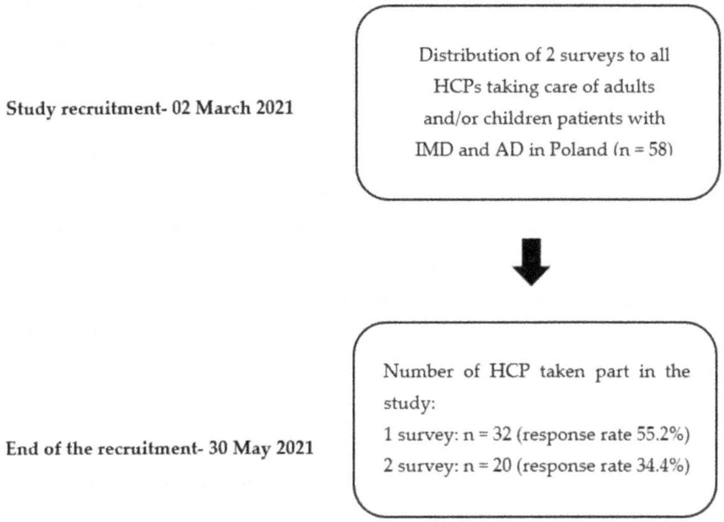

Study recruitment- 02 March 2021

Distribution of 2 surveys to all HCPs taking care of adults and/or children patients with IMD and AD in Poland (n = 58)

End of the recruitment- 30 May 2021

Number of HCP taken part in the study:
1 survey: n = 32 (response rate 55.2%)
2 survey: n = 20 (response rate 34.4%)

Figure 1. Flowchart of the study (HCP—health care providers; IMD—inherited metabolic disorders; AD—autoinflammatory diseases).

The multiple-choice and open-ended questions included three major topics: 1. Demographic data on patients, COVID-19 morbidity and its impact on patients health and follow-up (Survey S1). Additionally, the survey included a more detailed questionnaire on patients' whose therapy is reimbursed in Poland and who are hospitalised regularly (weekly or biweekly) according to a disease-specific therapeutic protocol: Gaucher disease (GD) type I and III, mucopolysaccharidosis (MPS) type I and II, Fabry disease, Pompe disease, tyrosinemia type I, IMDs requiring L-carnitine supplementation, hyperhomocysteinemia, and congenital autoinflammatory syndromes. 2. Organisational changes in health care units, including the implementation of telemedicine (Survey S1). 3. The impact of the pandemic on the diagnosis of new cases / routine admissions to a hospital (Survey S2).

The study protocol was approved by the Jagiellonian University Bioethical Committee and was in accordance with the Declaration of Helsinki. Informed consent was obtained from all individual participants included in the study.

IBM SPSS (Statistic for Windows, Version 25.0. IBM Corp, Armonk, NY, USA). was used for the data analysis.

3. Results

3.1. General Information

The response rate of the first survey was 55.2%. The data were collected from 32 HCP, including six strictly paediatric units, 21 centres providing healthcare only for adult patients, and five that follow both paediatric and adult patients. The majority of the clinics followed up 1–4 patients, and only four centres treated more than 50 patients (Table 1). Among all patients, 32.5% were adults, while 67.5% were pediatric patients.

In centers treating both children and adults, the percentage of pediatric patients varied from 69% to 91%. In total, all responders provided treatment to 1726 patients with rare inherited metabolic disorders and rare autoinflammatory diseases (Table 1). The patients received dedicated therapy: enzyme replacement therapy (ERT), substrate-reducing therapy, L-carnitine, anhydrous betaine, nitidinone, or anakinra. The cohort assessed in this study (whose therapy is reimbursed in Poland) included GD type I (40 patients), GD type III (12 patients), MPS I (3 patients), MPS II (18 patients), MPS IV (2 patients), Fabry disease (14 patients), Pompe disease (9 patients), tyrosinemia type I (17 patients), hyperhomocysteinemia (25 patients), diseases requiring L-carnitine supplementation (185 patients) and autoinflammatory diseases (30 patients). Sixty-nine percent of the cohort mentioned above were included in therapeutic programs treatment over some time from March 2020 to May 2021.

Table 1. Patients and healthcare units.

	No of Patients		
	Total	On Treatment	SARS-COV-2 (+)
Pediatric	1101	137	19
Adult	625	109	25
Group of IMD patients followed at the centre			
	No of healthcare units		
Only pediatric	6		
Only adult	21		
Both	5		
Number of treated patients in the centre			
	No of healthcare units		
1	12		
2 to 4	11		
5 to 50	5		
50 and more	4		

The response rate of the second survey was 34.4%. Only 20 HCP answered the questions about the pandemic impact on the diagnosis of new cases of IMD/AD. IMD, inherited metabolic disorders; AD, autoinflammatory diseases.

3.2. Health Care Units' Functioning during the Pandemic

Despite many restrictions and limitations during the COVID-19 pandemic, the majority of HCP (65%) reported that they could continue routine ambulatory visits of patients. Moreover, the continuity of visits was maintained in 7/9 units converted into temporary hospitals dedicated for SARS-COV-2 patients. The causes of postponement or cancellation of appointments in 12/32 cases are shown in Figure 2.

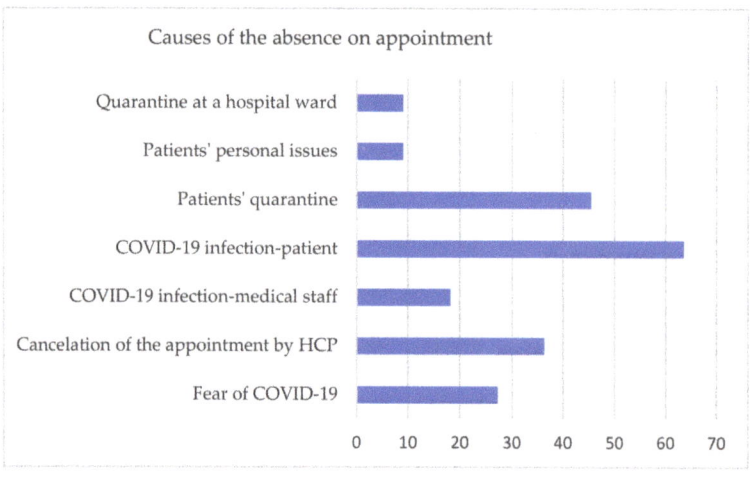

Figure 2. The causes of absence on appointments (HCP—health care providers).

For regular ambulatory visits, 56% (18/32) of HCP implemented remote visits as an alternative, and patients decided to use this form of consultation in 12/19 centres. Five HCP, which follow 1–4 patients each, did not introduce remote visits. The option of a remote visit was introduced in 50% (3/6) paediatric centers, 100% (5/5) units that treat both children and adults, and 52.4% (11/21) centres that follow adults only. The reasons why patients chose remote visits instead of face-to-face appointments are shown in Figure 3.

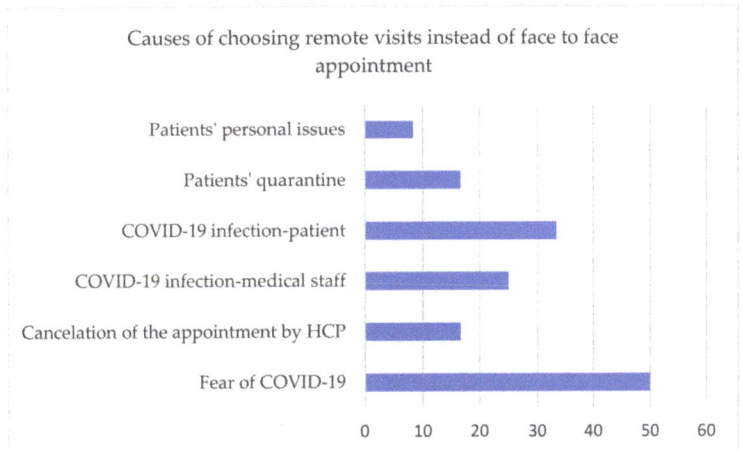

Figure 3. Causes of choosing telemedicine instead of "face-to-face" appointment (HCP—health care providers).

In 43.8% (14/32) of HCP, ERT administration was delayed for several reasons (Figure 4). The median time of delay was 17.5 days (7–56 days). In one hospital out of nine, which was converted into COVID-19 unit, there was a treatment delay caused by the cancellation of the visit by hospital authorities (21 days of delay). In another COVID-19 unit, disruptions were caused by fear of COVID-19 and patients' infection (maximum delay in this unit was 30 days). Other COVID-19 units (78%, 7/9) reported no treatment delay. Importantly, none of the healthcare units reported discontinuation of therapy during the COVID-19 pandemic.

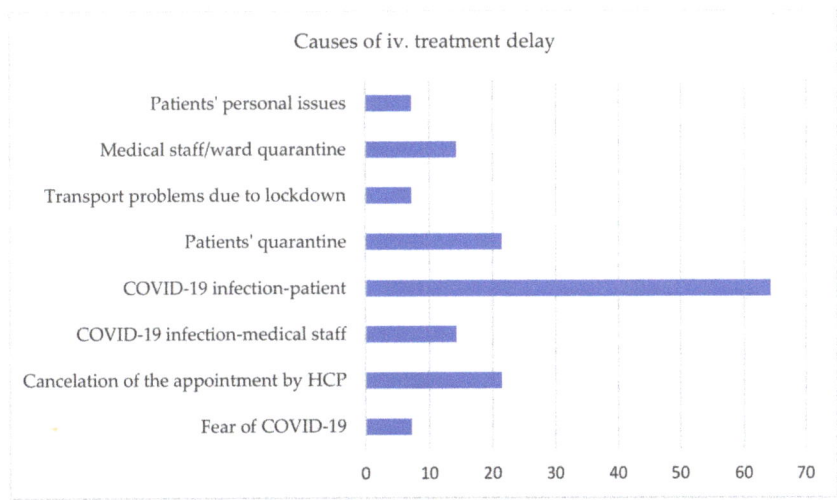

Figure 4. Causes of ERT delay (HCP—health care providers).

Two clinics reported that they succeeded in switching intravenous to oral therapy in two patients with GD. Also, two hospitals started home delivery of oral drugs for the first time in Poland.

3.3. Pandemic Impact on the Diagnosis of New Cases/Routine Admissions to Hospital

Only one hospital (1/20) reported that they experienced a delay in diagnosing new cases of rare diseases due to the pandemic. In the above case, the fear of infection resulted in postponing the planned hospitalisations. In the rest units (19/20), the number of new patients recently diagnosed or transferred from other hospitals was comparable with the time before the pandemic. This number includes all four hospitals with more than 50 rare disease patients. In 10% of healthcare units, fear of COVID-19 infection and patients' SARS-COV-2 infection resulted in the delay in qualifying patients for the treatment protocol.

Worsening of main disease symptoms, not related to SARS-COV-2 infection, was described in two cases of cystinosis. One patient experienced progression of ocular symptoms because of the postponement of a visit to the ophthalmology outpatient clinic. Another patient had eye complications, and kidney transplantation was delayed in this case.

3.4. Patients and SARS-COV-2 Infection

By the end of May 2021, 2.5% of all reported IMD and AD patients suffered from SARS-COV-2 infection confirmed by PCR test, including 25 adults and 19 children (Table 2). In 9 pediatric patients, data about the diagnosis of the main metabolic disease and on the course of infection are not complete. Therefore, these patients are excluded in further analysis.

Most patients reported fever (62.5%), rhinitis (59%), and general fatigue (56%) as the main symptoms. Four adult patients reported dyspnoea. In two cases it was associated with saturation decrease - one adult patient with Niemann Pick type C (NPC) required hospitalisation in the intensive care unit. Despite ventilator therapy, the patient died due to respiratory failure caused by massive bilateral pneumonia in the course of COVID-19. Additionally, one paediatric patient with very long-chain acyl-CoA dehydrogenase deficiency (VLADD) was hospitalised because of dehydration and metabolic decompensation during SARS-COV-2 infection. Two adult patients needed to be admitted to the hospital due to a thromboembolic event: massive deep vein thrombosis of lower limbs (a woman with Gaucher disease type 1) or ischaemic stroke (a man with Fabry disease type 1) (Table 2). The majority of reported COVID19 (+) patients (20 cases; 60%) received IMD/AD treatment. During SARS-COV-2 infection, nine of them did not have any delay in drug administration, whereas the other 11 had the treatment postponed from 7 up to 56 days (median: 17.5 days). Only one hospital reported worsening of the symptoms of the primary metabolic disease due to SARS-COV-2 infection. These were two cases of patients with NPC and one NPB disease. The first patient presented with psychomotor agitation during and after the infection. Two other patients, after a relatively mild course of COVID-19, revealed deterioration of motor abilities (less stable gait, slower speech, noticeably reduced concentration) in the absence of new MRI changes in the CNS.

Table 2. Characteristic of patients with COVID-19 infection.

Diagnosis	No of Adults	No of Children	Severity of COVID-19 Symptoms	No of Hospitalised Patients	Cause of Hospitalisation
MPS II	0	6	mild-6/6	0	n/a
MPS IV	1	0	moderate (dyspnea) 1/1	0	n/a
Gaucher disease t. I	4	0	mild-3/4, moderate 1/4 (dyspnea)	1	massive deep vein thrombosis (after SARS-COV-2 infection)
Gaucher disease t. III	0	1	mild 1/1	0	n/a
Fabry disease	3	2	mild 5/5	1 (adult)	ischemic stroke during SARS-COV-2 infection
Pompe disease	2	0	mild 2/2	0	n/a
NPC	4	0	mild 3/4 death 1/4	1	respiratory failure caused by massive bilateral pneumonia in the course of COVID-19
NPB	1	0	mild 1/1	0	n/a
Cystinosis	1	0	mild 1/1	0	n/a
VLCADD	0	1	moderate 1/1	1	dehydration and metabolic decompensation
Methylmalonic acidemia	1	0	moderate 1/1 (dyspnea, saturation decrease)	0	n/a
FCAS	3	0	mild 3/3	0	n/a
CAPS	3	0	mild 3/3	0	n/a
Schnitzler syndrome	2	0	mild 2/2	0	n/a

(MPS—mucopolysaccharidosis, NPC—Niemann Pick disease type C, NPB—Niemann Pick disease type B, VLCADD—Very long-chain acyl-CoA dehydrogenase deficiency, FCAS—Familial cold urticaria, CAPS—Cryopyrin associated periodic syndrome).

4. Discussion

Patients with rare diseases are a vulnerable group whose everyday functioning and access to healthcare drastically changed during the COVID-19 pandemic. For individuals receiving treatment in hospitals, every one or two weeks, the beginning of lockdown and the rising number of SARS-COV-2 patients caused the fear that their regular treatment would not be continued [16]. According to our data, in almost half of healthcare units (43.7%) that follow IMD and AD, the regular iv. infusions were disrupted. Those data are in line with the Italian study [8] concerning the same profile of patients (lysosomal storage disorders): 49% of patients (out of 102) ERT in hospitals experienced treatment disturbances. In another multicenter study regarding the impact of the COVID-19 pandemic on the diagnosis and management of IMD from a global perspective, the percentage of change of the total number of patients who received specialised treatment (particularly ERT) was 40% [17]. Moreover, a large study conducted by EURORDIS on rare disease patients in Europe revealed that a similar proportion of individuals (49.8% from 6945 patients) were unable to receive therapies such as infusions or chemotherapies [14]. Although the percentage of therapy disruptions was similar, their causes were surprisingly different. In this study, the main reason for treatment delay was a SARS-COV-2 infection, patient quarantine, or cancellation of the appointment by the hospital. Interestingly, fear of COVID-

19 infection as a reason for treatment delay was reported only in one hospital (1/32), which was converted into a strictly COVID-19 unit. The rest of the hospitals dedicated to patients with SARS-COV-2 (8/9) did not report treatment delay for that reason, and in all but one, they managed to create separate spaces for rare disease patients to maintain planned infusions without any delay. In similar questionnaires from other countries from the first months of 2020, fear of COVID-19 infection is listed as one of the main causes of therapy disruptions [8,13,18]. These differences may result from the fact that the first wave of the pandemic in Poland was relatively mild compared to other European countries. Therefore, hospitals had sufficient capacity to organise the administration of drugs so that patients felt safe and got used to the new situation until the next waves.

Many healthcare units outside Poland provided home therapy for people on i.v. treatments [5,8,15]. This solution was an excellent way to reduce the risk of treatment discontinuation during a pandemic [8]. Therefore, many HCP encouraged their patients to switch to that form of therapy [5,15]. In Poland, intravenous home therapy is not allowed in the case of rare metabolic diseases, even in the pandemic period. Only two hospitals reported that they started home delivery of oral drugs (tablets) after March 2020. A recent survey performed by the Polish Fabry Disease Collaboration Group [16] showed that 80% of patients with Fabry disease would prefer home infusions of ERT rather than in the hospital, and the majority would not change their preferences after the pandemic. Another way to make therapy more accessible during the pandemic is switching i.v. treatment into oral one as soon as this type of therapy is available, and the patient's clinical condition allows such a change. Such a possibility exists in the case of Gaucher and Fabry disease, where ERT therapy can be converted to a more convenient, oral substrate reduction/chaperone therapy. By May 2021, such a change in therapy was made in two adult patients with Gaucher disease in two independent hospitals. In both cases, it was done at the patient's request.

The number of healthcare units that reported disturbances in regular outpatient visits is lower than the number of hospitalisation disruptions (11 vs. 14). It is surprising when considering the fact that therapeutic programmes in Poland have strict organisational and administrative rules, and missed doses may have a serious health impact. On the other hand, patients might experience greater discomfort during hospitalisation than during a visit to the outpatient departments. In the MetaBERN study [5], 54,8% of health care providers of inherited rare metabolic diseases claimed to have a 75–100% of missing/postponed visits. However, there is a visible disproportion between health care units and patients' responses. In the same MetaBERN study, patient organisations responded that nearly 90% of the visits were postponed. In other similar surveys, the percentage of disrupted appointments based on answers of rare disease patients varied from 53% [11], through 67% [14] ,71% [9,19] up to 79% [12]. A probable reason for this disproportion is that healthcare providers answered only on behalf of their units, and patients visit disturbances might take place e.g. in GP/other specialist ambulatories. Considering the reasons for appointment disturbances, the most common were: patients SARS-COV-2 infection or quarantine (50%, 36%), cancellation of appointment by health care providers (29%), and fear of COVID-19 (21%). Unlike in other countries [14], fear of COVID-19 was not a crucial factor that caused patients to miss their appointments in Poland, and the survey results about remote visits confirm the results above. Only in 33% (6/18) of the centers allowing for remote visits, the patients chose this form because of fear of COVID-19 infection. Generally, access to telemedicine was provided by 56% of all responding physicians. It is less than in other countries, where the percentage of centres with telehealth options was 90% [5], and about 70% of patients experienced this form of consultations [6,9]. Both healthcare providers and patients claim telemedicine is a useful strategy and should continue in certain cases (e.g. electronic prescriptions) after the pandemic [6,9,13,16].

Patients with IMD, who often suffer from multiorgan dysfunctions, may be at risk of acute or chronic metabolic decompensation, and an infection may trigger even life-threatening episodes. At the beginning of the pandemic, rare disease experts were concerned about the impact of SARS-COV-2 infection on those patients [5]. In this survey, all healthcare providers reported 42 cases of COVID-19 infections of their patients. The coronavirus morbidity in investigated population is much lower than in the general population of Poland in the period from March 2020 to May 2021 (24.7/1000 vs. 76.25/1000) [20]. Those numbers might be underestimated because, in some cases, patients might have limited access to SARS-COV-2 diagnostic tests, even when they developed typical coronavirus symptoms. Moreover, paediatric patients are the majority of the described population, and testing in this age group was uncommon. Additionally, patients who are not receiving i.v./s.c. treatment in hospitals might not always contact their treatment centre in case of infection.

Almost all patients with infection reported mild, typical COVID-19 symptoms [21]. Those observations are in line with reports from other health care units worldwide [5,9,22–25]. Only in three cases, the worsening of primary disease symptoms was observed (two patients with NPC and one NPB: psychomotor agitation or deterioration of motor abilities), despite the continuation of symptomatic treatment during infection.

Coagulation abnormalities leading to thromboembolic complications are observed widely in patients with coronavirus infection [26,27]. One patient with Fabry disease was admitted to the hospital because of ischemic stroke symptoms, and routine tests revealed that he had a SARS-COV-2 infection. People with Fabry disease have a greater risk of developing an ischemic or hemorrhagic stroke [28] due to complex pathophysiology mechanisms leading to endothelial dysfunction and the development of chronic inflammation [29]. Therefore, the association between SARS-COV-2 and stroke is uncertain in this case. Another hospitalised patient was a woman with Gaucher disease type I, who developed massive deep vein thrombosis, probably related to coronavirus infection.

One patient with NPC revealed rapid respiratory failure caused by massive bilateral pneumonia in the course of COVID-19 and died. The observed worsening of primary disease symptoms and the severe course of coronavirus infection in patients with NPC opposes the hypothesis, claiming that inhibiting NPC1 enables a multistep blockade of viral entry and might be the treatment target for SARS-COV-2 [30,31]. That is a preliminary observation and requires further investigation. Nevertheless, our report draws attention to the group of adult NPC patients as those whose symptoms may worsen in SARS-COV-2 infection.

Interestingly, a large representation of adult patients with AD suffered from COVID-19 (8/30)—all of them with a mild course of the disease. This observation conforms to other studies, suggesting that the anti-inflammatory treatment may ameliorate the symptoms of COVID-19 infection [32,33].

Restrictions during the pandemic had an impact on already diagnosed patients and on diagnosing new ones. In Italy, the number of newly diagnosed patients with rare diseases in the first four months of 2020 was significantly lower than in 2019 and 2018 [15]. Similarly, a significant reduction (76%) of a number of established new IMD diagnoses was reported globally [17]. According to the records from the surveys, in Poland, only one hospital experienced a delay in diagnosing and two reported disturbances in starting i.v. therapy. All four hospitals that follow more than 50 patients reported that the process of diagnosis and qualification for therapy in 2020 was similar to 2019, and the number of diagnosed patients in both years was comparable. However, only 20/32 health care providers answered questions related to that topic. Moreover, 11/20 of those healthcare units followed only one patient and did not perform diagnosis or treatment qualification for years. Therefore, coronavirus pandemic's real impact in Poland on undiagnosed patients with IMD and AD remains unclear.

The study has several limitations. The survey focuses on physicians' points of view, highlighting the organisational aspect and general statistics. A special questionnaire dedicated to patients and caregivers of patients with inherited rare metabolic diseases would be crucial. It would help to assess healthcare availability outside main healthcare providers or causes of absence on appointments and, e.g. mental health problems during the pandemic or access to information about COVID-19. Secondly, not all hospitals that provide healthcare to patients with IMD and AD completed the entire survey. However, the response rate of 55.2% of the first survey makes the results of this study representative.

To conclude, although most hospitals managed to maintain the regularity of visits during the pandemic, wider implementation of remote visits and switch to oral therapy or home infusions would be a good solution to improve patients' health status.

Supplementary Materials: The following are available online at https://www.mdpi.com/2077-038 3/10/21/4862/s1, Survey S1: COVID-19 and rare metabolic diseases -PART I; Survey S2: COVID-19 and rare metabolic diseases -PART II.

Author Contributions: Conceptualization, B.K.-W.; Investigation, E.T.-Ś., J.S.-C., M.B.-M., M.W., D.R., Ł.K., J.W., M.P., K.J.-R., E.W.-S.; Methodology, E.T.-Ś., J.S.-C., M.B.-M., M.W., D.R., Ł.K., J.W., M.P., K.J.-R., E.W.-S.; Formal Analysis, E.T.-Ś.; Writing—Original Draft Preparation, E.T.-Ś.; Writing—Review & Editing, M.B.-M., J.S.-C., B.K.-W.; Supervision, B.K.-W., M.B.-M., J.S.-C.; Funding Acquisition, J.S.-C., M.W. All authors have read and agreed to the published version of the manuscript.

Funding: This research received no external funding.

Institutional Review Board Statement: The study was conducted according to the guidelines of the Declaration of Helsinki, and approved by the Ethics Committee of Jagiellonian University, Cracow (protocol code No 1072.6120.72.2021 and date of approval 21 April 2021).

Informed Consent Statement: Informed consent was obtained from all subjects involved in the study.

Data Availability Statement: The data presented in this study are available upon request from the corresponding author. The data are not publicly available due the specificity of the study, which concerns only Poland. This is a questionnaire survey and there are no standardized and generally available databases on this topic.

Acknowledgments: The authors wish to acknowledge all health professionals who kindly participated in this study and answered the questionnaire. The authors of the article would like to express their gratitude to Irmina Latko and Martyna Bandoch, who work in the Office of the Coordination Team for Ultra Rare Diseases, without whom the project could not be implemented.

Conflicts of Interest: The authors declare no conflict of interest.

Abbreviations

Abbreviations	
IMD	rare inherited metabolic disorders
AD	rare autoinflammatory diseases
HCP	health care providers
GD	Gaucher disease
MPS	mucopolysaccharidosis
ERT	enzyme replacement therapy
NPC	Niemann Pick disease type C
NPB	Niemann Pick disease type B
VLCADD	Very long-chain acyl-CoA dehydrogenase deficiency
FCAS	Familial cold urticaria
CAPS	Cryopyrin associated periodic syndrome

References

1. EURORDIS. *2017 Juggling Care and Daily Life: The Balancing Act of the Rare Disease Community*; EURORDIS: Paris, France, 2017.
2. Archived: WHO Timeline—COVID-19. Available online: https://www.who.int/news/item/27-04-2020-who-timeline---covid-19 (accessed on 21 June 2021).
3. Siegler, J.E.; Heslin, M.E.; Thau, L.; Smith, A.; Jovin, T.G. Falling Stroke Rates during COVID-19 Pandemic at a Comprehensive Stroke Center. *J. Stroke Cerebrovasc. Dis.* **2020**, *29*, 104953. [CrossRef]
4. Tam, C.-C.F.; Cheung, K.-S.; Lam, S.; Wong, A.; Yung, A.; Sze, M.; Lam, Y.-M.; Chan, C.; Tsang, T.-C.; Tsui, M.; et al. Impact of Coronavirus Disease 2019 (COVID-19) Outbreak on ST-Segment–Elevation Myocardial Infarction Care in Hong Kong, China. *Circ. Cardiovasc. Qual. Outcomes* **2020**, *13*, e006631. [CrossRef] [PubMed]

5. MetabERN Collaboration Group; Lampe, C.; Dionisi-Vici, C.; Bellettato, C.M.; Paneghetti, L.; van Lingen, C.; Bond, S.; Brown, C.; Finglas, A.; Francisco, R.; et al. The Impact of COVID-19 on Rare Metabolic Patients and Healthcare Providers: Results from Two MetabERN Surveys. *Orphanet J. Rare Dis.* **2020**, *15*, 341. [CrossRef] [PubMed]
6. Chung, C.C.Y.; Ng, Y.N.C.; Jain, R.; Chung, B.H.Y. A Thematic Study: Impact of COVID-19 Pandemic on Rare Disease Organisations and Patients across Ten Jurisdictions in the Asia Pacific Region. *Orphanet J. Rare Dis.* **2021**, *16*, 119. [CrossRef]
7. Castro, R.; Berjonneau, E.; Courbier, S. Learning from the Pandemic to Improve Care for Vulnerable Communities: The Perspectives and Recommendations from the Rare Disease Community. *Int. J. Integr. Care* **2021**, *21*, 12. [CrossRef]
8. Sechi, A.; Macor, D.; Valent, S.; Da Riol, R.M.; Zanatta, M.; Spinelli, A.; Bianchi, K.; Bertossi, N.; Dardis, A.; Valent, F.; et al. Impact of COVID-19 Related Healthcare Crisis on Treatments for Patients with Lysosomal Storage Disorders, the First Italian Experience. *Mol. Genet. Metab.* **2020**, *130*, 170–171. [CrossRef]
9. Schwartz, I.V.D.; Randon, D.N.; Monsores, N.; Moura de Souza, C.F.; Horovitz, D.D.G.; Wilke, M.V.M.B.; Brunoni, D. SARS-CoV-2 Pandemic in the Brazilian Community of Rare Diseases: A Patient Reported Survey. *Am. J. Med. Genet.* **2021**, *187*, 301–311. [CrossRef]
10. Canadian Organization for Rare Disorders. *Applying Lessons from COVID-19 to Better Healthcare for Rare Diseases*; Canadian Organization for Rare Disorders: Toronto, ON, Canada, 2020.
11. Rare Diseases Ireland. *Living with a Rare Disease in Ireland during the COVID-19 Pandemic*; Rare Diseases Ireland: Dublin, Ireland, 2020.
12. National Organisation for Rare Disorders. *COVID-19 Community Followup Survey Report: 92% of Rare Disease Patients Still Affected*; National Organisation for Rare Disorders: Danbury, CT, USA, 2020.
13. EURORDIS. *Rare Disease Patients' Experience of COVID-19*; EURORDIS: Paris, France, 2020.
14. EURORDIS. *How Has COVID-19 Impacted People with Rare Diseases?* EURORDIS: Paris, France, 2020.
15. Limongelli, G.; Iucolano, S.; Monda, E.; Elefante, P.; De Stasio, C.; Lubrano, I.; Caiazza, M.; Mazzella, M.; Fimiani, F.; Galdo, M.; et al. Diagnostic Issues Faced by a Rare Disease Healthcare Network during COVID-19 Outbreak: Data from the Campania Rare Disease Registry. *J. Public Health* **2021**, fdab137. [CrossRef]
16. Kusztal, M.; Kłopotowski, M.; Bazan-Socha, S.; Błażejewska-Hyżorek, B.; Pawlaczyk, K.; Oko, A.; Krajewska, M.; Nowicki, M. Is Home-Based Therapy in Fabry Disease the Answer to Compelling Patients' Needs during the COVID-19 Pandemic? *Survey Results from the Polish FD Collaborative Group. Adv. Clin. Exp. Med.* **2021**, *30*, 449–454. [CrossRef]
17. Elmonem, M.A.; Belanger-Quintana, A.; Bordugo, A.; Boruah, R.; Cortès-Saladelafont, E.; Endrakanti, M.; Giraldo, P.; Grünert, S.C.; Gupta, N.; Kabra, M.; et al. The Impact of COVID-19 Pandemic on the Diagnosis and Management of T Inborn Errors of Metabolism: A Global Perspective. *Mol. Genet. Metab.* **2020**, *131*, 285–288. [CrossRef] [PubMed]
18. Andrade-Campos, M.; Escuder-Azuara, B.; de Frutos, L.L.; Serrano-Gonzalo, I.; Giraldo, P. Direct and Indirect Effects of the SARS-CoV-2 Pandemic on Gaucher Disease Patients in Spain: Time to Reconsider Home-Based Therapies? *Blood Cells Mol. Dis.* **2020**, *85*, 102478. [CrossRef]
19. Chung, C.C.Y.; Wong, W.H.S.; Fung, J.L.F.; Hong Kong, R.D.; Chung, B.H.Y. Impact of COVID-19 Pandemic on Patients with Rare Disease in Hong Kong. *Eur. J. Med Genet.* **2020**, *63*, 104062. [CrossRef]
20. Koronawirus w Niedzielę 30 Maja. Niespełna 600 Zakażeń i 56 Zgonów. Available online: https://biqdata.wyborcza.pl/biqdata/7,159116,27143472,koronawirus-w-niedziele-30-maja-niespelna-600-zakazen-i-56.html (accessed on 22 June 2021).
21. Huang, C.; Wang, Y.; Li, X.; Ren, L.; Zhao, J.; Hu, Y.; Zhang, L.; Fan, G.; Xu, J.; Gu, X.; et al. Clinical Features of Patients Infected with 2019 Novel Coronavirus in Wuhan, China. *Lancet* **2020**, *395*, 497–506. [CrossRef]
22. Fierro, L.; Nesheiwat, N.; Naik, H.; Narayanan, P.; Mistry, P.K.; Balwani, M. Gaucher Disease and SARS-CoV-2 Infection: Experience from 181 Patients in New York. *Mol. Genet. Metab.* **2021**, *132*, 44–48. [CrossRef]
23. Pierzynowska, K.; Gaffke, L.; Węgrzyn, G. Transcriptomic Analyses Suggest That Mucopolysaccharidosis Patients May Be Less Susceptible to COVID-19. *FEBS Lett.* **2020**, *594*, 3363–3370. [CrossRef]
24. Gómez-Luján, M.; Cruzalegui, C.; Aguilar, C.; Alvarez-Vargas, M.; Segura-Saldaña, P. When Frequent (Pandemic) Occurs in a Non-Frequent Disease: COVID-19 and Fabry Disease: Report of Two Cases. *Jpn. J. Infect. Dis.* **2021**, *74*, 228–232. [CrossRef] [PubMed]
25. Zimran, A.; Szer, J.; Revel-Vilk, S. Impact of Gaucher Disease on COVID-19. *Intern. Med. J.* **2020**, *50*, 894–895. [CrossRef]
26. Al-Samkari, H.; Karp Leaf, R.S.; Dzik, W.H.; Carlson, J.C.T.; Fogerty, A.E.; Waheed, A.; Goodarzi, K.; Bendapudi, P.K.; Bornikova, L.; Gupta, S.; et al. COVID-19 and Coagulation: Bleeding and Thrombotic Manifestations of SARS-CoV-2 Infection. *Blood* **2020**, *136*, 489–500. [CrossRef]
27. Lazzaroni, M.G.; Piantoni, S.; Masneri, S.; Garrafa, E.; Martini, G.; Tincani, A.; Andreoli, L.; Franceschini, F. Coagulation Dysfunction in COVID-19: The Interplay between Inflammation, Viral Infection and the Coagulation System. *Blood Rev.* **2021**, *46*, 100745. [CrossRef] [PubMed]
28. Mehta, A.; Ginsberg, L. Natural History of the Cerebrovascular Complications of Fabry Disease: Cerebrovascular Complications of Fabry Disease. *Acta Paediatr.* **2007**, *94*, 24–27. [CrossRef] [PubMed]
29. Reisin, R.C.; Rozenfeld, P.; Bonardo, P. Fabry Disease Patients Have an Increased Risk of Stroke in the COVID-19 ERA. A Hypothesis. *Med. Hypotheses* **2020**, *144*, 110282. [CrossRef]

30. Sturley, S.L.; Rajakumar, T.; Hammond, N.; Higaki, K.; Márka, Z.; Márka, S.; Munkacsi, A.B. Potential COVID-19 Therapeutics from a Rare Disease: Weaponizing Lipid Dysregulation to Combat Viral Infectivity. *J. Lipid Res.* **2020**, *61*, 972–982. [CrossRef] [PubMed]
31. Ballout, R.A.; Sviridov, D.; Bukrinsky, M.I.; Remaley, A.T. The Lysosome: A Potential Juncture between SARS-CoV-2 Infectivity and Niemann-Pick Disease Type C, with Therapeutic Implications. *FASEB J.* **2020**, *34*, 7253–7264. [CrossRef] [PubMed]
32. Moutsopoulos, H.M. Anti-Inflammatory Therapy May Ameliorate the Clinical Picture of COVID-19. *Ann. Rheum. Dis.* **2020**, *79*, 1253–1254. [CrossRef] [PubMed]
33. Haslak, F.; Yildiz, M.; Adrovic, A.; Sahin, S.; Koker, O.; Aliyeva, A.; Barut, K.; Kasapcopur, O. Management of Childhood-Onset Autoinflammatory Diseases during the COVID-19 Pandemic. *Rheumatol. Int.* **2020**, *40*, 1423–1431. [CrossRef] [PubMed]

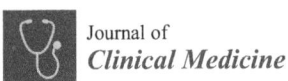

Article

Plasma Neurofilament Light (NfL) in Patients Affected by Niemann–Pick Type C Disease (NPCD)

Andrea Dardis [1,*], Eleonora Pavan [1], Martina Fabris [2], Rosalia Maria Da Riol [1], Annalisa Sechi [1], Agata Fiumara [3], Lucia Santoro [4], Maximiliano Ormazabal [1], Romina Milanic [2], Stefania Zampieri [1], Jessica Biasizzo [2] and Maurizio Scarpa [1]

[1] Regional Coordinator Centre for Rare Diseases, University Hospital of Udine, 33100 Udine, Italy; pavan.eleonora@gmail.com (E.P.); rosalia.dariol@asufc.sanita.fvg.itr (R.M.D.R.); annalisa.sechi@asufc.sanita.fvg.it (A.S.); maxi.ormazabal@gmail.com (M.O.); stefania.zampieri@asufc.sanita.fvg.it (S.Z.); maurizio.scarpa@asufc.sanita.fvg.it (M.S.)
[2] Institute of Clinical Pathology, Department of Laboratory Medicine, University Hospital of Udine, 33100 Udine, Italy; martina.fabris@asufc.sanita.fvg.it (M.F.); romina.milanic@asufc.sanita.fvg.it (R.M.); jessica.biasizzo@asufc.sanita.fvg.it (J.B.)
[3] Regional Referral Center for Inherited Metabolic Disease, Department of Pediatrics, University of Catania, 95131 Catania, Italy; agatafiumara@yahoo.it
[4] Division of Pediatrics, Department of Clinical Sciences, Polytechnic University of Marche, Ospedali Riuniti, 60123 Ancona, Italy; dott.luciasantoro@gmail.com
* Correspondence: andrea.dardis@asufc.sanita.fvg.it

Abstract: (1) Background: Niemann–Pick type C disease (NPCD) is an autosomal recessive lysosomal storage disorder caused by mutations in the NPC1 or NPC2 genes. The clinical presentation is characterized by visceral and neurological involvement. Apart from a small group of patients presenting a severe perinatal form, all patients develop progressive and fatal neurological disease with an extremely variable age of onset. Different biomarkers have been identified; however, they poorly correlate with neurological disease. In this study we assessed the possible role of plasma NfL as a neurological disease-associated biomarker in NPCD. (2) Methods: Plasma NfL levels were measured in 75 healthy controls and 26 patients affected by NPCD (24 NPC1 and 2 NPC2; 39 samples). (3) Results: Plasma NfL levels in healthy controls correlated with age and were significantly lower in pediatric patients as compared to adult subjects ($p = 0.0017$). In both pediatric and adult NPCD patients, the plasma levels of NfL were significantly higher than in age-matched controls ($p < 0.0001$). Most importantly, plasma NfL levels in NPCD patients with neurological involvement were significantly higher than the levels found in patients free of neurological signs at the time of sampling, both in the pediatric and the adult group ($p = 0.0076$; $p = 0.0032$, respectively). Furthermore, in adults the NfL levels in non-neurological patients were comparable with those found in age-matched controls. No correlations between plasma NfL levels and NPCD patient age at sampling or plasma levels of cholestan 3β-5α-6β-triol were found. (4) Conclusions: These data suggest a promising role of plasma NfL as a possible neurological disease-associated biomarker in NPCD.

Keywords: Niemann–Pick C; neurofilament light; biomarkers; neurological disease

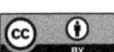

1. Introduction

Niemann–Pick type C disease (NPCD-MIM 257220; MIM607625) is an autosomal recessive neurovisceral lysosomal storage disorder due to mutations in the NPC1 (95% of patients) or NPC2 genes, encoding two proteins involved in the intracellular trafficking of cholesterol and other lipids. The deficiency of either of them leads to the accumulation of endocytosed unesterified cholesterol and other lipids within the lysosome/late endosome compartment [1].

The clinical presentation of the disease is extremely variable and the age at onset ranges from the perinatal period to adulthood. The disease is typically characterized by visceral and neurological signs and symptoms that follow an independent clinical course. When visceral involvement is present, it is characterized by hepatosplenomegaly that precedes the onset of neurological signs. Apart from a small group of patients presenting a severe perinatal form leading to death due to liver or respiratory failure within the first months of age, and a few mildly affected adult cases, all patients develop progressive and fatal neurological disease [2–4]. Indeed, NPCD has been classically classified on the basis of age at onset of neurological symptoms, irrespective of the age of first visceral symptoms [1].

Miglustat, a glucosylceramide synthase inhibitor, is the only therapeutic option approved for the treatment of neurological symptoms of NPCD. However, other approaches such us the use of arimoclomol (a co-inducer of the heat shock response) and 2-hydroxypropyl-β-cyclodextrin (HP-β-CD) are currently under clinical investigation [5]. In addition, a recent study supports the efficacy and safety of Tanganil (N-acetyl-L-Leucine) for the symptomatic treatment of NPCD [6].

To date, several molecules have been proposed and validated as biomarkers of NPCD to support the diagnosis and follow up of affected patients [7–19]. Among them, the plasma levels of cholestan-3β,5α,6β-triol (3β,5α,6β-triol) and 7-ketocholesterol (7-KC) are the most widely used in clinical settings [13–19]. However, a relatively weak correlation with severity or age at onset of neurological involvement has been found [13,20]. Therefore, new biomarkers that better correlate with neurological involvement, which represents the most devastating aspect of the disease, are needed.

Neurofilaments are major structural elements of neurons. They are composed of four subunits: a triplet of NF light (NfL), NF medium (NfM) and NF heavy (NfH) chains, and either α-internexin or peripherin in the central and peripheral nervous systems, respectively [21]. Nfs can be detected in the cerebrospinal fluid (CSL) as surrogate markers of axonal injury, degeneration, and loss [22]. As such, increased levels of NfL, the most abundant subunit, have been reported in the CSF of patients affected by several neurological diseases [23–28].

Although NfL has not been systematically studied in NPCD patients, elevated levels in CSF have been described in two case report studies [29,30].

Recently, highly sensitive assays have been developed for the detection of NfL in blood. Most importantly, a strong correlation between serum and CSF NfL levels has been demonstrated in several disorders [24,31–38].

Based on this evidence, plasma levels of NfL have already been investigated and found to be elevated in patients affected by two neurodegenerative lysosomal disorders: mucopolysaccharidosis II and neuronal ceroid lipofuscinosis type 2 [39,40].

Given the reports of elevated NfL levels in CSF or plasma in genetic, inflammatory, and other neurodegenerative diseases [23–40], NfL in body fluids appears to be a general, not disease-specific, but sensitive marker of neurodegeneration due to the loss of neurons and axons. This has led to the present study on the possible role of NfL in plasma as a biomarker for the neurological disease associated with NPCD.

2. Materials and Methods

2.1. Patients

Plasma samples from patients affected by NPCD were obtained during the diagnostic work-up at the Regional Coordinator Centre for Rare Diseases. Patient phenotype classification was based on the age at onset of neurological symptoms as follows: severe infantile (SI, age at onset <2 years), late infantile (LI, age at onset 2–6 years), juvenile (J, age at onset 6–15 years), and adult (A, age at onset >15 years) [41]. Patients who died during the first 6 month of life due to liver or respiratory insufficiency without signs of neurological involvement were classified as having the early infantile systemic lethal form (EISL). Asymptomatic patients and patients who did not present clinical or imaging signs of neurological involvement at last follow-up were considered non-classifiable (NC).

Control samples were obtained from 75 healthy age-matched subjects. Adult samples were obtained from healthy blood donors, while pediatric samples were recovered from material used for routine investigations, without further sampling, of children with normal neurological and liver function. The study was conducted in accordance with the ethical standards of 1964 Helsinki Declaration and its later amendments and written informed consent was obtained from all subjects or care/guardians on behalf of the minors.

NPCD diagnosis was established by NPC1 and NPC2 genotyping. Biochemical confirmation by the analysis of intracellular cholesterol accumulation by filipin staining was done in all patients presenting at least 1 allele carrying a variant of unknown significance (VUS) and whenever available in cases with pathogenetic variants of both alleles [42] (Table S1). Patients presenting at least 1 VUS and a variant biochemical phenotype presented high levels of NPCD biomarkers: oxysterols and/or N-palmitoyl-O-phosphocholineserine (PPCS). Genotype was confirmed in relatives whenever possible.

2.2. Neurofilament Light (NfL)

Plasma NfL was assessed using a microfluidic Simple PlexTM NfL Assay (ProteinSimple, San José, CA, USA) on an EllaTM instrument according to the manufacturers' instructions. The instrument was calibrated using the in-cartridge factory standard curve. All samples were measured after a single thaw, with a 1:2 dilution.

2.3. Plasma Cholestane-3β,5α,6β-triol Concentration

The concentration of cholestane-3β,5α,6β-triol was determined as previously described [16]. Briefly, internal standard/protein precipitation solution (250 µL) was added to 50 µL of samples. After centrifugation, the supernatant was dried under a stream of nitrogen and then derivatized with N,N-dimethyilglycine (DMG) in the presence of both 1-ethyl-3-(3-dimethylaminopropyl)cabodiimide (ECD) and 4-(N,N-dimethylaminopyrididine) (DMAP). After quenching the reaction with 20 µL of methanol, tubes were dried with nitrogen stream and reconstituted with 200 µL of methanol–water (4:1). Sample analysis was performed by HPLC-MS/MS using a Prominence UFLCXR system (Shimadzu Scientific Instruments, Columbia, MD, USA) and a 4000 Qtrap MASS SPECTROMETER (ABSciex, Framingham, MA, USA).

2.4. Statistical Analysis

Descriptive statistics were used to describe the patients' demographic and clinical characteristics at the time of sampling.

The nonparametric Mann–Whitney test was used to assess the significance of plasma NfL differences between groups. Relationships between plasma NfL and oxysterols or age were evaluated by Pearson's correlation test. Analysis was performed using the GraphPad Prism v8 (GraphPad Soft-ware, San Diego, CA, USA).

3. Results

Plasma NfL levels were measured in 75 healthy controls and 26 patients affected by NPCD (24 NPC1 and 2 NPC2). Patients were classified according to the age at onset of neurological symptoms as previously described [1]. Serial samples obtained during regular follow-up visits were available for 8/26 NPCD patients. In total, 39 NPCD samples were analyzed. Details on the clinical phenotype, age at NfL assessment, and neurological involvement at the time of NfL assessment are summarized in Table 1 and Table S1. In total, 3 patients died during follow up: 2 of them, affected by the EISL phenotype (NP1 and NP2; Table S1), died from respiratory insufficiency and liver failure, respectively, before 6 months of age; and 1, affected by the EI clinical form, died from neurological disease at the age of 3 years (NP4; Table S1).

As already reported [43], plasma NfL levels in healthy controls correlated with age (Pearson's correlation coefficient = 0.4313; p = 0.0097) and were significantly lower in the pediatric population (<18 years of age; n = 39; median: 7.94 pg/mL; IQR: 6.4–9.8 pg/mL) than in adults (≥18 years; n = 36; median: 11.2 pg/mL; IQR: 8.3–15.3 pg/mL) p = 0.0017. Therefore, to compare the NfL levels found in NPCD patients vs. healthy controls, samples were divided in 2 groups according to the age at the time of NfL assessment: <18 years of age and ≥18 years of age. As shown in Table 2 and Figure 1, in both pediatric and adult NPCD patients the plasma levels of NfL were significantly higher when compared with age-matched controls ($p < 0.0001$).

Table 1. Characteristics of the studied cohort.

	Pediatric NPCD Patients ($n = 12$)	Adult NPCD Patients ($n = 14$)
Gender		
Male	6	5
Female	6	9
Clinical phenotype		
EISL	2 *	0
EI	2 (1+)	0
LI	4	0
J	2	4
A	0	6
NC	2	4
Number of analyzed samples		
	15	24
Age at sampling (years)		
Mean	4.8	29.4
Range	0.08–13.08	21.58–53.08
Presence of Neurological involvement at sampling		
	6	14

EISL: early infantile severe lethal; EI: early infantile; LI: late infantile; J: juvenile; A: adult; NC: nonclassified because of lack of neurological involvement at last follow-up [41] Two J patients were twins and 2 adults were siblings, as were 2 J, 1 A, and 2 NC patients. * deceased due to liver failure and respiratory insufficiency, respectively. + deceased at 3 years of age due to neurological disease.

Table 2. Plasma levels of NfL (pg/mL).

	Pediatric		Adults	
	Healthy Controls ($n = 39$)	NPCD ($n = 15$)	Healthy Controls ($n = 36$)	NPCD ($n = 24$)
Median	7.94	28.97 ****	11.2	25.6 ****
IQ range	6.38–9.75	15.83–70.21	8.265–15.26	15.9–34.75
Range	4.56–21.2	8.82–581.4	4.01–33.97	7.59–62.5

**** $p < 0.0001$.

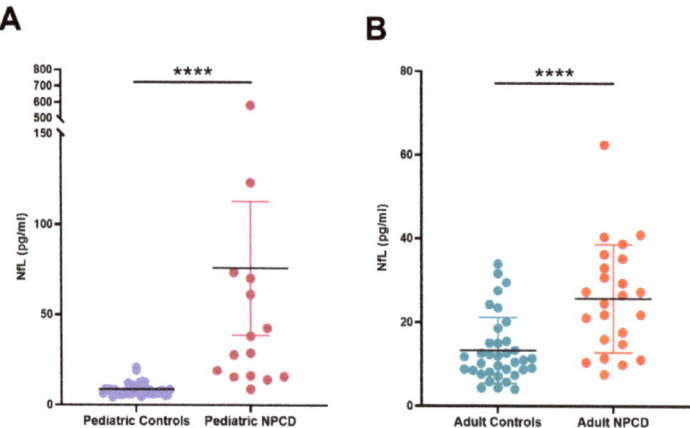

Figure 1. NfL concentrations in plasma of NPCD patients. (**A**) Pediatric NPCD patients vs. healthy controls. (**B**) Adult NPCD patients vs. healthy controls. **** $p < 0.0001$.

However, since 10/24 adult and 9/15 pediatric samples were obtained from NPCD patients free of neurological signs and symptoms at the time of sampling (Table S1), we divided both groups according to the presence or absence of neurological involvement and compared their NfL levels. As shown in Figure 2, NfL levels in NPCD patients with neurological involvement were significantly higher than the levels found in non-neurological patients, both in the pediatric and the adult group ($p = 0.0076$; $p = 0.0032$, respectively). Furthermore, in adults the NfL levels found in non-neurological patients were comparable with those found in age matched healthy subjects. Among pediatric NPCD patients, only two non-neurological patients displayed NfL values that overlap with those found in neurological patients (Figure 2). It is worth noting that these two patients were affected by the EISL clinical form, an extremely severe phenotype rapidly leading to death due to liver failure and respiratory insufficiency, before the development of neurological disease.

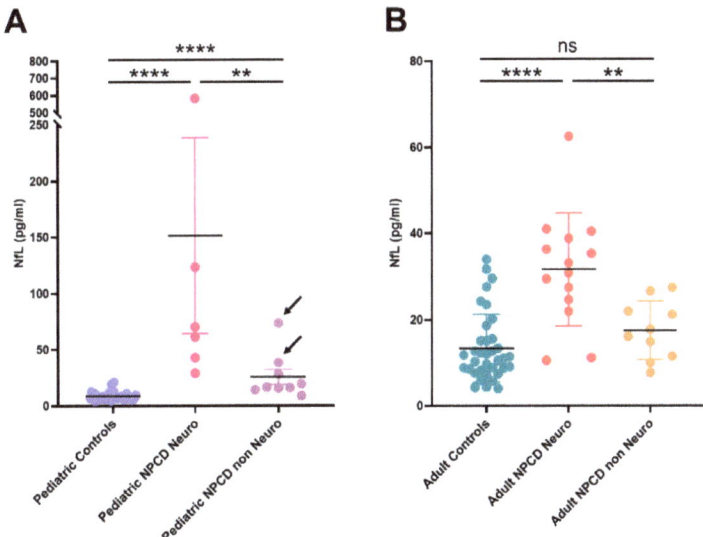

Figure 2. NfL concentration in plasma from neurological and non-neurological NPCD patients. (**A**) Pediatric patients. Arrows indicate NPCD patients affected by the EISL phenotype. (**B**) Adult patients. **** $p < 0.0001$; ** $p < 0.01$; NS: non-significant.

Since a possible bias in the presented results might have been introduced due to the inclusion of NfL values obtained in serial samples of the same patient in the NPCD group, we performed the analysis considering only one sample per patient (obtained during the first visit). As shown in Table 3, also excluding serial samples from the analysis, both pediatric and adult NPCD patients displayed significant increased levels of NfL when compared with age-matched controls, and patients with neurological involvement presented significantly higher levels of plasma NfL than non-neurological patients.

In two neurological patients (NP8 and NP21; Table S1), plasma NfL was assessed just after starting treatment with miglustat, while in other two neurological adult patients, plasma NfL were measured before and after starting miglustat therapy (NP18; NP18sib). In these last patients, plasma NfL levels remained stable or slightly decreased (Table S1).

In contrast to healthy controls, no correlation between plasma NfL levels and age at sampling was found in NPCD patients (Pearson's correlation coefficient = -0.2658; $p = 0.102$) (Figure 3A).

Table 3. Plasma levels of NfL (pg/mL).

	Pediatric				Adults			
	Healthy Controls ($n = 39$)	NPCD ($n = 12$)	NPCD Neuro ($n = 4$)	NPCD Non Neuro ($n = 7$)	Healthy Controls ($n = 36$)	NPCD ($n = 14$)	NPCD Neuro ($n = 9$)	NPCD Non Neuro ($n = 5$)
Median	7.94	33.07 ****	65.75	19.26 *	11.20	27.02 ***	33.10	16.07 *
IQ range	6.38–9.75	15.78–67.98	47.35–453.60	14.12–38.24	8.20–15.47	14.91–36.18	27.02–39.63	9.51–19.43
Range	4.56–21.20	8.82–581.40	42.70–581.40	8.82–73.50	4.01–33.97	7.59–62.50	11.12–62.50	7.59–21.15

**** $p < 0.0001$; *** $p < 0.001$ NPCD patients vs. healthy age matched controls. * $p < 0.05$ NPCD neurological vs. non-neurological patients.

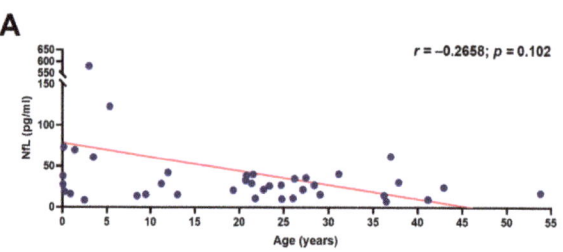

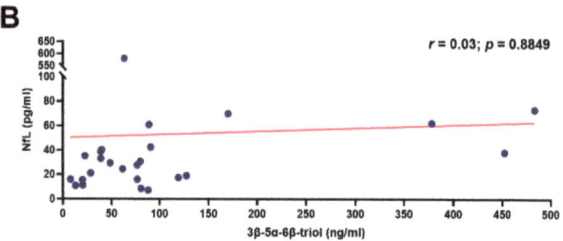

Figure 3. Association of NfL concentrations in the plasma of NPCD patients with age (**A**) and 3β,5α,6β-triol (**B**). Correlations were assessed by Pearson's linear regression correlation test.

Plasma levels of cholestan 3β-5α-6β-triol were measured in samples taken during the first visit in 25 out of 26 patients, and no correlation between plasma levels of this oxysterol and those of NfL was found (Pearson's correlation coefficient = 0.03; $p = 0.8849$) (Figure 3B).

4. Discussion

NPCD is a rare neurovisceral lysosomal storage disorder characterized by a wide spectrum of clinical phenotypes. However, almost all patients ultimately develop progressive and fatal neurological disease, even if the age at onset of neurological symptoms is extremely variable, ranging from early infancy to adulthood. To date, miglustat is the only approved treatment for the neurological manifestations of the disease in adult and pediatric NPCD patients. Although miglustat does not prevent the development of neurological symptoms [44], experience with hundreds of treated patients over the last decade demonstrates its effectiveness in reducing the rate of disease progression and stabilizing the neurological disease [45–47]. However, treatment should be started as soon as the first neurological signs become evident [4,46]. This evidence highlights the crucial role of neurological disease-associated biomarkers to monitor disease progression and optimize care in NPCD patients.

Several studies have reported an association between CSF levels of NfL and neuronal death and axonal degeneration in various neurodegenerative diseases. Although extremely useful, the downside of the CSF biomarkers is the requirement of invasive sampling. Recently, the development of highly sensitive immunometric methods able to reliable detect low levels of proteins in plasma has opened new opportunities in the field of neurodegenerative disease-associated biomarkers. Indeed, the use of plasma NfL and GFAP levels in patients at different landmarks of multiple sclerosis (NeurofilMS) is currently being studied in a clinical trial [48].

In this work we explored the role of plasma NfL as a possible biomarker in NPCD.

We showed that plasma levels of NfL are significantly increased in patients affected by NPCD compared with age-matched healthy controls. Furthermore, plasma NfL are significantly higher in NPCD patients presenting neurological disease compared with patients free of neurological involvement. Although these results should be confirmed in larger cohorts, the presented data strongly suggest that plasma levels of NfL might be a potential biomarker of neurological disease in NPCD. This hypothesis is supported by the observation that all NPCD patients, who were either asymptomatic or presented visceral involvement without neurological disease, showed levels of plasma NfL comparable with those found in age-matched controls. Conversely, levels of $3\beta,5\alpha,6\beta$-triol, a widely used biomarker of NPCD, were increased (above the cut off value) in most of them (75%). Furthermore, no correlation between plasma NfL and $3\beta,5\alpha,6\beta$-triol was found. These data confirmed a poor correlation between oxysterols levels and neurological disease in NPCD.

It is interesting to look at the results obtained in the two patients affected by the EISL phenotype. These patients presented the highest values of $3\beta,5\alpha,6\beta$-triol, reflecting the extremely severe visceral disease that led to death within the first year of life. It has been extensively documented that apart from patients affected by this clinical phenotype and exceptional adult cases, all NPCD patients ultimately develop progressive and fatal neurological disease. Therefore, it is possible to hypothesize that even though neurological symptoms are subtle in patients affected by the EISL phenotype, they died from liver failure or respiratory insufficiency before neurological involvement become evident and if they had survived, they probably would have developed severe neurological disease [49]. Indeed, the two patients affected by the EISL phenotype were the only pediatric non-neurological patients displaying levels of plasma NfL that overlapped with those found in neurological patients. However, it is important to acknowledge that EISL patients were 1 and 2 months old, respectively, at the time of NfL assessment, while the pediatric healthy controls were older than 1 year. Therefore, a different behavior due to age could not be ruled out in these patients and further studies should be done to clarify the role of NfL in this particular clinical phenotype.

It should be noted that the highest levels of plasma NfL (581.4 pg/mL) were found in the most severely affected neurological patient in the studied cohort (NP4; Table S1) who presented the EI phenotype and died at 3 years of age, while the lowest value (7.59 pg/mL) was observed in an adult patient diagnosed at 36 years due to mild splenomegaly (NP25; Table S1). Furthermore, two patients developed neurological disease during follow-up and their NfL levels increased 2- and 4-fold, respectively. Although the number of patients is too low to draw definitive conclusion, these data further support the possible association between NfL levels and neurological disease. It would be interesting to follow the development of plasma NfL levels during the further natural course of the NPCD in single patients over months or even years.

It is important to point out the low specificity of plasma NfL levels, which make them unsuitable for NPCD diagnosis, in contrast to their possible high sensitivity and valuable use for assessing and monitoring the neurological course once the diagnosis is definitively established by means of biochemical or molecular methods.

In two patients, samples before and after miglustat treatment were assessed. Both neurological disease and NfL remained stable in one of them while in the other a slightly decrease in NfL levels and an amelioration of symptoms were observed. However, the possible utility of this marker in monitoring the response to therapy remains to be addressed.

5. Conclusions

In conclusion, this study shows that plasma levels of NfL are increased in NPCD patients and correlate with the presence of neurological disease, suggesting a possible role of this molecule as a neurological disease biomarker in NPCD. Based on these promising results, studies aimed at evaluating the levels of NfL during long-term follow-up and in response to treatment in larger cohorts should be undertaken.

Supplementary Materials: The following are available online at https://www.mdpi.com/2077-0383/10/20/4796/s1, Table S1: Plasma NfL in individual NPCD patients.

Author Contributions: Conceptualization, M.S. and A.D.; methodology, E.P., M.F., R.M., J.B.; formal analysis, E.P., M.O., A.D.; investigation, E.P., M.F., A.S., R.M.D.R., A.F., L.S., R.M., M.O., S.Z., J.B.; supervision: A.D.; writing—original draft preparation, A.D.; writing—review and editing, E.P., M.F., A.S., R.M.D.R., A.F., J.B., M.S. All authors have read and agreed to the published version of the manuscript.

Funding: This research received no external funding.

Institutional Review Board Statement: The study was conducted according to the guidelines of the Declaration of Helsinki. Ethical review and approval were waived for this study since analyses were performed as part of diagnostic workup and/or samples were recovered from material used for routine investigations without further sampling.

Informed Consent Statement: Informed consent was obtained from all subjects involved in the study.

Data Availability Statement: The data presented in this study are available on request from the corresponding author. The data are not publicly available due to privacy issues.

Conflicts of Interest: A.D. received speaker fees and travel grants from Sanofi-Genzyme and Takeda, participated at advisory boards from Amicus and Actelion, and received research grants from Actelion, Orphazyme, and Amicus. E.P. received a fellowship funded by Sanofi-Genzyme. A.S. received speaker fees and travel grants from Sanofi-Genzyme, Takeda, Actelion, and Amicus. L.C. received speaker fees and travel/research grants from Sanofi-Genzyme and Chiesi. A.F. participated in advisory boards from Sanofi-Genzyme and Biomarin, and received travel grants from Sanofi-Genzyme, Takeda-Shire, and Biomarin. M.S. receives a research grant and honoraria for lecturing and travel from Alexion, Sanofi-Genzyme, Takeda, Ultragenix, Chiesi, Orphazyme, Azafaros, and Orchard. M.F., R.M.D.R., M.O., R.M., J.B., S.Z. have no conflicts to declare.

References

1. Vanier, M.T. Niemann-Pick Disease Type C. *Orphanet. J. Rare Dis.* **2010**, *5*, 1–18. [CrossRef]
2. Walterfang, M.; Fietz, M.; Fahey, M.; Sullivan, D.; Leane, P.; Lubman, D.I.; Velakoulis, D. The Neuropsychiatry of Niemann-Pick Type C Disease in Adulthood. *J. Neuropsychiatry Clin. Neurosci.* **2006**, *18*, 158–170. [CrossRef]
3. Patterson, M.C.; Hendriksz, C.J.; Walterfang, M.; Sedel, F.; Vanier, M.T.; Wijburg, F. Recommendations for the Diagnosis and Management of Niemann–Pick Disease Type C: An Update. *Mol. Genet. Metab.* **2012**, *106*, 330–344. [CrossRef]
4. Mengel, E.; Klünemann, H.-H.; Lourenço, C.M.; Hendriksz, C.J.; Sedel, F.; Walterfang, M.; Kolb, S.A. Niemann-Pick Disease Type C Symptomatology: An Expert-Based Clinical Description. *Orphanet. J. Rare Dis.* **2013**, *8*, 166. [CrossRef]
5. ClinicalTrials.Gov. Available online: https://clinicaltrials.gov/ (accessed on 13 September 2021).
6. Bremova-Ertl, T.; Claassen, J.; Foltan, T.; Gascon-Bayarri, J.; Gissen, P.; Hahn, A.; Hassan, A.; Hennig, A.; Jones, S.A.; Kolnikova, M.; et al. Efficacy and Safety of N-Acetyl-l-Leucine in Niemann–Pick Disease Type C. *J. Neurol.* **2021**, *1*, 1.
7. Jiang, X.; Sidhu, R.; Porter, F.D.; Yanjanin, N.M.; Speak, A.O.; te Vruchte, D.T.; Platt, F.M.; Fujiwara, H.; Scherrer, D.E.; Zhang, J.; et al. A Sensitive and Specific LC-MS/MS Method for Rapid Diagnosis of Niemann-Pick C1 Disease from Human Plasma. *J. Lipid Res.* **2011**, *52*, 1435–1445. [CrossRef]
8. Maekawa, M.; Misawa, Y.; Sotoura, A.; Yamaguchi, H.; Togawa, M.; Ohno, K.; Nittono, H.; Kakiyama, G.; Iida, T.; Hofmann, A.F.; et al. LC/ESI-MS/MS Analysis of Urinary 3β-Sulfooxy-7β-N-Acetylglucosaminyl-5-Cholen-24-Oic Acid and Its Amides: New Biomarkers for the Detection of Niemann–Pick Type C Disease. *Steroids* **2013**, *78*, 967–972. [CrossRef]
9. Liu, N.; Tengstrand, E.A.; Chourb, L.; Hsieh, F.Y. Di-22:6-Bis(Monoacylglycerol)Phosphate: A Clinical Biomarker of Drug-Induced Phospholipidosis for Drug Development and Safety Assessment. *Toxicol. Appl. Pharmacol.* **2014**, *279*, 467–476. [CrossRef]
10. Giese, A.-K.; Mascher, H.; Grittner, U.; Eichler, S.; Kramp, G.; Lukas, J.; te Vruchte, D.; al Eisa, N.; Cortina-Borja, M.; Porter, F.D.; et al. A Novel, Highly Sensitive and Specific Biomarker for Niemann-Pick Type C1 Disease. *Orphanet. J. Rare Dis.* **2015**, *10*, 1–8. [CrossRef] [PubMed]

11. Mazzacuva, F.; Mills, P.; Mills, K.; Camuzeaux, S.; Gissen, P.; Nicoli, E.; Wassif, C.; Vruchte, D.; Porter, F.D.; Maekawa, M.; et al. Identification of Novel Bile Acids as Biomarkers for the Early Diagnosis of Niemann-Pick C Disease. *FEBS Lett.* **2016**, *590*, 1651. [CrossRef] [PubMed]
12. Marques, A.R.A.; Gabriel, T.L.; Aten, J.; Roomen, C.P.A.A.; van Ottenhoff, R.; Claessen, N.; Alfonso, P.; Irún, P.; Giraldo, P.; Aerts, J.M.F.G.; et al. Gpnmb Is a Potential Marker for the Visceral Pathology in Niemann-Pick Type C Disease. *PLoS ONE* **2016**, *11*, 0147208. [CrossRef] [PubMed]
13. Porter, F.D.; Scherrer, D.E.; Lanier, M.H.; Langmade, S.J.; Molugu, V.; Gale, S.E.; Olzeski, D.; Sidhu, R.; Dietzen, D.J.; Fu, R.; et al. Cholesterol Oxidation Products Are Sensitive and Specific Blood-Based Biomarkers for Niemann-Pick C1 Disease. *Sci. Transl. Med.* **2010**, *2*, 56ra81. [CrossRef]
14. Boenzi, S.; Deodato, F.; Taurisano, R.; Martinelli, D.; Verrigni, D.; Carrozzo, R.; Bertini, E.; Pastore, A.; Dionisi-Vici, C.; Johnson, D.W. A New Simple and Rapid LC–ESI-MS/MS Method for Quantification of Plasma Oxysterols as Dimethylaminobutyrate Esters. Its Successful Use for the Diagnosis of Niemann–Pick Type C Disease. *Clin. Chim. Acta* **2014**, *437*, 93–100. [CrossRef] [PubMed]
15. Reunert, J.; Fobker, M.; Kannenberg, F.; du Chesne, I.; Plate, M.; Wellhausen, J.; Rust, S.; Marquardt, T. Rapid Diagnosis of 83 Patients with Niemann Pick Type C Disease and Related Cholesterol Transport Disorders by Cholestantriol Screening. *EBioMedicine* **2016**, *4*, 170–175. [CrossRef] [PubMed]
16. Romanello, M.; Zampieri, S.; Bortolotti, N.; Deroma, L.; Sechi, A.; Fiumara, A.; Parini, R.; Borroni, B.; Brancati, F.; Bruni, A.; et al. Comprehensive Evaluation of Plasma 7-Ketocholesterol and Cholestan-3β,5α,6β-Triol in an Italian Cohort of Patients Affected by Niemann-Pick Disease Due to NPC1 and SMPD1 Mutations. *Clin. Chim. Acta* **2016**, *455*, 39–45. [CrossRef]
17. Polo, G.; Burlina, A.P.; Kolamunnage, T.B.; Zampieri, M.; Dionisi-Vici, C.; Strisciuglio, P.; Zaninotto, M.; Plebani, M.; Burlina, A.B. Diagnosis of Sphingolipidoses: A New Simultaneous Measurement of Lysosphingolipids by LC-MS/MS. *Clin. Chem. Lab. Med.* **2017**, *55*, 403–414. [CrossRef]
18. Pettazzoni, M.; Froissart, R.; Pagan, C.; Vanier, M.T.; Ruet, S.; Latour, P.; Guffon, N.; Fouilhoux, A.; Germain, D.P.; Levade, T.; et al. LC-MS/MS Multiplex Analysis of Lysosphingolipids in Plasma and Amniotic Fluid: A Novel Tool for the Screening of Sphingolipidoses and Niemann-Pick Type C Disease. *PLoS ONE* **2017**, *12*, e0181700. [CrossRef]
19. Wu, C.; Iwamoto, T.; Hossain, M.A.; Akiyama, K.; Igarashi, J.; Miyajima, T.; Eto, Y. A Combination of 7-Ketocholesterol, Lysosphingomyelin and Bile Acid-408 to Diagnose Niemann-Pick Disease Type C Using LC-MS/MS. *PLoS ONE* **2020**, *15*, e0238624. [CrossRef]
20. Pajares, S.; Arias, A.; García-Villoria, J.; MacÍas-Vidal, J.; Ros, E.; de Las Heras, J.; Girós, M.; Coll, M.J.; Ribes, A. Cholestane-3β,5α,6β-Triol: High Levels in Niemann-Pick Type C, Cerebrotendinous Xanthomatosis, and Lysosomal Acid Lipase Deficiency. *J. Lipid Res.* **2015**, *56*, 1926–1935. [CrossRef]
21. Lee, M.; Cleveland, D. Neuronal Intermediate Filaments. *Ann. Rev. Neurosci.* **1996**, *19*, 187–217. [CrossRef]
22. Petzold, A. Neurofilament Phosphoforms: Surrogate Markers for Axonal Injury, Degeneration and Loss. *J. Neurol. Sci.* **2005**, *233*, 183–198. [CrossRef] [PubMed]
23. Petzold, A.; Eikelenboom, M.J.; Keir, G.; Grant, D.; Lazeron, R.H.C.; Polman, C.H.; Uitdehaag, B.M.J.; Thompson, E.J.; Giovannoni, G. Axonal Damage Accumulates in the Progressive Phase of Multiple Sclerosis: Three Year Follow up Study. *J. Neurol. Neurosurg. Psychiatry* **2005**, *76*, 206–211. [CrossRef] [PubMed]
24. Lu, C.-H.; Macdonald-Wallis, C.; Gray, E.; Pearce, N.; Petzold, A.; Norgren, N.; Giovannoni, G.; Fratta, P.; Sidle, K.; Fish, M.; et al. Neurofilament Light Chain: A Prognostic Biomarker in Amyotrophic Lateral Sclerosis. *Neurology* **2015**, *84*, 2247. [CrossRef]
25. Zetterberg, H.; Skillbäck, T.; Mattsson, N.; Trojanowski, J.Q.; Portelius, E.; Shaw, L.M.; Weiner, M.W.; Blennow, K.; Alzheimer's Disease Neuroimaging Initiative. Association of Cerebrospinal Fluid Neurofilament Light Concentration With Alzheimer Disease Progression. *JAMA Neurol.* **2016**, *73*, 60. [CrossRef]
26. Meeter, L.H.; Dopper, E.G.; Jiskoot, L.C.; Sanchez-Valle, R.; Graff, C.; Benussi, L.; Ghidoni, R.; Pijnenburg, Y.A.; Borroni, B.; Galimberti, D.; et al. Neurofilament Light Chain: A Biomarker for Genetic Frontotemporal Dementia. *Ann. Clin. Tansl. Neurol.* **2016**, *3*, 623. [CrossRef]
27. Rojas, J.C.; Bang, J.; Lobach, I.V.; Tsai, R.M.; Rabinovici, G.D.; Miller, B.L.; Boxer, A.L. CSF Neurofilament Light Chain and Phosphorylated Tau 181 Predict Disease Progression in PSP. *Neurology* **2018**, *90*, e273. [CrossRef] [PubMed]
28. Martin, S.-J.; McGlasson, S.; Hunt, D.; Overell, J. Cerebrospinal Fluid Neurofilament Light Chain in Multiple Sclerosis and Its Subtypes: A Meta-Analysis of Case–Control Studies. *J. Neurol. Neurosurg. Psychiatry* **2019**, *90*, 1059–1067. [CrossRef]
29. Eratne, D.; Loi, S.M.; Li, Q.-X.; Varghese, S.; McGlade, A.; Collins, S.; Masters, C.L.; Velakoulis, D.; Walterfang, M. Cerebrospinal Fluid Neurofilament Light Chain Is Elevated in Niemann–Pick Type C Compared to Psychiatric Disorders and Healthy Controls and May Be a Marker of Treatment Response. *Aust. N. Z. J. Psychiatry* **2019**, *54*, 648–649. [CrossRef]
30. Bountouvi, E.; Giorgi, M.; Papadopoulou, A.; Blennow, K.; Björkhem, I.; Tsirouda, M.; Kanellakis, S.; Fryganas, A.; Spanou, M.; Georgaki, I.; et al. Longitudinal Data in Patients with Niemann-Pick Type C Disease Under Combined High Intrathecal and Low Intravenous Dose of 2-Hydroxypropyl-β-Cyclodextrin. *Innov. Clin. Neurosci.* **2021**, *18*, 11. [PubMed]
31. Gaiottino, J.; Norgren, N.; Dobson, R.; Topping, J.; Nissim, A.; Malaspina, A.; Bestwick, J.P.; Monsch, A.U.; Regeniter, A.; Lindberg, R.L.; et al. Increased Neurofilament Light Chain Blood Levels in Neurodegenerative Neurological Diseases. *PLoS ONE* **2013**, *8*, 75091. [CrossRef]

32. Wilke, C.; Preische, O.; Deuschle, C.; Roeben, B.; Apel, A.; Barro, C.; Maia, L.; Maetzler, W.; Kuhle, J.; Synofzik, M. Neurofilament Light Chain in FTD Is Elevated Not Only in Cerebrospinal Fluid, but Also in Serum. *J. Neurol. Neurosurg. Psychiatry* **2016**, *87*, 1270–1272. [CrossRef]
33. Kuhle, J.; Barro, C.; Disanto, G.; Mathias, A.; Soneson, C.; Bonnier, G.; Yaldizli, Ö.; Regeniter, A.; Derfuss, T.; Canales, M.; et al. Serum Neurofilament Light Chain in Early Relapsing Remitting MS Is Increased and Correlates with CSF Levels and with MRI Measures of Disease Severity. *Mult. Scler.* **2016**, *22*, 1550–1559. [CrossRef] [PubMed]
34. Novakova, L.; Zetterberg, H.; Sundström, P.; Axelsson, M.; Khademi, M.; Gunnarsson, M.; Malmeström, C.; Svenningsson, A.; Olsson, T.; Piehl, F.; et al. Monitoring Disease Activity in Multiple Sclerosis Using Serum Neurofilament Light Protein. *Neurology* **2017**, *89*, 2230. [CrossRef] [PubMed]
35. Disanto, G.; Barro, C.; Benkert, P.; Naegelin, Y.; Schädelin, S.; Giardiello, A.; Zecca, C.; Blennow, K.; Zetterberg, H.; Leppert, D.; et al. Serum Neurofilament Light: A Biomarker of Neuronal Damage in Multiple Sclerosis. *Ann. Neurol.* **2017**, *81*, 857. [CrossRef]
36. Piehl, F.; Kockum, I.; Khademi, M.; Blennow, K.; Lycke, J.; Zetterberg, H.; Olsson, T. Plasma Neurofilament Light Chain Levels in Patients with MS Switching from Injectable Therapies to Fingolimod. *Mult. Scler.* **2017**, *24*, 1046–1054. [CrossRef]
37. Mattsson, N.; Andreasson, U.; Zetterberg, H.; Blennow, K. Association of Plasma Neurofilament Light With Neurodegeneration in Patients With Alzheimer Disease. *JAMA Neurol.* **2017**, *74*, 557. [CrossRef] [PubMed]
38. Andersson, E.; Janelidze, S.; Lampinen, B.; Nilsson, M.; Leuzy, A.; Stomrud, E.; Blennow, K.; Zetterberg, H.; Hansson, O. Blood and Cerebrospinal Fluid Neurofilament Light Differentially Detect Neurodegeneration in Early Alzheimer's Disease. *Neurobiol. Aging* **2020**, *95*, 143. [CrossRef]
39. Ru, Y.; Corado, C.; Soon, R.K.J.; Melton, A.C.; Harris, A.; Yu, G.K.; Pryer, N.; Sinclair, J.R.; Katz, M.L.; Ajayi, T.; et al. Neurofilament Light Is a Treatment-responsive Biomarker in CLN2 Disease. *Ann. Clin. Tansl. Neurol.* **2019**, *6*, 2437. [CrossRef]
40. Bhalla, A.; Ravi, R.; Fang, M.; Arguello, A.; Davis, S.S.; Chiu, C.-L.; Blumenfeld, J.R.; Nguyen, H.N.; Earr, T.K.; Wang, J.; et al. Characterization of Fluid Biomarkers Reveals Lysosome Dysfunction and Neurodegeneration in Neuronopathic MPS II Patients. *Int. J. Mol. Sci.* **2020**, *21*, 5188. [CrossRef] [PubMed]
41. Geberhiwot, T.; Moro, A.; Dardis, A.; Ramaswami, U.; Sirrs, S.; Marfa, M.P.; Vanier, M.T.; Walterfang, M.; Bolton, S.; Dawson, C.; et al. Consensus Clinical Management Guidelines for Niemann-Pick Disease Type C. *Orphanet J. Rare Dis.* **2018**, *13*, 1–19. [CrossRef] [PubMed]
42. Dardis, A.; Zampieri, S.; Gellera, C.; Carrozzo, R.; Cattarossi, S.; Peruzzo, P.; Dariol, R.; Sechi, A.; Deodato, F.; Caccia, C.; et al. Molecular Genetics of Niemann–Pick Type C Disease in Italy: An Update on 105 Patients and Description of 18 NPC1 Novel Variants. *J. Clin. Med.* **2020**, *9*, 679. [CrossRef]
43. Gauthier, A.; Viel, S.; Perret, M.; Brocard, G.; Casey, R.; Lombard, C.; Laurent-Chabalier, S.; Debouverie, M.; Edan, G.; Vukusic, S.; et al. Comparison of Simoa TM and Ella TM to Assess Serum Neurofilament-Light Chain in Multiple Sclerosis. *Ann. Clin. Tansl. Neurol.* **2021**, *8*, 1141–1150. [CrossRef] [PubMed]
44. di Rocco, M.; Barone, R.; Madeo, A.; Fiumara, A. Miglustat Does Not Prevent Neurological Involvement in Niemann Pick C Disease. *Pediatr. Neurol.* **2015**, *53*, e15. [CrossRef]
45. Pineda, M.; Walterfang, M.; Patterson, M.C. Miglustat in Niemann-Pick Disease Type C Patients: A Review. *Orphanet J. Rare Dis.* **2018**, *13*, 1–21. [CrossRef] [PubMed]
46. Rego, T.; Farrand, S.; Goh, A.M.Y.; Eratne, D.; Kelso, W.; Mangelsdorf, S.; Velakoulis, D.; Walterfang, M. Psychiatric and Cognitive Symptoms Associated with Niemann-Pick Type C Disease: Neurobiology and Management. *CNS Drugs* **2019**, *33*, 125–142. [CrossRef] [PubMed]
47. Patterson, M.C.; Mengel, E.; Vanier, M.T.; Moneuse, P.; Rosenberg, D.; Pineda, M. Treatment Outcomes Following Continuous Miglustat Therapy in Patients with Niemann-Pick Disease Type C: A Final Report of the NPC Registry. *Orphanet J. Rare Dis.* **2020**, *15*, 1–10. [CrossRef] [PubMed]
48. Serum Neurofilament-Light Chain and GFAP Levels in Patients From the OFSEP Cohort at Different Landmarks of Multiple Sclerosis—ClinicalTrials.Gov. Available online: https://clinicaltrials.gov/ct2/show/NCT03981003 (accessed on 13 September 2021).
49. Yamada, N.; Inui, A.; Sanada, Y.; Ihara, Y.; Urahashi, T.; Fukuda, A.; Sakamoto, S.; Kasahara, M.; Yoshizawa, A.; Okamoto, S.; et al. Pediatric Liver Transplantation for Neonatal-Onset Niemann-Pick Disease Type C: Japanese Multicenter Experience. *Pediatr. Transplant.* **2019**, *23*, e13462. [CrossRef]

Review

Atherosclerosis in Fabry Disease—A Contemporary Review

Ashwin Roy [1,2,*], Hamza Umar [1,3], Antonio Ochoa-Ferraro [1], Adrian Warfield [1], Nigel Lewis [4], Tarekegn Geberhiwot [1,5] and Richard Steeds [1,2]

[1] University Hospitals Birmingham NHS Foundation Trust, Birmingham B15 2TT, UK; hamza.umar@uhb.nhs.uk (H.U.); antonio.ochoa-ferraro@uhb.nhs.uk (A.O.-F.); adrian.warfield@uhb.nhs.uk (A.W.); tarekegn.geberhiwot@uhb.nhs.uk (T.G.); rick.steeds@uhb.nhs.uk (R.S.)
[2] Institute of Cardiovascular Sciences, College of Medical and Dental Sciences, University of Birmingham, Birmingham B15 2TT, UK
[3] University of Birmingham Medical School, Birmingham B15 2TT, UK
[4] Sheffield Teaching Hospitals NHS Foundation Trust, Sheffield S10 2JF, UK; Nigel.lewis1@nhs.net
[5] Institute of Metabolism and System Research, College of Medical and Dental Sciences, University of Birmingham, Birmingham B15 2TT, UK
* Correspondence: ashwinroy@nhs.net

Abstract: Fabry disease (FD) is a lysosomal storage disorder characterised by a deficiency in the enzyme α-galactosidase A resulting in sphingolipid deposition which causes progressive cardiac, renal, and cerebral manifestations. The case illustrates a patient with FD who died suddenly, and medical examination demonstrated myocardial scarring and prior infarction. Angina is a frequent symptom in FD. Our own data are consistent with registry data indicating a high prevalence of risk factors for coronary artery disease (CAD) in FD that may accelerate conventional atherosclerosis. Patients with FD also have a higher high-density lipoprotein (HDL)/total cholesterol (T-Chol) ratio which may further accelerate atherosclerosis through expression of early atherosclerotic markers. Patients with FD may develop CAD both via classical atherosclerosis and through formation of thickened fibrocellular intima containing fibroblasts with storage of sphingolipids. Both mechanisms occurring together may accelerate coronary stenosis, as well as alter myocardial blood flow. Our data supports limited data that, although coronary flow may be reduced, the prevalence of epicardial coronary stenosis is low in FD. Microvascular dysfunction and arterial wall stress from sphingolipid deposition may form reactive oxygen species (ROS) and myeloperoxidase (MPO), key atherosclerotic mediators. Reduced myocardial blood flow in FD has also been demonstrated using numerous imaging modalities suggesting perfusion mismatch. This review describes the above mechanisms in detail, highlighting the importance of modifying cardiovascular risk factors in FD patients who likely develop accelerated atherosclerosis compared to the general population.

Keywords: Fabry; atherosclerosis; ischaemia; perfusion; angina

1. Case

A 69-year-old male was seen with a history of chest pain and palpitations. He had a background of Fabry disease (FD) with typical cardiomyopathy phenotype, hypertension, and hypercholesterolaemia. FD was diagnosed in 2012. The patient was hemizygous for the N215S variant mutation. He was first referred to the hypertrophic cardiomyopathy (HCM) clinic with symptoms of angina after a transthoracic echocardiogram (TTE) identified left ventricular hypertrophy (LVH). DNA testing for sarcomeric HCM was negative but alpha galactosidase—A levels were 0.45 µmol/L/hour (normal range 3–20 µmol/L/hour), and Sanger gene testing then confirmed homozygosity for the N215S variant mutation. As well as symptoms of angina, the patient also had pain and paraesthesia in the upper limbs, although nerve conduction studies were normal. In view of his symptoms of angina, he underwent invasive coronary angiography in 2012. This showed moderate mid left anterior descending (LAD) disease and significant ostial circumflex disease which was managed medically (Figures 1 and 2). His resting 12-lead electrocardiogram showed sinus rhythm with first degree atrio-ventricular block and right bundle branch block.

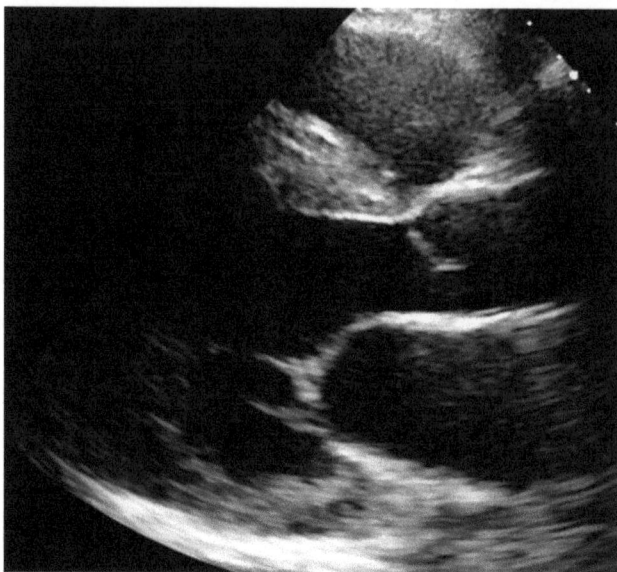

Figure 1. Transthoracic Echocardiogram (TTE) parasternal long axis view demonstrating left ventricular hypertrophy with thinning of the basal inferolateral wall, associated with impaired ventricular function that are typical changes in Fabry disease (FD) cardiomyopathy.

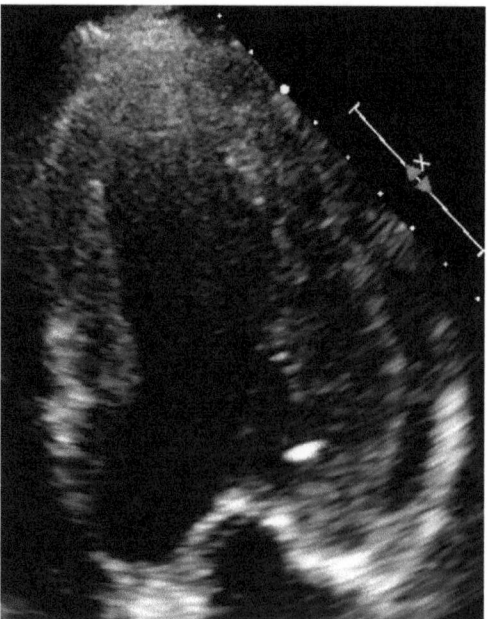

Figure 2. TTE apical 4-chamber view end-systole demonstrating concentric left ventricular hypertrophy (LVH).

In 2014, the patient underwent a further TTE which detected impaired left ventricular function with regional wall motion abnormalities and myocardial thinning, with an apical thrombus. Following gadolinium-based contrast on cardiac magnetic resonance imaging (CMR), thrombus was confirmed at the apex, with extensive subendocardial late gadolinium enhancement (LGE). Tissue characterisation with T1 and T2 mapping were not performed at time of presentation, and early enhancement images were not available (Figures 3 and 4). Increased wall thickness on CMR was concordant. He had a cerebral magnetic resonance imaging (MRI) scan which demonstrated scattered white matter changes and 24 h urinary protein confirmed microalbuminuria. The patient was commenced on enzyme replacement therapy (ERT) in 2012 (agalsidase alpha). This was switched briefly to oral chaperone therapy (Migalastat) in 2017 but he was recommenced on ERT in view of side effects (nausea). He was treated with optimal heart failure medications, including an angiotensin converting enzyme (ACE) inhibitor, beta blocker, and mineralocorticoid receptor antagonist (MRA). The ventricular thrombus was managed with anticoagulation in the form of warfarin and aspirin was discontinued.

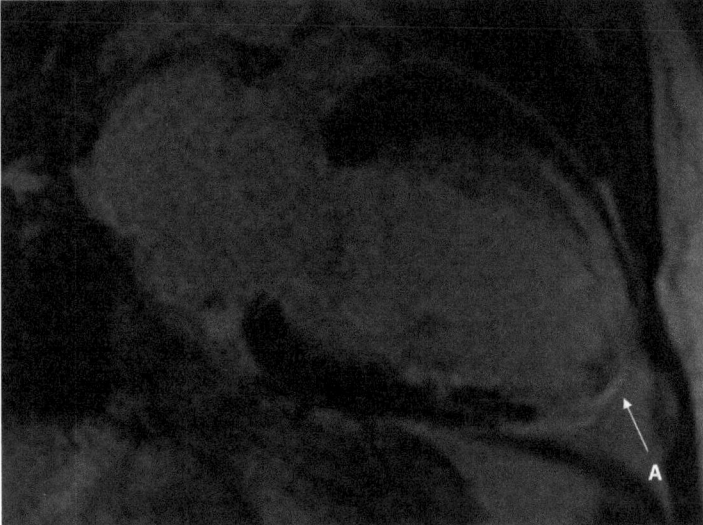

Figure 3. Cardiac magnetic resonance imaging (CMR) vertical long-axis view demonstrating extensive apical transmural late gadolinium enhancement in a region with myocardial thinning and akinesis, consistent with completed myocardial infarction (A).

In September 2016, the patient had an acute admission to hospital with sustained ventricular tachycardia (VT). In view of this, he underwent repeat invasive coronary angiography which was similar to that performed in 2012, with persistent, moderate mid-LAD disease and significant ostial Cx disease. A decision was made to implant a dual chamber implantable cardioverter defibrillator (ICD). In 2018, he was admitted following ICD shocks for ventricular arrhythmia without evidence of heart failure, ischaemia, or electrolyte disturbance. Despite anti-arrhythmic medication and VT ablation, he continued to have VT, deteriorated, and subsequently died. Examination of the heart and histological assessment demonstrated chronic myocardial scarring corresponding to previous healed regional myocardial infarction that was consistent with the regional wall motion abnormality in a coronary artery distribution, with myocardial thinning and late enhancement imaging that had been performed pre-mortem (Figures 5–8). This case illustrates the point that, as Fabry patients live longer, they are susceptible to acquired heart disease in the same way as the general population.

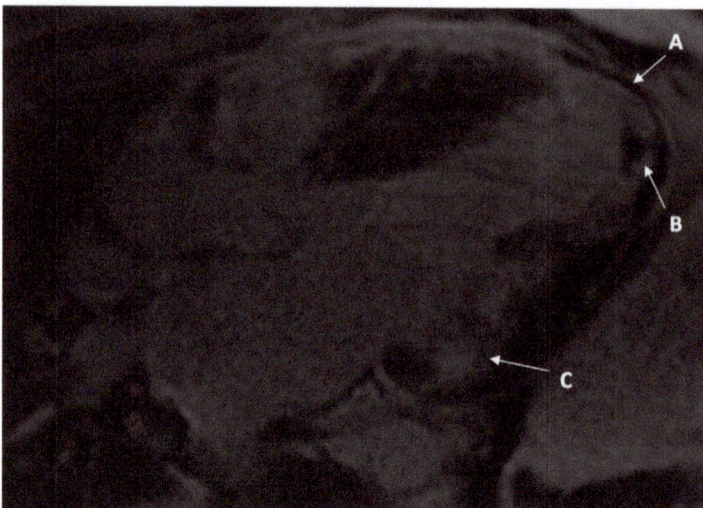

Figure 4. CMR three-chamber view demonstrating extensive apical transmural late gadolinium enhancement in a region with myocardial thinning and akinesis (A), which could be explained by FD with cardiomyopathy but most likely consistent with completed myocardial infarction in the LAD and circumflex territory that was confirmed on histology. In addition, there is an apical thrombus visible (B). There is also the region of thinning in the basal inferolateral wall with late enhancement (C), consistent with typical fibrosis seen in FD.

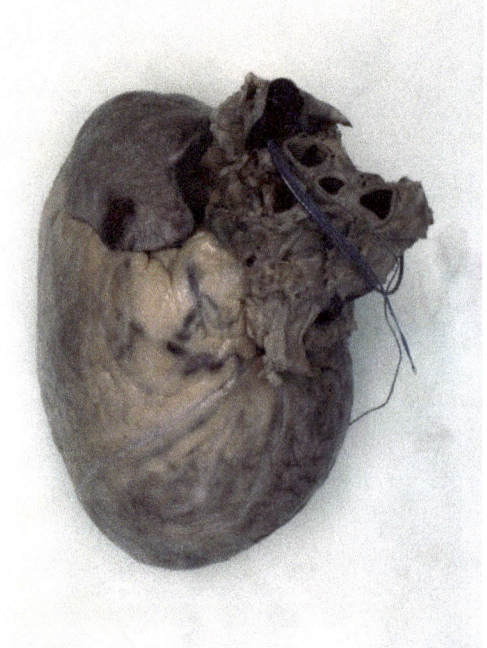

Figure 5. Anterior view of embalmed intact heart prior to dissection—there is global massive cardiomegaly (empty heart weight 950 g). Severed remnants of the ICD wires are visualised around the base of the heart.

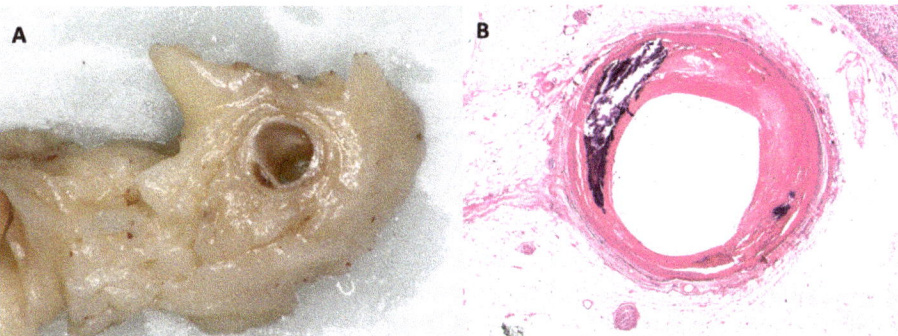

Figure 6. (**A**) Cross sectional slice through mid-right main coronary artery demonstrating eccentric atherosclerotic plaque with localised medial calcification. (**B**) Corresponding histological section of mid right main coronary artery depicting fibro-intimal atheromatous thickening and multi-centric fractured mineralisation of tunica media (haematoxylin and eosin stain; original magnification ×1.25).

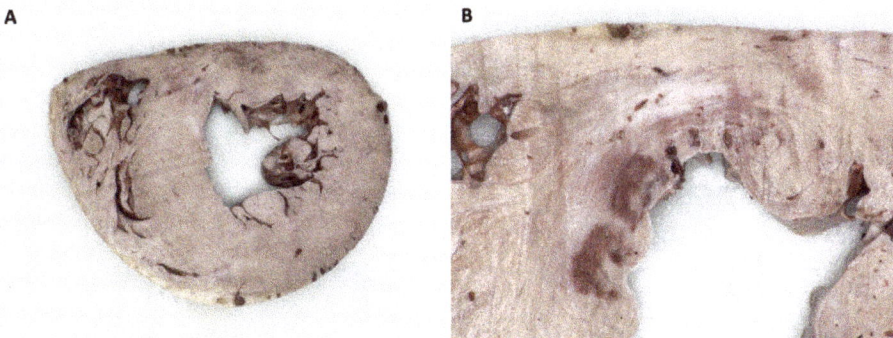

Figure 7. (**A**) Short axis mid-septal ventricular slice through the embalmed heart showing very considerable asymmetrical septum/anterior wall predominant left ventricular hypertrophy (up to 32 mm thick) and right ventricular hypertrophy (up to 8 mm thick). (**B**) Close-up view of healed postero-septal sub-endocardial myocardial infarct scar (the blood clot is an artefact of embalmment; there was no microscopical evidence of more recent acute infarct extension in this region).

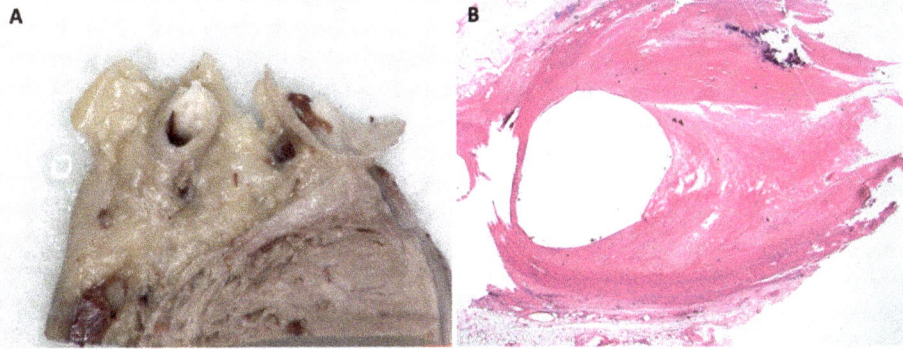

Figure 8. (**A**) Transverse slice through proximal left anterior descending coronary artery illustrating significant luminal stenosis by eccentric atherosclerotic plaque. (**B**) Corresponding histological section through left anterior descending coronary artery showing severe fibrous intimal encroachment into the lumen plus fractured focal calcification (haematoxylin and eosin stain; original magnification ×1.25).

2. Introduction

Fabry disease (FD) is an X-linked multisystem lysosomal storage disorder caused by a deficiency in the enzyme α-galactosidase A [1]. This results in the accumulation of sphingolipids, including globotriaosylceramide (Gb3), and globotriaosylsphingosine (lyso-Gb3) [2]. Progressive accumulation ultimately leads to end-organ damage and subsequent life-threatening renal, cardiac, and cerebrovascular manifestations [3]. Over time, renal failure has been replaced by cardiovascular disease as the most common cause of morbidity and mortality in FD, with relative rates differing according to the source of data and definitions of endpoints. The Fabry Outcomes Survey reported 38% deaths due to cardiovascular disease, compared to 7% attributed to renal disease and 9.5% to cerebrovascular disease [4]. In comparison, the Fabry Registry identified the cause of death to be cardiovascular in 53%, renal in 10.6%, and cerebrovascular in 12% reported cases [5]. Life expectancy in FD is limited to an average 58 years in males and 75 years in females, although 10-year follow-up registry data suggest a modifying effect of enzyme replacement therapy (ERT) on serious organ complications and survival [6,7]. Traditionally, atherosclerotic coronary CAD has been considered an uncommon occurrence in FD, and symptoms such as chest pain and shortness of breath are often attributed to microvascular dysfunction, altered oxygen supply-demand mismatch in left ventricular hypertrophy and reduced arterial compliance. Figures 5–8 however, show the post-mortem findings of a 69-year old male diagnosed with FD in 2013 and treated with ERT, which confirmed myocardial infarction as a result of occlusive thrombus complicating atherosclerotic CAD. The aim of this article is to review symptoms, risk factors, and evidence behind the relative risks of atherosclerotic CAD and the disease-specific causes for chest pain, myocardial ischaemia, and death in FD. As patients live longer, clinicians caring for patients with FD need to take into account susceptibility to the risk factors and presentations of cardiovascular morbidity and mortality that are found in the general population.

3. Angina

Sphingolipid accumulation can take place in all cardiac cell types leading to left ventricular hypertrophy (LVH), arterial stiffness, conduction abnormalities, and valvular disease [4,8]. Cardiac symptoms are common and include angina, dyspnoea and palpitations. Angina affects between 22–23% patients at a mean age 36–42 years, a frequency that is similar in both genders but with an onset that is typically earlier in males. Symptoms are more common in those patients on treatment than those not on treatment, presumably reflecting more advanced disease and, in particular, greater LVH [9]. Angina is severe enough in these cases to limit quality of life, with the majority affected having greater than or equal to Class II limitation using the Canadian Cardiovascular Society (CCS) grading, which means that the patient develops chest pain on vigorous activity such as walking quickly up a flight of stairs, walking after eating or on a windy day [10]. Prevalence of cardiac symptoms increases with age and although more common in those on ERT, appears to be stable in the majority (26/42; 63%) when on long-term therapy for 10 years or more [9].

Although direct comparisons have not been performed, these data contrast with the occurrence and severity of angina in the general population. For example, the large multinational, multicentre Clarify registry included 32,703 patients with chronic coronary syndrome from 45 countries, of whom 7212 (22.1%) had angina [11]. The mean age of adults with angina was 64.2 + 10.5 year, with the large majority being male (78%) [11]. In those 7212 patients with angina, 29% had only Class I limitation, with the rest having Class II or higher symptoms.

In our case, the patient presenting with angina and was found to have coronary artery disease that was treated medically, at the same time as investigations revealed LVH that was subsequently confirmed due to FD. In summary, angina seems to occur with a similar frequency in FD as those with chronic coronary syndromes in the general population but is more often found in women, impacts on quality of life at an earlier age and with a higher proportion limited by more disabling symptoms. The diagnostic approach in patient with

FD and angina should follow conventional methods of assessing patients with chest pain of suspected cardiac origin with the aim to exclude conventional coronary artery disease as a cause of symptoms [12]. In our practice, this involves clinical assessment of the nature of the pain—whether typical, atypical, or non-anginal; consideration of the likelihood of coronary artery disease taking into account risk factor profile; and a preference for use of non-invasive CT coronary angiography with calcium scoring, given the limitations of ischaemia testing in FD [13].

4. Conventional Risk Factors

The likelihood of conventional atherosclerosis increases with age, particularly in men [14]. The large majority of major adverse coronary artery events in the general population are explained by the presence of conventional risk for atherosclerosis—beyond increasing age—including hypertension, hypercholesterolaemia, smoking, diabetes, renal impairment, and obesity [15]. Registry data in FD shows that the prevalence of hypertension is 57% in men and 47% in females [16], with hypercholesterolaemia also being frequent at 33% [17]. The prevalence of chronic kidney disease (CKD) in FD can be as high as 42% [18], with registry data showing 26% suffer from CKD stage 3–5, and proteinuria presenting in 44% males and 33% females [19].

Our own data support this frequency of classical risk factors in FD or active treatment thereof (see Table 1) In a retrospective analysis of our Fabry cohort of 47 patients on enzyme replacement therapy (average age 52.4 years; 47% female), 32/47 (68%) were on anti-hypertensive medication, 18/47 (38%) were on a statin, and 12/47 (26%) had a total Cholesterol (T-Chol) > 5 mmol/L. In total, 13/47 (28%) patients had stage 3–5 CKD and 14/47 (30%) with stage 2 CKD. Moreover, 30/47 (63%) had proteinuria defined as an albumin: creatinine ratio (ACR) > 3 mg/mmol. Given the high frequency of conventional risk factors in adults with FD observed in registry and our own data, it is likely that these accelerate atherosclerosis via a conventional pathophysiological process.

Table 1. Baseline characteristics of cardiovascular risk factors in a cohort of patients on ERT in a UK-based FD centre.

Characteristic	N = 47 (%)
Gender	Male: 25 (53.2) Female: 22 (46.8)
Age (mean)	Male 51.4 Female 53.6 Overall 52.4
Enzyme replacement therapy/oral chaperone therapy	Fabrazyme: 10 (21.3) Migalastat: 20 (42.6) Replagal: 17 (36.1)
Anti-hypertensive medication	0 anti-hypertensives 15 (31.9) 1 anti-hypertensive 20 (42.6) 2 anti-hypertensives 7 (14.9) 3 anti-hypertensives 5 (10.6)
Angiotensin converting enzyme inhibitor/angiotensin receptor blocker	27 (57.4)
Statin therapy	18 (38.3)
T-Chol (mmol/L)	≤5 mmol/L: 35 (74.5) >5 mmol/L: 12 (25.5)
Systolic blood pressure (mmHg)	>140: 16 (34.0) <140: 31 (66.0)
eGFR (mLmin)	>90: 11 (23.4) 60–89: 23 (48.9) 45–59: 10 (21.3) 30–44: 1 (2.1) 15–29: 1 (2.1) <15: 1 (2.1)
ACR (mg/mmol)	<3: 15 (31.9) 3–30: 19 (40.4) >30: 11 (23.4) Not available: 2 (4.3)

Abbreviations: mmol/L—millimoles per litre; eGFR—estimated glomerular filtration rate; mmHg—millimetres of mercury); mL/min—millilitres per minute; mg/mmol—milligrams per millimole; ACR—albumin:creatinine ratio.

An interesting finding is that high levels of high-density lipoprotein cholesterol (HDL-C)/T-Chol ratio have been observed in FD [20,21]. In the general population, this finding has been associated with a lower cardiovascular risk, certainly in comparison to a raised low-density lipoprotein cholesterol (LDL-C)/T-Chol ratio which is associated with higher cardiovascular risk [22]. In FD however, the reverse may be true because a high HDL-C/T-Chol ratio has been linked with high levels of vascular endothelial growth factor (VEGF) and intracellular adhesion molecule-1 (ICAM-1) [23], both markers of early stages of atherosclerosis [24,25]. The same study showed that patients with raised HDL-C/T-Chol ratio and VEGF/ICAM-1 had a greater number of ocular vascular lesions identified on ophthalmic examination (including arteriolar tortuosity, arteriolar narrowing, broadening of the light reflex with minimal arteriolovenous compression in fundic vessels), although no direct examination of the coronary arteries was performed in this study. Of interest, HDL-C level did not change with enzyme replacement therapy [23]. KCa3.1 (calcium-activated potassium channel expressed in vascular endothelial cells) is downregulated with sphingolipid accumulation which causes endothelial dysfunction [26], suggesting that the high HDL-C/T-Chol ratio may be due to endocytosis of LDL-C to the endothelial cells [23] (sphingolipid accumulation may increase LDL-receptor expression [27]).

In our case, the patient was diagnosed with FD at the age of 69 years, following appropriate invasive investigations for CAD given an adverse risk profile, including both hypertension and hypercholesterolaemia. Conventional risk factors for atherosclerosis are common in FD patients. Although different pathological processes may be driving atherosclerosis, arteriosclerosis, and microvascular disease in FD, it seems logical for aggressive risk factor modification though lifestyle and pharmacological therapy to be promoted to minimise cardiovascular risk.

5. Histopathology

Endomyocardial biopsies in patients with FD shows the presence of perinuclear vacuoles within cardiac cells representing sphingolipid accumulation. Myocardial fibrosis surrounding severely narrowed intramural coronary arteries was also observed, suggesting this as a primary mechanism for myocardial ischaemia [28]. Hypertrophy of smooth muscle and proliferation of endothelial cells with accumulated sphingolipids may cause small vessel obstruction and subsequent ischaemia. Replacement fibrosis seen on microscopy with cardiomyocyte loss has been shown to be more common in FD patients with angina compared to those without [28].

Classic atherosclerosis is characterised by formation of atheromatous plaques, which are lesions caused by combinations of fibrous tissue and cholesterol-rich lipids. In contrast, case reports and post-mortem findings in FD have hitherto emphasised the formation of a thickened fibrocellular intima, which contain fibroblasts with storage of Gb3, together with fibrosis and calcification of the media [29]. The latter has conventionally been characterised as a different process to the formation of atherosclerotic plaques, and more akin to fibromuscular dysplasia or arteriosclerosis. Furthermore, there is also evidence of narrowing of myocardial capillaries due to GL-3 inclusion bodies that contribute to a unique coronary artery pathology in FD [30]. These data however were acquired from endomyocardial biopsies of FD patients with an average age of 32 years, before conventional atherosclerotic plaque, may be common.

In summary, given the frequency of conventional risk factors in FD patients—considering the extended life expectancy of contemporary, treated patients—it is conceivable that both sphingolipid accumulation and associated fibrosis, as well as classical atherosclerosis may develop and contribute to increased risk in FD. In our case, histology documented typical atherosclerotic plaque, together with evidence of chronic myocardial infarction, alongside classical histological and cellular changes reflecting sphingolipid deposition. The myocardial changes in our case, including both prior myocardial infarction and hypertrophy with fibrosis, could be potential causes of a terminal arrhythmia in our case, although downloads from the ICD device were not available for examination.

6. Calcification, Computed Tomography, and Invasive Angiography

The frequency of epicardial coronary stenosis has not been explored in large scale studies of patients with FD. There are published case reports that described the presence of atherosclerotic coronary artery disease in patients with FD [31–33], although invasive coronary angiography in single centre studies have tended to demonstrate a low frequency of epicardial stenosis. In a small, single-centre study of 10 male patients with genetically confirmed FD, average age 54 years, and no risk factors for CAD, none were found to have significant epicardial coronary stenosis on invasive coronary angiography (ICA) [34]. This result was replicated in a study of 38 FD patients without conventional risk factors at an average age of 43 years (15 (39%) female; 25 (66%) asymptomatic). None were found to have epicardial coronary stenosis on invasive coronary angiography, although coronary flow was reduced using thrombolysis in myocardial infarction (TIMI) frame count [28]. These studies included patients both younger (aged 69 years) and without the conventional risk factors (hypertension and hypercholesterolaemia) seen in our case.

Our own data relating to computed tomography and invasive coronary angiography are consistent with these findings, following investigation for recent or active symptoms (see Table 2). Within our cohort, 25/47 (53%) patients have had a formal assessment of their coronary arteries having experienced symptoms of chest pain. 12/47 (26%) underwent an ICA and 13/47 (28%) underwent a non-invasive computed tomography coronary angiogram (CTCA). Of those who underwent an ICA, 7/12 (58%) had no flow-limiting coronary artery disease but 3/12 required coronary artery bypass grafting (CABG) and 2 required percutaneous coronary intervention (PCI). Although none of the patients studied by CTCA had flow-limiting or severe coronary artery stenosis, 7/13(54%) had either mild or moderate coronary atheroma. 9/13 (69%) had normal calcium scores with no coronary calcium. In contrast to the two earlier studies, the cohort studied for clinical indications at our centre were mostly male (68%) and were older (average age 60), suggesting that atherosclerotic coronary artery disease should be considered in the differential diagnosis of these patients as they age.

Table 2. ICA and CTCA findings in adults with FD in a UK-based FD centre including associated cardiovascular risk factors. Abbreviations: mmol/L (millimoles per litre).

Characteristic	ICA n = 12 (%)	CTCA n = 13 (%)	Total n = 25 (%)
Gender/Age	M: 9 (75) F: 3 (25) mean age 65	M: 8 (61.5) F: 5 (38.5) mean age 54	M: 17 (68) F: 8 (32) mean age 60
Angiography findings	Normal: 5 (41.7) Mild coronary disease: 2 (16.6) CABG with patent grafts: 3 (25) PCI with patent stents: 2 (16.6) Significant coronary disease (including occluded grafts/stents): 0 (0)	No coronary stenosis: 6 (46.2) Mild coronary stenosis: 6 (46.2) Moderate coronary stenosis 1(7.6) Significant coronary stenosis 0 (0)	No coronary disease: 11 (44) Mild/moderate coronary disease: 9 (36) Coronary disease with patent grafts/stents: 5 (20) Significant/Severe coronary disease: 0 (0)
Hypertension	5 (41.7)	3 (23.1)	8 (32)
Diabetes	0 (0)	0 (0)	0 (0)
Cholesterol	<4 mmol/L: 7 (58.3) 4–5 mmol/L: 3 (25) >5 mmol/L: 2 (16.7)	<4 mmol/L: 3 (23.1) 4–5 mmol/L: 7 (53.8) >5 mmol/L: 3 (23.1)	<4 mmol/L: 10 (40) 4–5 mmol/L: 10 (40) >5 mmol/L: 5 (10)
Family History	2 (16.7)	2 (15.4)	4 (16)
Smoking History	1 (8.3)	6 (46.2)	7 (28)

Consistent with this evidence from ICA and CTCA, there is supportive evidence of accelerated atherosclerosis in FD. Autopsy studies of FD patients show plaques that are more concentric with a white discolouration [35]. It is theorised that the microvascular endothelial dysfunction and arterial wall stress from sphingolipid infiltration results in the formation of reactive oxygen species (ROS) [36]. ROS may increase the risk of vascular dysfunction including superimposed atherosclerosis [37]. Myeloperoxidase (MPO) is a peroxidase enzyme secreted by neutrophils during degranulation and is a key component within atherosclerotic plaques [38]. Its presence within plaques is associated with lesion apoptosis, erosion, and rupture. Elevated MPO levels have been observed in patients with FD suggesting this could be a mediator of accelerated atherosclerosis in the FD cohort [39]. Furthermore, in mouse models, α-galactosidase A deficiency was associated with accelerated atherosclerosis due potentially to nitrous oxide (NO) dysregulation. Excess NO accumulated in the atherosclerotic vessels of mice with GLA deficiency may enhance atherogenesis [40]. The high incidence of myocardial infarction, early stroke, and transient ischaemic attack (TIA) in FD suggest a pro-thrombotic state in those with FD [41,42]. Furthermore, due to progressive sphingolipid accumulation within the kidneys, patients with FD often have CKD which in itself further increases thrombotic risk [43]. An interesting observation is the concurrence of FD with the pro-thrombotic Factor V Leiden (FVL) mutation and subsequent heightened risk of thrombosis observed (5-fold higher risk of stroke with FD and FVL) [44].

In summary, consistent with case reports of acute coronary events, although atherosclerotic lesions are not an explanation of chest pain in younger, female FD patients, in an older, predominantly male cohort, atheroma that requires revascularisation can be found as in our case. In those without occlusive disease, as in adults from the general population with angina and no evidence of angiographic stenosis, symptoms may be attributed to abnormal coronary flow reserve. Many of these subjects in the general population have been shown to have subclinical coronary atherosclerosis on intravascular ultrasound (IVUS), which has never been performed in FD patients [45]. Mechanisms underpinning coronary flow are multifaceted with varying physiology, and those that may affect patients with FD are highlighted in Figure 9. Supportive evidence of their impact has been found in non-invasive imaging studies.

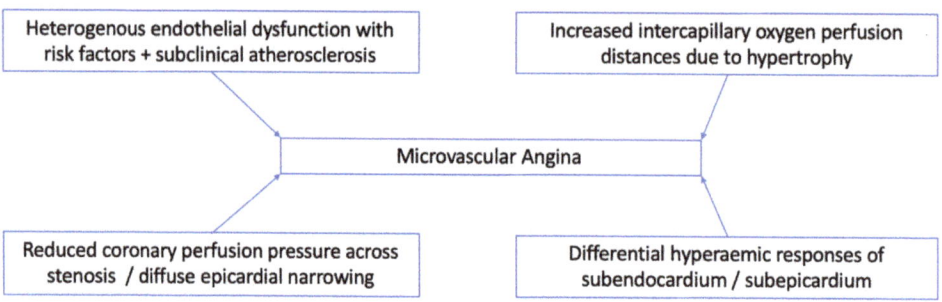

Figure 9. Mechanisms underpinning coronary flow in the absence of angiographic coronary stenosis [46–48].

7. Non-Invasive Imaging: Ischaemia

In the study of 38 patients studied using ICA, those with FD exhibited slow flow and slow run off angiographically with delayed opacification of distal vasculature [28]. This slow flow did not correlate with age, gender, or degree of LVH (all patients in the study had LVH). The extent of small vessel disease, however, did correlate with slow coronary flow and myocardial replacement fibrosis. The presence of slow flow in the FD group and absence in control is consistent with microvascular disease and abnormal coronary resistance vessels [49]. In the same study, when exposed to exercise stress, patients with FD developed ST-depression in association with angina. During myocardial perfusion tomography, all patients with angina had an ischaemic response to stress identified by perfusion mismatch.

Abnormal coronary flow in FD was confirmed in a study of 10 adult FD males using gold-standard positron emission tomography (PET) to measure coronary flow reserve (CFR) [34]. Nine patients had symptoms of myocardial ischaemia and underwent ICA to exclude coronary disease as a cause. Interestingly, compared with controls, serum T-Chol and HDL-C was higher in the FD group as has been observed in previously described studies. Resting and hyperaemic CFR and myocardial blood flow (MBF) were both significantly reduced compared with controls with no changes with enzyme replacement therapy. The authors suggested that myocyte hypertrophy and fibrosis secondary to Gb3 deposition could cause increased vascular resistance and subsequent myocardial oxygen demand. This supports the mechanism of microvascular angina due to demand–supply oxygen perfusion mismatch due to hypertrophy in FD (Figure 9). This mechanism is different to that of hypertrophic cardiomyopathy where myocardial ischaemia is usually a result of intramural arteriole remodelling [50,51].

Another study in 10 adults with FD on ERT for a duration of 12 months assessed myocardial perfusion and perfusion reserve using PET [52]. Though coronary disease was not excluded by ICA, none of the patients had angina or signs of ischaemia on ECG or TTE. In all patients, low levels of hyperaemic myocardial blood flow and flow reserve were recorded at baseline and persisted despite treatment with ERT. This supports the mechanism of differing levels of hyperaemia causing microvascular ischaemia in FD.

Work has also been conducted assessing myocardial blood flow (MBF) using multiparametric CMR [53]. In a study of 44 adults with FD, 24 (55%) had LVH, 23 (52%) had evidence of LGE, and 30 (44%) were on treatment (enzyme replacement therapy/oral chaperone therapy). Compared with controls, global stress MBF was lower in FD with no significant differences in rest MBF. Stress MBF was lower when LVH was present but, compared with controls, the LVH-negative cohort had lower stress MBF. These patients had a variety of symptoms (chest pain, breathlessness, and palpitations) which could be explained by reduced stress MBF representing early microvascular dysfunction. The findings suggest that microvascular perfusion abnormalities may precede cardiomyocyte storage and thus be the earliest feature of cardiac involvement in FD. These changes reflect what is observed in studies looking at endomyocardial biopsies of those with FD and angina where endothelial cells were swollen due to sphingolipid storage with arteriolar luminal narrowing due to hypertrophy and fibrosis [28]. The results of this study show that areas with the greatest degree of hypertrophy and sphingolipid deposition (seen as low T1) and fibrosis (high ECV and presence of LGE) are those with lowest MBF. This supports the mechanisms of endothelial dysfunction as a trigger for microvascular angina in FD (see Figure 9). The study also demonstrated greater perfusion abnormalities within the sub-endocardium suggesting that chronic fibrosis predominantly affecting the sub-endocardium over sub-epicardium may result in more perfusion defects in FD patients with LVH.

In our own cohort of FD patients, five underwent a myocardial perfusion scan (MPS) in view of symptoms of chest pain to assess for perfusion defects. Three of the MPS were normal. One was in a patient with known ischaemic heart disease with a previous CABG. Interestingly the MPS demonstrated fixed perfusion defects in two segments coinciding with basal inferolateral wall LGE on CMR reflecting FD fibrotic change and not ischaemic cardiomyopathy (see Figure 10). The final MPS demonstrated reduced tracer uptake in the anterior wall on stress with improvement at rest in a patient who underwent ICA, demonstrating non-flow limiting disease within the coronary arteries.

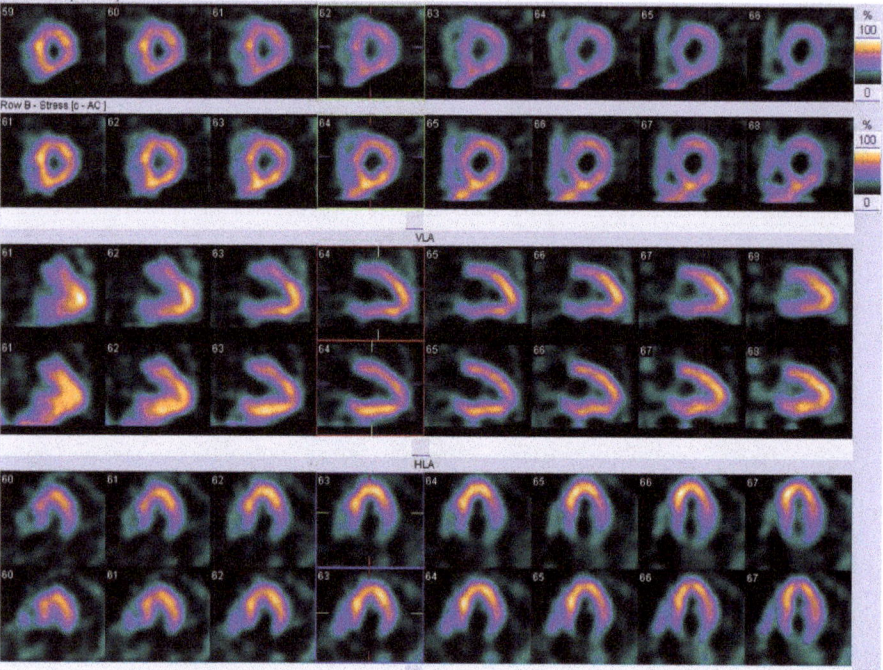

Figure 10. MPS of an adult with FD demonstrating fixed perfusion defects in the basal inferolateral wall of the left ventricle under stress which is typically seen in FD.

8. Treatment of Angina in FD

There is no clear evidence that treating symptoms of chest pain or risk factors lowers risk of cardiovascular events in FD patients. There is limited evidence of the effectiveness of conventional angina therapy in FD and future work should aim to explore this in more detail. The use of enzyme replacement therapy has not been shown to improve symptoms of angina or myocardial blood flow after over 12 months of treatment [28,34]. Medical management can be particularly challenging due to the progressive nature of the disease. Added to this, the prevalence of cognitive impairment as well as depression is high in the FD cohort compared with the general population [54] which can affect perception of symptoms and compliance with medications. Arrythmia is a likely cause for many cardiovascular related deaths in FD and ICD implantation is frequent. However, as illustrated in the case, due to the progressive nature of the disease, many patients continue to have sustained arrhythmia that requires advanced treatment. Moreover, the efficacy of some of these therapies including cardiac resynchronisation therapy (CRT) and ICD, do not have an evidence-base in FD.

The main aim of treatment in FD is to minimise end-organ damage. While there is no evidence specifically in FD patients, it is widely accepted that aggressive management of conventional risk factors for atherosclerosis (including lipid lowering therapy, tight control of hypertension and good glycemic control) should be encouraged as well as smoking cessation and regular physical exercise [55]. Aggressive blood pressure control may reduce progression of LVH and use of angiotensin converting (ACE) inhibitors are often used due to renal dysfunction in FD [56]. There is limited evidence that patients with FD who have renal impairment develop accelerated LVH compared to FD patients without renal disease, and that therefore there may be genetic or other modifying factors that work in an incremental fashion on myocyte hypertrophy. Whether this effect is limited to renal dysfunction and whether hypertension is a further modifier of LVH is not known, but it seems reasonable to ensure optimal control of hypertension to minimise risk.

9. Conclusions

Angina is a prevalent cardiac symptom in FD and is due to ischaemia that may be secondary to diverse mechanisms, including microvascular disease, altered coronary vasoreactivity, and perfusion mismatch due to sphingolipid deposition within cardiomyocytes and consequent LVH. Ischaemia may also be due to the phenomenon of accelerated atherosclerosis which may be seen in FD and lead to CAD which may result in occlusive thrombus causing myocardial infarction and subsequent death. Patients with FD also demonstrate an increased prevalence of conventional risk factors for CAD and so may develop atherosclerosis though conventional mechanisms as a result of having these risk factors. However, the effect of FD and atherosclerosis is still not completely understood and further research is therefore needed in this area in order to better understand the disease mechanisms involved with the aim of reducing cardiovascular mortality in FD. In patients with FD that have chest pain, whilst this may be due to microvascular dysfunction, it is important to ensure macrovascular CAD is excluded, in particular in the older, male cohort.

Author Contributions: Idea and conceptualization, R.S. and T.G. Methodology, validation, data analysis and writing up of manuscript, A.R., H.U., A.W., N.L. Review and editing of the manuscript, R.S., T.G., N.L., A.W., A.O.-F., A.R., H.U. All authors have read and agreed to the published version of the manuscript.

Funding: This research reviewed no external funding.

Institutional Review Board Statement: Ethical approval was not required for this study as it was a case report, registered audit and literature review.

Informed Consent Statement: Informed consent was taken in advance and the descedent bequeathed the embalmed and undissected heart to medical science.

Acknowledgments: R.S. acknowledges part-funding from the NIHR West Midlands Senior Clinical Scholarship.

Conflicts of Interest: The authors declare no conflict of interest.

Abbreviations

FD	Fabry disease
CAD	coronary artery disease
HDL	high-density lipoprotein
T-Chol	total cholesterol
ROS	reactive oxygen species
MPO	myeloperoxidase
HCM	hypertrophic cardiomyopathy
TTE	transthoracic echocardiogram
LVH	left ventricular hypertrophy
DNA	deoxyribose nucleic acid
LAD	left anterior descending artery
CMR	cardiac magnetic resonance imaging
LGE	late gadolinium enhancement
MRI	magnetic resonance imaging
ERT	enzyme replacement therapy
ACE	angiotensin converting enzyme
MR	mineralocorticoid receptor antagonist
VT	ventricular tachycardia

ICD	implantable cardioverter defibrillator
ATP	anti-tachycardia pacing
Gb3	globotriaosylceramide
lysoGv3	globotriaosylsphingosine
CCS	Canadian Cardiovascular Society
CT	computed tomography
CKD	chronic kidney disease
ACR	albumin:creatinine ratio
HDL-C	high-density lipoprotein cholesterol
LDL-C	low-density lipoprotein cholesterol
VEGF	vascular endothelial growth factor
ICAM-1	intracellular adhesion molecule 1
ICA	invasive coronary angiography
TIMI	thrombolysis in myocardial infarction
CTCA	computed tomography coronary angiogram
CABG	coronary artery bypass grafting
PCI	percutaneous coronary intervention
GLA	galactosidase alpha
NO	nitrous oxide
TIA	transient ischaemic attack
FVL	factor V Leiden
PET	positron emission tomography
CFR	coronary flow reserve
MBF	myocardial blood flow
ECG	electrocardiogram
ECV	extracellular volume
MPS	myocardial perfusion scan
CRT	cardiac resynchronisation therapy

References

1. Desnick, R.J.; Brady, R.; Barranger, J.; Collins, A.J.; Germain, D.P.; Goldman, M.; Grabowski, G.; Packman, S.; Wilcox, W.R. Fabry disease, an under-recognized multisystemic disorder: Expert recommendations for diagnosis, management, and enzyme replacement therapy. *Ann. Intern. Med.* **2003**, *138*, 338–346. [CrossRef]
2. Sweeley, C.C.; Klionsky, B. Fabry's Disease: Classification as a sphingolipidosis and partial characterization of a novel glycolipid. *J. Biol. Chem.* **1963**, *238*, 3148–3150. [CrossRef]
3. Mehta, A.; Beck, M.; Eyskens, F.; Feliciani, C.; Kantola, I.; Ramaswami, U.; Rolfs, A.; Rivera, A.; Waldek, S.; Germain, D.P. Fabry disease: A review of current management strategies. *QJM* **2010**, *103*, 641–659. [CrossRef] [PubMed]
4. Mehta, A.; Clarke, J.T.; Giugliani, R.; Elliott, P.; Linhart, A.; Beck, M.; Sunder-Plassmann, G. Natural course of Fabry disease: Changing pattern of causes of death in FOS-Fabry Outcome Survey. *J. Med. Genet.* **2009**, *46*, 548–552. [CrossRef]
5. Waldek, S.; Patel, M.R.; Banikazemi, M.; Lemay, R.; Lee, P. Life expectancy and cause of death in males and females with Fabry disease: Findings from the Fabry Registry. *Genet. Med.* **2009**, *11*, 790–796. [CrossRef] [PubMed]
6. Germain, D.P.; Charrow, J.; Desnick, R.J.; Guffon, N.; Kempf, J.; Lachmann, R.H.; Lemay, R.; Linthorst, G.E.; Packman, S.; Scott, C.R.; et al. Ten-year outcome of enzyme replacement therapy with agalsidase beta in patients with Fabry disease. *J. Med. Genet.* **2015**, *52*, 353–358. [CrossRef]
7. Beck, M.; Hughes, D.; Kampmann, C.; Larroque, S.; Mehta, A.; Pintos-Morell, G.; Ramaswami, U.; West, M.; Wijatyk, A.; Giugliani, R.; et al. Long-term effectiveness of agalsidase alfa enzyme replacement in Fabry disease: A Fabry Outcome Survey analysis. *Mol. Genet. Metab. Rep.* **2015**, *3*, 21–27. [CrossRef]
8. Linhart, A.; Lubanda, J.C.; Palecek, T.; Bultas, J.; Karetová, D.; Ledvinová, J.; Elleder, M.; Aschermann, M. Cardiac manifestations in Fabry disease. *J. Inherit. Metab. Dis.* **2001**, *24* (Suppl. 2), 75–83; discussion 65. [CrossRef]
9. Linhart, A.; Kampmann, C.; Zamorano, J.L.; Sunder-Plassmann, G.; Beck, M.; Mehta, A.; Elliott, P.M.; Investigators, E.F. Cardiac manifestations of Anderson-Fabry disease: Results from the international Fabry outcome survey. *Eur. Heart J.* **2007**, *28*, 1228–1235. [CrossRef] [PubMed]
10. Kampmann, C.; Perrin, A.; Beck, M. Effectiveness of agalsidase alfa enzyme replacement in Fabry disease: Cardiac outcomes after 10 years' treatment. *Orphanet J. Rare Dis.* **2015**, *10*, 125. [CrossRef]
11. Sorbets, E.; Fox, K.M.; Elbez, Y.; Danchin, N.; Dorian, P.; Ferrari, R.; Ford, I.; Greenlaw, N.; Kalra, P.R.; Parma, Z.; et al. Long-term outcomes of chronic coronary syndrome worldwide: Insights from the international CLARIFY registry. *Eur. Heart J.* **2020**, *41*, 347–356. [CrossRef] [PubMed]

12. NICE. Stable Angina: Management. Available online: www.nice.org.uk/guidance/CG126 (accessed on 28 July 2021).
13. Linhart, A.; Germain, D.P.; Olivotto, I.; Akhtar, M.M.; Anastasakis, A.; Hughes, D.; Namdar, M.; Pieroni, M.; Hagège, A.; Cecchi, F.; et al. An expert consensus document on the management of cardiovascular manifestations of Fabry disease. *Eur. J. Heart Fail.* 2020, *22*, 1076–1096. [CrossRef]
14. Head, T.; Daunert, S.; Goldschmidt-Clermont, P.J. The Aging Risk and Atherosclerosis: A Fresh Look at Arterial Homeostasis. *Front. Genet.* 2017, *8*, 216. [CrossRef]
15. Herrington, W.; Lacey, B.; Sherliker, P.; Armitage, J.; Lewington, S. Epidemiology of Atherosclerosis and the Potential to Reduce the Global Burden of Atherothrombotic Disease. *Circ. Res.* 2016, *118*, 535–546. [CrossRef] [PubMed]
16. Kleinert, J.; Dehout, F.; Schwarting, A.; de Lorenzo, A.G.; Ricci, R.; Kampmann, C.; Beck, M.; Ramaswami, U.; Linhart, A.; Gal, A.; et al. Prevalence of uncontrolled hypertension in patients with Fabry disease. *Am. J. Hypertens.* 2006, *19*, 782–787. [CrossRef]
17. Patel, M.R.; Cecchi, F.; Cizmarik, M.; Kantola, I.; Linhart, A.; Nicholls, K.; Strotmann, J.; Tallaj, J.; Tran, T.C.; West, M.L.; et al. Cardiovascular events in patients with fabry disease natural history data from the fabry registry. *J. Am. Coll. Cardiol.* 2011, *57*, 1093–1099. [CrossRef] [PubMed]
18. Jaurretche, S.; Antogiovanni, N.; Perretta, F. Prevalence of chronic kidney disease in fabry disease patients: Multicenter cross sectional study in Argentina. *Mol. Genet. Metab. Rep.* 2017, *12*, 41–43. [CrossRef] [PubMed]
19. Mehta, A.; Ricci, R.; Widmer, U.; Dehout, F.; Garcia de Lorenzo, A.; Kampmann, C.; Linhart, A.; Sunder-Plassmann, G.; Ries, M.; Beck, M. Fabry disease defined: Baseline clinical manifestations of 366 patients in the Fabry Outcome Survey. *Eur. J. Clin. Investig.* 2004, *34*, 236–242. [CrossRef] [PubMed]
20. Cartwright, D.J.; Cole, A.L.; Cousins, A.J.; Lee, P.J. Raised HDL cholesterol in Fabry disease: Response to enzyme replacement therapy. *J. Inherit. Metab. Dis.* 2004, *27*, 791–793. [CrossRef]
21. Stepien, K.M.; Hendriksz, C.J. Lipid profile in adult patients with Fabry disease-Ten-year follow up. *Mol. Genet. Metab. Rep.* 2017, *13*, 3–6. [CrossRef] [PubMed]
22. Sacks, F.M.; Cholesterol, E.G.o.H. The role of high-density lipoprotein (HDL) cholesterol in the prevention and treatment of coronary heart disease: Expert group recommendations. *Am. J. Cardiol.* 2002, *90*, 139–143. [CrossRef]
23. Katsuta, H.; Tsuboi, K.; Yamamoto, H.; Goto, H. Correlations Between Serum Cholesterol and Vascular Lesions in Fabry Disease Patients. *Circ. J.* 2018, *82*, 3058–3063. [CrossRef] [PubMed]
24. Tsai, W.C.; Li, Y.H.; Huang, Y.Y.; Lin, C.C.; Chao, T.H.; Chen, J.H. Plasma vascular endothelial growth factor as a marker for early vascular damage in hypertension. *Clin. Sci.* 2005, *109*, 39–43. [CrossRef] [PubMed]
25. Kitagawa, K.; Matsumoto, M.; Sasaki, T.; Hashimoto, H.; Kuwabara, K.; Ohtsuki, T.; Hori, M. Involvement of ICAM-1 in the progression of atherosclerosis in APOE-knockout mice. *Atherosclerosis* 2002, *160*, 305–310. [CrossRef]
26. Park, S.; Kim, J.A.; Joo, K.Y.; Choi, S.; Choi, E.N.; Shin, J.A.; Han, K.H.; Jung, S.C.; Suh, S.H. Globotriaosylceramide leads to K(Ca)3.1 channel dysfunction: A new insight into endothelial dysfunction in Fabry disease. *Cardiovasc. Res.* 2011, *89*, 290–299. [CrossRef]
27. Altarescu, G.; Moore, D.F.; Pursley, R.; Campia, U.; Goldstein, S.; Bryant, M.; Panza, J.A.; Schiffmann, R. Enhanced endothelium-dependent vasodilation in Fabry disease. *Stroke* 2001, *32*, 1559–1562. [CrossRef]
28. Chimenti, C.; Morgante, E.; Tanzilli, G.; Mangieri, E.; Critelli, G.; Gaudio, C.; Russo, M.A.; Frustaci, A. Angina in fabry disease reflects coronary small vessel disease. *Circ. Heart Fail.* 2008, *1*, 161–169. [CrossRef]
29. Buja, L.M. Evaluation of recombinant alpha-galactosidase A therapy for amelioration of the cardiovascular manifestations of Fabry disease: An important role for endomyocardial biopsy. *Circulation* 2009, *119*, 2539–2541. [CrossRef]
30. Thurberg, B.L.; Fallon, J.T.; Mitchell, R.; Aretz, T.; Gordon, R.E.; O'Callaghan, M.W. Cardiac microvascular pathology in Fabry disease: Evaluation of endomyocardial biopsies before and after enzyme replacement therapy. *Circulation* 2009, *119*, 2561–2567. [CrossRef]
31. Schiffmann, R.; Rapkiewicz, A.; Abu-Asab, M.; Ries, M.; Askari, H.; Tsokos, M.; Quezado, M. Pathological findings in a patient with Fabry disease who died after 2.5 years of enzyme replacement. *Virchows Arch.* 2006, *448*, 337–343. [CrossRef]
32. Kotnik, J.; Kotnik, F.; Desnick, R.J. Fabry disease. A case report. *Acta Derm. Alp. Pannonica Adriat.* 2005, *14*, 15–19.
33. Fisher, E.A.; Desnick, R.J.; Gordon, R.E.; Eng, C.M.; Griepp, R.; Goldman, M.E. Fabry disease: An unusual cause of severe coronary disease in a young man. *Ann. Intern. Med.* 1992, *117*, 221–223. [CrossRef] [PubMed]
34. Elliott, P.M.; Kindler, H.; Shah, J.S.; Sachdev, B.; Rimoldi, O.E.; Thaman, R.; Tome, M.T.; McKenna, W.J.; Lee, P.; Camici, P.G. Coronary microvascular dysfunction in male patients with Anderson-Fabry disease and the effect of treatment with alpha galactosidase A. *Heart* 2006, *92*, 357–360. [CrossRef] [PubMed]
35. Case records of the Massachusetts General Hospital. Weekly clinicopathological exercises. Case 2-1984. A 47-year-old man with coronary-artery disease and variable neurologic abnormalities. *N. Engl. J. Med.* 1984, *310*, 106–114. [CrossRef] [PubMed]
36. Simoncini, C.; Torri, S.; Montano, V.; Chico, L.; Gruosso, F.; Tuttolomondo, A.; Pinto, A.; Simonetta, I.; Cianci, V.; Salviati, A.; et al. Oxidative stress biomarkers in Fabry disease: Is there a room for them? *J. Neurol.* 2020, *267*, 3741–3752. [CrossRef] [PubMed]
37. Laurindo, F.R.; Pedro, M.e.A.; Barbeiro, H.V.; Pileggi, F.; Carvalho, M.H.; Augusto, O.; da Luz, P.L. Vascular free radical release. Ex vivo and in vivo evidence for a flow-dependent endothelial mechanism. *Circ. Res.* 1994, *74*, 700–709. [CrossRef]
38. Senders, M.L.; Mulder, W.J.M. Targeting myeloperoxidase in inflammatory atherosclerosis. *Eur. Heart J.* 2018, *39*, 3311–3313. [CrossRef]

39. Kaneski, C.R.; Moore, D.F.; Ries, M.; Zirzow, G.C.; Schiffmann, R. Myeloperoxidase predicts risk of vasculopathic events in hemizgygous males with Fabry disease. *Neurology* **2006**, *67*, 2045–2047. [CrossRef]
40. Bodary, P.F.; Shen, Y.; Vargas, F.B.; Bi, X.; Ostenso, K.A.; Gu, S.; Shayman, J.A.; Eitzman, D.T. Alpha-galactosidase A deficiency accelerates atherosclerosis in mice with apolipoprotein E deficiency. *Circulation* **2005**, *111*, 629–632. [CrossRef]
41. Moore, D.F.; Kaneski, C.R.; Askari, H.; Schiffmann, R. The cerebral vasculopathy of Fabry disease. *J. Neurol. Sci.* **2007**, *257*, 258–263. [CrossRef]
42. Feldt-Rasmussen, U. Fabry disease and early stroke. *Stroke Res. Treat.* **2011**, *2011*, 615218. [CrossRef] [PubMed]
43. Wattanakit, K.; Cushman, M.; Stehman-Breen, C.; Heckbert, S.R.; Folsom, A.R. Chronic kidney disease increases risk for venous thromboembolism. *J. Am. Soc. Nephrol.* **2008**, *19*, 135–140. [CrossRef]
44. Lenders, M.; Karabul, N.; Duning, T.; Schmitz, B.; Schelleckes, M.; Mesters, R.; Hense, H.W.; Beck, M.; Brand, S.M.; Brand, E. Thromboembolic events in Fabry disease and the impact of factor V Leiden. *Neurology* **2015**, *84*, 1009–1016. [CrossRef]
45. Lee, B.K.; Lim, H.S.; Fearon, W.F.; Yong, A.S.; Yamada, R.; Tanaka, S.; Lee, D.P.; Yeung, A.C.; Tremmel, J.A. Invasive evaluation of patients with angina in the absence of obstructive coronary artery disease. *Circulation* **2015**, *131*, 1054–1060. [CrossRef] [PubMed]
46. el-Tamimi, H.; Mansour, M.; Wargovich, T.J.; Hill, J.A.; Kerensky, R.A.; Conti, C.R.; Pepine, C.J. Constrictor and dilator responses to intracoronary acetylcholine in adjacent segments of the same coronary artery in patients with coronary artery disease. Endothelial function revisited. *Circulation* **1994**, *89*, 45–51. [CrossRef] [PubMed]
47. Lipscomb, K.; Gould, K.L. Mechanism of the effect of coronary artery stenosis on coronary flow in the dog. *Am. Heart J.* **1975**, *89*, 60–67. [CrossRef]
48. Downey, H.F.; Crystal, G.J.; Bashour, F.A. Asynchronous transmural perfusion during coronary reactive hyperaemia. *Cardiovasc Res.* **1983**, *17*, 200–206. [CrossRef] [PubMed]
49. Beltrame, J.F.; Limaye, S.B.; Horowitz, J.D. The coronary slow flow phenomenon—A new coronary microvascular disorder. *Cardiology* **2002**, *97*, 197–202. [CrossRef]
50. Camici, P.; Chiriatti, G.; Lorenzoni, R.; Bellina, R.C.; Gistri, R.; Italiani, G.; Parodi, O.; Salvadori, P.A.; Nista, N.; Papi, L. Coronary vasodilation is impaired in both hypertrophied and nonhypertrophied myocardium of patients with hypertrophic cardiomyopathy: A study with nitrogen-13 ammonia and positron emission tomography. *J. Am. Coll. Cardiol.* **1991**, *17*, 879–886. [CrossRef]
51. Maron, B.J.; Wolfson, J.K.; Epstein, S.E.; Roberts, W.C. Intramural ("small vessel") coronary artery disease in hypertrophic cardiomyopathy. *J. Am. Coll. Cardiol.* **1986**, *8*, 545–557. [CrossRef]
52. Kalliokoski, R.J.; Kantola, I.; Kalliokoski, K.K.; Engblom, E.; Sundell, J.; Hannukainen, J.C.; Janatuinen, T.; Raitakari, O.T.; Knuuti, J.; Penttinen, M.; et al. The effect of 12-month enzyme replacement therapy on myocardial perfusion in patients with Fabry disease. *J. Inherit. Metab. Dis.* **2006**, *29*, 112–118. [CrossRef]
53. Knott, K.D.; Augusto, J.B.; Nordin, S.; Kozor, R.; Camaioni, C.; Xue, H.; Hughes, R.K.; Manisty, C.; Brown, L.A.E.; Kellman, P.; et al. Quantitative Myocardial Perfusion in Fabry Disease. *Circ. Cardiovasc. Imaging* **2019**, *12*, e008872. [CrossRef] [PubMed]
54. Körver, S.; Geurtsen, G.J.; Hollak, C.E.M.; van Schaik, I.N.; Longo, M.G.F.; Lima, M.R.; Vedolin, L.; Dijkgraaf, M.G.W.; Langeveld, M. Predictors of objective cognitive impairment and subjective cognitive complaints in patients with Fabry disease. *Sci. Rep.* **2019**, *9*, 188. [CrossRef]
55. Baig, S.; Vijapurapu, R.; Alharbi, F.; Nordin, S.; Kozor, R.; Moon, J.; Bembi, B.; Geberhiwot, T.; Steeds, R.P. Diagnosis and treatment of the cardiovascular consequences of Fabry disease. *QJM* **2019**, *112*, 3–9. [CrossRef] [PubMed]
56. Krämer, J.; Bijnens, B.; Störk, S.; Ritter, C.O.; Liu, D.; Ertl, G.; Wanner, C.; Weidemann, F. Left Ventricular Geometry and Blood Pressure as Predictors of Adverse Progression of Fabry Cardiomyopathy. *PLoS ONE* **2015**, *10*, e0140627. [CrossRef]

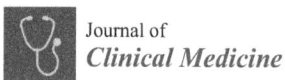

Article

Disease Manifestations in Mucopolysaccharidoses and Their Impact on Anaesthesia-Related Complications—A Retrospective Analysis of 99 Patients

Luise Sophie Ammer [1,*,†], Thorsten Dohrmann [2,†], Nicole Maria Muschol [1], Annika Lang [1,‡], Sandra Rafaela Breyer [1,3,4], Ann-Kathrin Ozga [5] and Martin Petzoldt [2]

[1] Department of Paediatrics, International Centre for Lysosomal Disorders (ICLD), University Medical Centre Hamburg-Eppendorf, 20246 Hamburg, Germany; muschol@uke.de (N.M.M.); annika.lang@stud.uke.uni-hamburg.de (A.L.); s.breyer@uke.de (S.R.B.)
[2] Department of Anaesthesiology, University Medical Centre Hamburg-Eppendorf, 20246 Hamburg, Germany; t.dohrmann@uke.de (T.D.); m.petzoldt@uke.de (M.P.)
[3] Department of Paediatric Orthopaedics, Children's Hospital Altona, 22763 Hamburg, Germany
[4] Department of Orthopaedics, University Medical Centre Hamburg-Eppendorf, 20246 Hamburg, Germany
[5] Department of Medical Biometry and Epidemiology, University Medical Centre Hamburg-Eppendorf, 20246 Hamburg, Germany; a.ozga@uke.de
* Correspondence: l.ammer@uke.de; Tel.: +49-40-7410-53714
† These authors contributed equally to this work.
‡ This work is part of the doctoral thesis of Annika Lang.

Abstract: Patients with mucopolysaccharidoses (MPS) frequently require anaesthesia for diagnostic or surgical interventions and thereby experience high morbidity. This study aimed to develop a multivariable prediction model for anaesthesia-related complications in MPS. This two-centred study was performed by retrospective chart review of children and adults with MPS undergoing anaesthesia from 2002 until 2018. We retrieved the patients' demographics, medical history, clinical manifestations, and indication by each anaesthesia. Multivariable mixed-effects logistic regression was calculated for a clinical model based on preoperative predictors preselected by lasso regression and another model based on disease subtypes only. Of the 484 anaesthesia cases in 99 patients, 22.7% experienced at least one adverse event. The clinical model resulted in a better forecast performance than the subtype-model (AICc 460.4 vs. 467.7). The most relevant predictors were hepatosplenomegaly (OR 3.10, CI 1.54–6.26), immobility (OR 3.80, CI 0.98–14.73), and planned major surgery (OR 6.64, CI 2.25–19.55), while disease-specific therapies, i.e., haematopoietic stem cell transplantation (OR 0.45, CI 0.20–1.03), produced a protective effect. Anaesthetic complications can best be predicted by surrogates for advanced disease stages and protective therapeutic factors. Further model validation in different cohorts is needed.

Keywords: mucopolysaccharidosis; MPS; disease manifestations; symptoms; morbidity; spine disease; anaesthesia; airway; perioperative complications; surgery

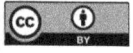

1. Introduction

Mucopolysaccharidoses (MPS), a group of inherited rare lysosomal storage disorders, are caused by reduced enzyme activity of lysosomal enzymes involved in the degradation of glycosaminoglycans (GAGs). In MPS, partially degraded GAGs accumulate in multiple organs and impair cellular function. Depending on the specific GAGs stored, MPS divide into eleven subtypes (I, II, IIIA-D, IVA and B, VI, VII and IX), each with a predominant phenotype. MPS manifests as a progressive disease and may involve craniofacial dysmorphism, cardiac and respiratory pathologies, obstructive or central sleep apnoea, hepatosplenomegaly, skeletal deformities, and neurocognitive affection [1,2]. An approved enzyme replacement therapy (ERT) exists for MPS Types I, II, IVA, VI, and VII.

Hematopoietic stem cell transplantation (HSCT) is the therapy of choice in patients with MPSIH (Hurler-syndrome) below 2.5 years of age [3]. New and supplementary therapeutic approaches (e.g., gene therapy, anti-inflammatory drugs) are being tested within clinical trials.

Due to the multi-systemic morbidity, MPS patients frequently require anaesthesia for diagnostic or surgical interventions. To exemplify this, 44% of MPSI patients have undergone at least two surgeries by four years of age [4]. Simultaneously, MPS patients experience a high perioperative risk of morbidity and mortality [5–7]. Registry data on MPSI patients revealed a perioperative morbidity rate of up to 30% [8] and a risk of death of 0.7% within 30 days after surgery [9]. A high rate of failed direct laryngoscopy and respiratory events prove an especially difficult airway and call for advanced airway management in these patients [5,10]. We recently published that the anaesthetic risk is higher in patients with MPS types I or II than with MPSIII and suggested using indirect intubation techniques as the first-line airway approach in individuals with MPS [11].

While perioperative event rate and procedure-related risk factors have already been analysed in MPS, it has never been investigated, which disease manifestations prone for complications and to what extent. Such data are essential considering the clinical variability not only between the different MPS types but also within one type [12]. Indirect intubation techniques such as fibreoptic intubation with guidance by a supraglottic conduit are considered to be safe for the management of difficult paediatric airway [10,13], but an a priori approach may not be necessary for all MPS patients. A better prediction of the anaesthetic risk may enable a more appropriate, patient-based pre-anaesthesia strategy as well as precautionary measures and a more personalized perioperative patient management. This study aimed to develop a multivariable prediction model of anaesthesia-related complications in MPS based on available preoperative patient-specific information.

2. Patients and Methods

2.1. Study Sites and Patients

This study was performed by retrospective chart review of patients of the International Centre for Lysosomal Disorders (ICLD) located at the University Medical Centre Hamburg-Eppendorf (UKE), Hamburg, Germany. Inclusion criteria were biochemically or molecular genetically confirmed diagnosis of MPS and at least one anaesthesia procedure (procedural sedation, regional anaesthesia, general anaesthesia) performed within the framework of the clinical routine between April 2002 and October 2018, either at the UKE or the Children's Hospital Altona (AKK), Hamburg, Germany.

2.2. Data Acquisition

Retrospective data acquisition was performed by systematic review of analogue and electronic patient folders (Soarian™ Health Archive, Release 3.04 SP12, Siemens Healthcare, Erlangen, Germany). The latter were introduced in 2009. Of each included patient, data on the sex, the underlying subtype and the age at diagnosis were collected. The patient folders were systematically screened for information regarding the following aspects at the time of each anaesthesia (study case): body measurements, MPS-typical disease manifestations and medical history. As a surrogate parameter for the increasing experience with the disease, we also included the date and patient age at each anaesthesia.

As part of the medical history, data were collected on whether ERT (if applicable, also the age at ERT-start) or HSCT (if applicable, also the age at successful) had been performed. This study aimed to focus on anaesthesia-relevant disease manifestations, precisely, macroglossia, tonsil hyperplasia, short neck, thorax deformities (as per reports of physical examinations), spine deformities (as per reports of radiological examinations), impaired lung function (as by pulmonary function testing), sleep apnoea, respiratory infection within two weeks prior to the anaesthesia, apparent dysphagia, cardiac pathologies, relevant organomegaly (by standard deviation of the index for body length), persistent seizures, shunt-supported hydrocephalus, cognitive impairment, reduced mobility, and facial dysmorphia as an apparent symptom. Cardiac pathologies were graded as: unremarkable (incl. incomplete right bundle branch block; s/p septum defects), mild (plump valves; valvular heart defects Grades I/I–II; small septum defects; small pericardial effusion; atrioventricular block Grade I; left bundle branch block; arterial hypertension), moderate (valvular heart defects Grade II; discrete cardiac hypertrophy or dilative cardiomyopathy) and severe (valvular heart defects Grade III/IV; any manifestation requiring cardiac medication or intervention). Motor and cognitive function was graded according to the four-point scoring system (FPSS) by Meyer et al. [14]. For describing patient characteristics, the most pathologic finding counted from repeated anaesthesia procedures.

We furthermore collected anaesthesia procedure-related information. The reasons for anaesthesia were each categorised as diagnostics only, intervention, minor surgery, surgery affecting the airway, or major surgery. If anaesthesia was performed due to different reasons, the most invasive one determined classification. Punctures/injections (e.g., intravenous, catheter, lumbar), stitching, endoscopy, arthrography, change of tracheal cannulas or gastric tubes and cast installations counted as interventions. Minor surgeries comprised dental, ear and ophthalmological surgeries, catheter and gastric tube implantations, removals and revisions, herniotomies, lung and liver biopsies, abscess cleavage, circumcision, carpal tunnel syndrome releases, and surgical interventions of the lower extremities (e.g., temporary epiphysiodesis). Because of the cardiorespiratory risk, surgeries affecting the airway (e.g., tracheotomy, tonsillotomy, adenotomy) were counted as more invasive, excelled by major surgeries (i.e., thorax, cardiac, neurosurgery).

The primary endpoint "anaesthesia-related complications" was a composite of difficult airway management, respiratory events, cardiocirculatory events, and other postoperative complications and thus comprised any anaesthesia-related complication until hospital discharge. The airway management, respiratory and cardiocirculatory endpoint measures were defined as recently described [11].

2.3. Statistics

Data were collected in Microsoft Excel (Version 2011, Microsoft Corporation, Redmont, WA, USA) and analysed in R 4.0.3 (R core team, Vienna, Austria). Demographic data, disease manifestations, procedure-related factors and outcome data were stratified by disease type and summarised as frequencies and percentages for categorical variables and as medians and ranges or means and standard deviations (SD) for continuous variables as appropriate.

We used multivariable mixed-effects logistic regression to identify disease-specific risk factors for the composite binary endpoint "anaesthesia-related complications". The model included one random effect to account for multiple anaesthesia procedures within one patient. Potentially eligible factors were identified by literature research, clinical implications, and descriptive and graphical analysis of the data. For variable selection least absolute shrinkage selector operator (lasso) regression was calculated [15]. The shrinkage parameter was estimated by five-fold cross-validation. For the starting model, the following variables were included for fixed effects: subtype, height, weight, age, sex, HSCT, ERT, macroglossia, tonsil hyperplasia, short neck, respiratory infection, obstructive and restrictive lung disease, sleep apnoea, cardiac manifestation, thorax deformity, hepatosplenomegaly, dysphagia, cervical spine stenosis, cervical spine immobility, spine deformity, seizures, shunt-supported hydrocephalus, cognitive and motor function impairment, reason for anaesthesia. Missing data were not imputed and cases with at least one missing value were excluded (listwise deletion). The resulting model was compared to a model, which included only the disease types (I, II, III, IV and VI) as predictors. This model was fitted by optimising the restricted maximum likelihood (REML) criterion using an iterative nonlinear optimisation algorithm as described by Bates et al., 2015 [16] and implemented in the "lme4" package for R. Odds ratios (OR) for the fixed effects are presented and respective 95% confidence intervals (CI) were calculated by Wald approximation. For categorical variables, the OR was calculated by using the category with the lowest expected event rate as reference, for example, MPSIII for the disease types. The model performance was evaluated by comparing the Akaike information criterion (AICc) and the area under the receiver operator curve (AUC). As this is an explorative study, neither model validation nor adjustment for multiple testing were performed.

3. Results

3.1. Data Acquisition and Quality

Two hundred twenty patients with MPS were screened, of which 99 underwent at least one anaesthetic procedure and were enrolled. Four cases were excluded because the anaesthesia protocol was either unreadable ($n = 1$) or unavailable ($n = 3$), adding up to 484 cases. The data quality was sufficient, with an overall missing rate of 0.75%. However, in four cases, the primary endpoint could not be defined due to insufficient data quality. Further three cases were missing primary endpoints and in 12 cases local anaesthesia was performed by a surgeon, only with anaesthesia standby. These cases had to be excluded from multivariable modelling, leaving 469 cases for the outcome analysis (Figure 1).

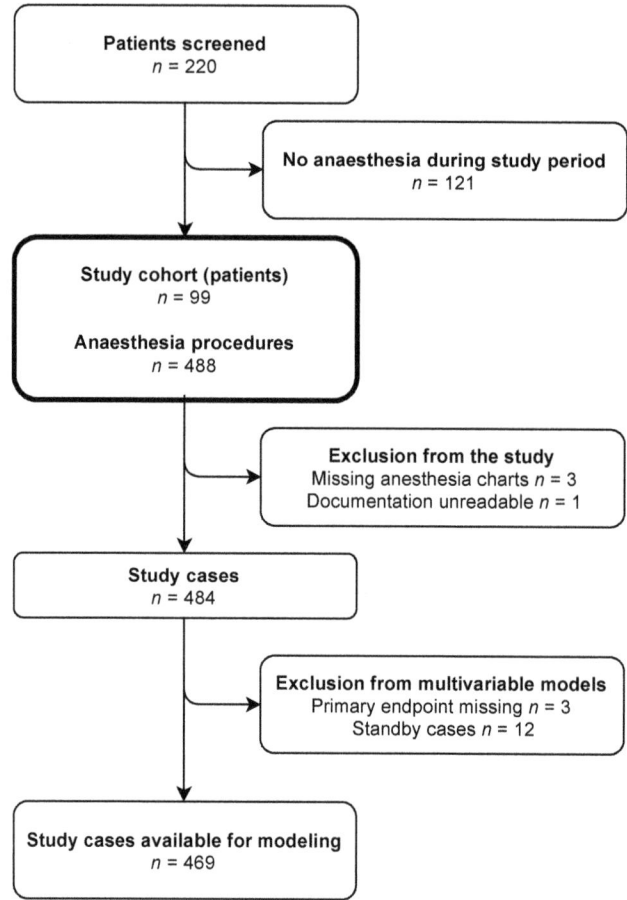

Figure 1. Flowchart of the study inclusion process.

3.2. Patient Characteristics

The 99 study patients underwent a median of three anaesthetic procedures per patient (range 1–19). Sex distribution was slightly unbalanced with 71 male cases (72%). Overall, the patients were diagnosed at a median age of 3.1 years (range 0.0–29 years). The median age at first anaesthesia was 4.8 years (range 0.7–38.3 years), the median age at the last one was 9.7 years (range 0.8–38.7 years). Of the 99 patients, 35 patients had MPSI (35%), of whom 32 had MPSIH and 3 MPSIS (Scheie-syndrome). Of the 32 MPSIH patients, 22 (69%) had undergone HSCT, of whom 2 had graft failure. Another 16 patients suffered from MPSII (16%), 37 from MPSIII (37%; 27 MPSIIIA, 7 MPS IIIB, 3 MPS IIIC), 7 from MPSIV (7%; all MPS IVA) and 4 from MPSVI (4%). Overall, 36 patients received ERT (median age at start: 6.2 years, range 0.2–29 years) and 28 patients HSCT (22 MPSIH, 3 MPSII, 3 MPSIIIA; median age at HSCT: 1.3 years, range 0.4–1.8 years).

Clinical patient characteristics are described by disease type (Table 1). The most frequent symptom was facial dysmorphism (92%). Macroglossia was documented in 52% of the patients, tonsil hyperplasia in 45% and a short neck in 85%. Concerning the respiratory manifestations, 51% of the patients had impaired lung function, 39% obstructive sleep apnoea, and 26% thorax deformity. Dysphagia was apparent in 29% of the patients and 60% had at least one relevant organomegaly. Cardiac manifestations were present in 71% of the patients, of whom more than half (53%) had only mild cardiac pathologies. Overall, cervical spine pathologies were manifest in 46% of the patients and thoracolumbar spine deformity in 65%. A detailed table of cervical spine pathologies is shown in the supplement (Table S1). Seizures persisted in 19% of the MPS patients, 5% had a shunt-supported hydrocephalus, 75% a cognitive impairment and 86% reduced mobility. Manifestations of different types overlap, especially of MPSI and II. However, the types have dominant features, particularly neurological features (seizures, cognitive impairment, immobility) in MPSIII. However, patients with MPSIII also manifest peripheral symptoms, namely, facial dysmorphism (95%), macroglossia (43%), tonsil hyperplasia (41%), short neck (78%), obstructed lung disease (32%), sleep apnoea (19%), cardiac pathologies (49%, foremost mild ones), at least one organomegaly (65%), cervical spine pathology (11%), and spine deformity (32%; foremost kyphosis and kyphoscoliosis).

3.3. Characteristics of Anaesthesia Procedures

Anaesthesia care was provided for 484 cases. The median age at anaesthesia was 6.1 years (IQR 3.7–11.1 years). General anaesthesia was administered in 383 cases (80%). In total, 85 patients (18%) underwent procedural sedation, with MPSIII being the type with the highest rate of procedural sedation (31%). Procedural sedation was the most common anaesthesia method for small interventions (59%). In contrast, for diagnostics (mostly magnetic resonance imaging, MRI), general anaesthesia was preferred (55.7%), while procedural sedation was less common (32%). As management was at discretion of the handling anaesthetist, the airway management was heterogeneous. Tracheal intubation was used in 69.5% of the general anaesthesia cases and a laryngeal mask airway was used in 23.6%. Tracheal intubation was facilitated by indirect methods such as videolaryngoscopy or fibreoptic intubation with or without guidance via supraglottic conduits in 71.5%. The main indications for anaesthesia were diagnostics (22%), small interventions (12%) and a broad variety of surgeries (66.5%). The anaesthesia-associated details are described by disease type in the supplement (Table S2).

Table 1. Patient characteristics stratified by MPS disease types.

Characteristics	Overall N = 99	MPSIH N = 32	MPSIS N = 3	MPSII N = 16	MPSIII N = 37	MPSIV N = 7	MPSVI N = 4
Demographic characteristics							
Sex, male, n (%)	71 (71.7)	20 (62.5)	1 (33.3)	16 (100.0)	27 (73.10)	4 (57.1)	3 (75.0)
Min. age at anaesthesia (years) *	4.8 (0.7–38.3)	1.9 (0.8–20.8)	13.9 (7.1–29.1)	7.8 (0.7–29.7)	5.8 (1.1–38.3)	8.6 (4.1–18.6)	10.4 (7.5–24.2)
Max. age at anaesthesia (years) *	9.7 (0.8–38.7)	8.6 (0.8–23.8)	24.0 (7.1–29.1)	12.2 (2.5–32.1)	8.9 (3.5–38.7)	15.7 (6.1–18.6)	21.6 (8.5–38.2)
Medical history							
Age at diagnosis (years) *	3.1 (0.0–29.0)	1.2 (0.0–8.0)	6.6 (3.8–29.0)	4.5 (0.1–15.8)	3.7 (0.5–16.8)	4.3 (0.9–8.6)	4.4 (1.6–11.5)
Total no. of anaesthesias	3.0 (1.0–19.0)	5.0 (1.0–19.0)	1.0 (1.0–18.0)	3.0 (1.0–10.0)	2.5 (1.0–12.0)	3.0 (1.0–9.0)	5.5 (1.0–11.0)
HSCT, n (%)	28 (28.3)	22 (68.8)	-	3 (18.8)	3 (8.1)	-	-
Age at HSCT (years) *	1.3 (0.4–1.8)	1.4 (1.1–1.8)	N/A	0.4 (0.4–0.4)	4.7 (3.0–5.7)	N/A	N/A
ERT, n (%)	36 (36.4)	15 (46.9)	3 (100.0)	11 (68.8)	-	5 (71.4)	3 (75.0)
Age at ERT-start (years) *	6.2 (0.2–29.0)	1.0 (0.7–6.4)	7.0 (6.7–29.0)	8.2 (0.2–22.1)	N/A	12.0 (4.6–14.5)	11.5 (11.5–11.5)
Craniofacial pathologies							
Facial dysmorphism, n (%)	91 (91.9)	30 (93.8)	2 (66.7)	15 (93.8)	35 (94.6)	5 (71.4)	4 (100.0)
Macroglossia, n (%)	51 (51.5)	20 (62.5)	1 (33.3)	11 (68.8)	16 (43.2)	1 (14.3)	2 (50.0)
Tonsil hyperplasia, n (%)	45 (45.5)	17 (53.1)	-	6 (37.5)	15 (40.5)	4 (57.1)	3 (75.0)
Short neck, n (%)	84 (84.8)	27 (84.4)	2 (66.7)	16 (100.0)	29 (78.4)	6 (85.7)	4 (100.0)
Respiratory manifestations							
Lung function, n (%)							
Normal	49 (49.5)	13 (40.6)	2 (66.7)	4 (25.0)	25 (67.6)	4 (57.1)	1 (25.0)
Obstruction	23 (23.2)	6 (18.8)	-	4 (25.0)	12 (32.4)	1 (14.3)	-
Restriction	15 (15.2)	12 (37.5)	-	1 (6.2)	-	1 (14.3)	1 (25.0)
Both	12 (12.1)	1 (3.1)	1 (33.3)	7 (43.8)	-	1 (14.3)	2 (50.0)
Sleep apnoea, n (%)							
No	60 (60.6)	18 (56.2)	1 (33.3)	7 (43.8)	30 (81.1)	4 (57.1)	-
Suspected	17 (17.2)	5 (15.6)	-	4 (25.0)	5 (13.5)	1 (14.3)	2 (50.0)
Diagnosis	11 (11.1)	5 (15.6)	1 (33.3)	3 (18.8)	1 (2.7)	-	1 (25.0)
CPAP	11 (11.1)	4 (12.5)	1 (33.3)	2 (12.5)	1 (2.7)	2 (28.6)	1 (25.0)
Thorax deformity, n (%)	26 (26.3)	11 (34.4)	-	4 (25.0)	3 (8.1)	6 (85.7)	2 (50.0)

Table 1. Cont.

Characteristics	Overall N = 99	MPSIH N = 32	MPSIS N = 3	MPSII N = 16	MPSIII N = 37	MPSIV N = 7	MPSVI N = 4
Cardiac pathology, n (%)			Cardiac manifestations				
No	29 (29.3)	5 (15.6)	-	3 (18.8)	19 (51.4)	2 (28.6)	-
Mild	38 (38.4)	13 (40.6)	2 (66.7)	5 (31.2)	12 (32.4)	4 (57.1)	2 (50.0)
Moderate	15 (15.2)	4 (12.5)	1 (33.3)	5 (31.2)	3 (8.1)	1 (14.3)	1 (25.0)
Severe	17 (17.2)	10 (31.2)	-	3 (18.8)	3 (8.1)	-	1 (25.0)
			Gastrointestinal manifestations				
Organomegaly, n (%)							
No	40 (40.4)	11 (34.4)	2 (66.7)	5 (31.2)	13 (35.1)	7 (100.0)	2 (50.0)
Any	23 (23.2)	8 (25.0)	-	1 (6.2)	13 (35.1)	-	1 (25.0)
Hepatosplenomegaly	36 (36.4)	13 (40.6)	1 (33.3)	10 (62.5)	11 (29.7)	-	1 (25.0)
Dysphagia, n (%)	29 (29.3)	4 (12.5)	1 (33.3)	5 (31.2)	19 (51.4)	-	-
			Spine disease				
Cervical spine stability, n (%)							
Stable	75 (75.8)	18 (56.2)	3 (100.0)	13 (81.2)	37 (100)	3 (42.9)	1 (25.0)
Instable	19 (19.2)	11 (34.4)	-	3 (18.8)	-	3 (42.9)	2 (50.0)
Surgical Fusion	5 (5.1)	3 (9.4)	-	-	-	1 (14.3)	1 (25.0)
Cervical spine stenosis, n (%)							
No	57 (57.6)	11 (34.4)	1 (33.3)	11 (68.8)	33 (89.2)	1 (14.3)	-
Stenosis	25 (25.3)	12 (37.5)	-	3 (18.8)	4 (10.8)	4 (57.1)	2 (50.0)
Stenosis with myelopathy	6 (6.1)	3 (9.4)	1 (33.3)	2 (12.5)	-	-	-
Decompression surgery	11 (11.1)	6 (18.8)	1 (33.3)	-	-	2 (28.6)	2 (50.0)
Spine deformity, n (%)							
No	35 (35.4)	1 (3.1)	1 (33.3)	8 (50.0)	25 (67.6)	-	-
Scoliosis	10 (10.1)	2 (6.2)	-	5 (31.2)	2 (5.4)	-	1 (25.0)
Kyphosis	26 (26.3)	13 (40.6)	-	1 (6.2)	7 (18.9)	3 (42.9)	2 (50.0)
Both	28 (28.3)	16 (50.0)	2 (66.7)	2 (12.5)	3 (8.1)	4 (57.1)	1 (25.0)

Table 1. Cont.

Characteristics	Overall N = 99	MPSIH N = 32	MPSIS N = 3	MPSII N = 16	MPSIII N = 37	MPSIV N = 7	MPSVI N = 4
			Neurological manifestations				
Seizures, n (%)	19 (19.2)	3 (9.4)	-	2 (12.5)	14 (37.8)	-	-
Shunted hydrocephalus, n (%)	5 (5.1)	3 (9.4)	1 (33.3)	-	-	-	1 (25.0)
Cognitive function, n (%)							
Normal	25 (25.3)	11 (34.4)	2 (66.7)	5 (31.2)	-	5 (71.4)	2 (50.0)
Impaired	46 (46.5)	18 (56.2)	1 (33.3)	7 (43.8)	16 (34.2)	2 (28.6)	2 (50.0)
Regression	15 (15.2)	2 (6.2)	-	4 (25.0)	9 (24.3)	-	-
Unresponsiveness	13 (13.1)	1 (3.1)	-	-	12 (32.4)	-	-
Motor function, n (%)							
No impairment	14 (14.1)	1 (3.1)	-	5 (31.2)	8 (21.6)	-	-
Impaired	34 (34.3)	16 (50.0)	1 (33.3)	6 (37.5)	7 (18.9)	2 (28.6)	2 (50.0)
Constant help needed	23 (23.2)	7 (21.9)	1 (33.3)	1 (6.2)	11 (29.7)	3 (42.9)	-
Immobile	28 (28.3)	8 (25.0)	1 (33.3)	4 (25.0)	11 (29.7)	2 (28.6)	2 (50.0)

* Median (range). Abbreviations: CPAP, continuous positive airway pressure device; ERT, enzyme replacement therapy; HSCT, haematopoietic stem cell transplantation.

3.4. Anaesthesia-Related Complication

At least one anaesthesia-related complication occurred in 22.7% ($n = 109$) of the cases (Table 2). In 6.6% ($n = 32$) of the cases more than one event occurred during or after anaesthesia. The total number of events was 171 with the following event type distribution: 35.1% ($n = 60$) technically difficult airway management, 50.3% ($n = 86$) respiratory events, 7.0% ($n = 12$) cardiocirculatory events, and 7.6% ($n = 13$) other events. 45% ($n = 77$) of the events occurred during induction of anaesthesia, 17.5% ($n = 30$) during anaesthesia and 37.4% ($n = 64$) after anaesthesia. Patients with MPSIII had the lowest event rate (7.2%), whereas the highest event rate occurred in patients with MPSII (38.7%), MPSVI (31.8%), and MPSI (27.4%). Problems in airway management arose primarily due to difficult tracheal intubation (20%). Bag-mask-ventilation was described as difficult in 4.5% and the laryngeal mask placement or ventilation via laryngeal mask were problematic in 8.1% of the cases.

Table 2. Anaesthesia-related complications stratified by MPS disease types.

Characteristics	Overall N = 484	MPSIH N = 224	MPSIS N = 20	MPSII N = 62	MPSIII N = 126	MPSIV N = 29	MPSVI N = 23
Respiratory events, n (%)	86 (17.8)	38 (17.0)	6 (30.0)	25 (40.3)	7 (5.6)	2 (6.9)	8 (34.8)
Respiratory insufficiency	23 (4.8)	8 (3.6)	2 (10.0)	7 (11.3)	2 (1.6)	1 (3.4)	3 (13.0)
Hypoxemia	17 (3.5)	11 (4.9)	1 (5.0)	2 (3.2)	2 (1.6)	-	1 (5.0)
Airway obstruction	19 (3.9)	6 (2.7)	2 (10.0)	8 (12.9)	1 (0.8)	-	2 (10.0)
Increased ventilation pressure	8 (1.7)	2 (0.9)	-	4 (6.5)	-	1 (3.4)	1 (5.0)
Hypercapnia	7 (1.4)	7 (3.1)	-	-	-	-	-
Pneumonia	6 (1.2)	2 (0.9)	1 (5.0)	2 (3.2)	-	-	1 (5.0)
Atelectasis	4 (0.8)	2 (0.9)	-	-	2 (1.6)	-	-
Pneumothorax	1 (0.2)	-	-	1 (1.6)	-	-	-
Cardiocirculatory events, n (%)	12 (2.5)	3 (1.3)	-	1 (1.6)	4 (3.2)	-	4 (17.4)
Bradycardia/tachycardia	6 (1.2)	2 (0.9)	-	1 (1.6)	3 (2.4)	-	-
Hypotension	3 (0.6)	1 (0.4)	-	-	-	-	2 (8.7)
Heart failure	3 (0.6)	-	-	-	1 (0.8)	-	2 (8.7)
Difficult airway management, n (%)	60 (12.4)	37 (16.5)	5 (25.0)	13 (21.0)	2 (1.6)	-	3 (13.0)
Technique changes necessary	31 (6.4)	22 (9.8)	1 (5)	5 (8.1)	1 (0.8)	-	2 (8.7)
Blind intubation	12 (2.5)	7 (3.1)	1 (5)	3 (4.8)	1 (0.8)	-	-
Primary technique difficulty	11 (2.3)	7 (3.1)	2 (10)	2 (8.1)	-	-	-
Airway could not be secured	4 (0.8)	-	1 (5)	2 (8.1)	-	-	1 (4.3)
Prolonged ventilation due to difficult airway	2 (0.4)	1 (0.4)	-	1 (1.6)	-	-	-
Other Events, n (%)	13 (2.7)	5 (2.2)	1 (5.0)	4 (6.5)	2 (1.6)	-	1 (4.3)
Seizures	5 (1.0)	1 (0.4)	-	2 (3.2)	2 (1.6)	-	-
Fever	4 (0.8)	3 (1.3)	-	-	-	-	1 (4.3)
Delirium	2 (0.4)	-	1 (5.0)	1 (1.6)	-	-	-
Neurological residues	2 (0.4)	1 (0.4)	-	1 (1.6)	-	-	-

Until discharge, 64 postoperative events occurred in 39 study cases (22 patients) with more than one postoperative event in 41% ($n = 16$). The most frequent complications were respiratory insufficiency ($n = 21$), acute airway obstruction ($n = 15$; i.e., stridor $n = 9$, collapsed trachea $n = 2$, soft tissue swelling $n = 1$, glossoptosis $n = 1$, both-sided vocal cord paralysis $n = 1$, bronchospasm ($n = 1$), pneumonia ($n = 6$), seizures ($n = 5$), fever ($n = 4$) and atelectasis ($n = 3$). Other postoperative events comprised delirium ($n = 2$), heart failure ($n = 2$), tachycardia ($n = 1$), bronchospasm ($n = 1$), both-sided pneumothorax ($n = 1$), temporary neurological deficit ($n = 1$, MPSIH) and permanent tetraplegia ($n = 1$, MPSII). Anaesthesia-related postoperative death occurred in two cases (postoperative mortality rate: 0.4%), in both cases by cardiorespiratory decompensation on the backdrop of a difficult airway management. The first, previously described [11] patient was a 14-year-old boy with MPSII, who suffered from a severe fulminant laryngo-bronchospasm during fiberoptic intubation resulting in hypoxic cardiac arrest and death eight hours afterwards despite immediate cardiopulmonary resuscitation and emergency tracheotomy. The second patient was a 38-year-old woman with MPSVI who underwent emergency surgery of an incarcerated hernia. An extubation attempt on the first postoperative day resulted in re-intubation due to respiratory insufficiency. Tracheostomy was anatomically impossible, and weaning did not succeed. Ventilation became increasingly difficult, requiring high ventilation pressures due to a swollen and spastic airway. Based on severe aortic and mitral valve stenosis, the patient died of acute decompensated heart failure 25 days after surgery.

Within the study period of 16.7 years, the total number of anaesthesia measures increased each year, while the number of events stayed relatively stable (Figure 2). As a result, the probability of anaesthetic events decreased over time.

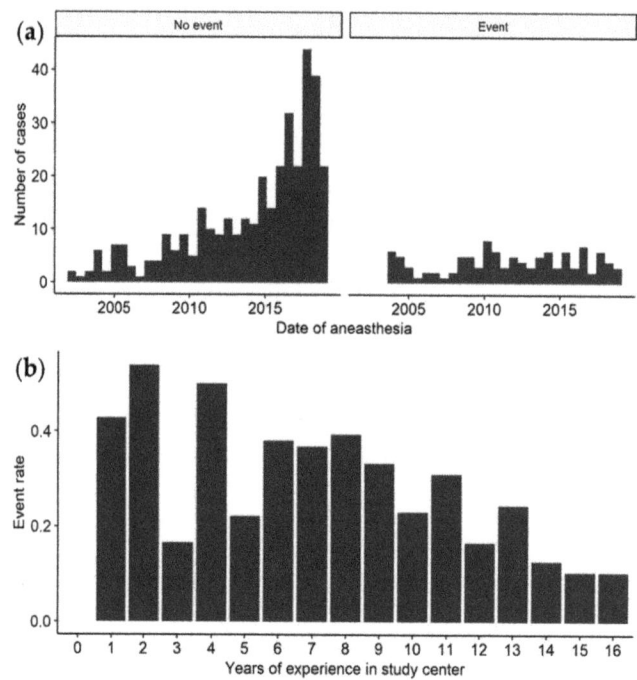

Figure 2. Centre experience. (**a**) Cases with and without events performed during the study period. (**b**) Event rates in different study intervals, calculated in years after inclusion of the first study patient.

3.5. Best Forecast Performance of Anaesthesia-Related Complications by a Model Based on Disease Manifestations, Disease-Specific Therapies and the Indication for Surgery

The clinical model, which was generated by means of automatic variable selection via lasso regression (Figure 3) included 469 observations. With a shrinkage parameter of 29, the model produced the following results: HSCT (OR 0.45, CI 0.20–1.03) and ERT (OR 0.74, CI 0.36–1.55) were associated with lower risk for events. Spine deformity (OR 1.94, CI 0.80–4.71), immobility (OR 3.80, CI 0.98–14.73), obstructive lung disease (OR 1.24, CI 0.59–2.61), hepatosplenomegaly (OR 3.10, CI 1.54–6.26) and scheduled major surgery (OR 6.64, CI 2.25–19.55) were associated with an increased risk and selected for model fitting. A comparison of the effect size and the confidence intervals distinguishes hepatosplenomegaly, immobility and a planned major surgery as the most relevant predictors for anaesthesia-related complications. All other variables that had been incorporated into the starting model, including the age, gender and subtype, were dismissed as predictors during the lasso selection process. The detailed model selection path is presented in the supplement (Figure S1). The model fit and predictive power were compared to the disease subtype-model (Figure 4). Patients with MPSIII had the lowest risk for anaesthesia-related complications. Patients with MPSIH (OR 5.16, CI 2.00–13.28), MPSIS (OR 8.52, CI 1.16–62.44), MPSII (OR 9.74, CI 3.15–30.15) and MPSVI (OR 20.60, CI 3.43–123.76) suffer from a substantially increased risk compared to MPSIII patients. However, in comparison of the clinical model with the subtype-model, the addition of patient-specific information in the starting models increases the model performance (AICc 460.4 vs. 467.7; AUC 0.880 vs. 0.834).

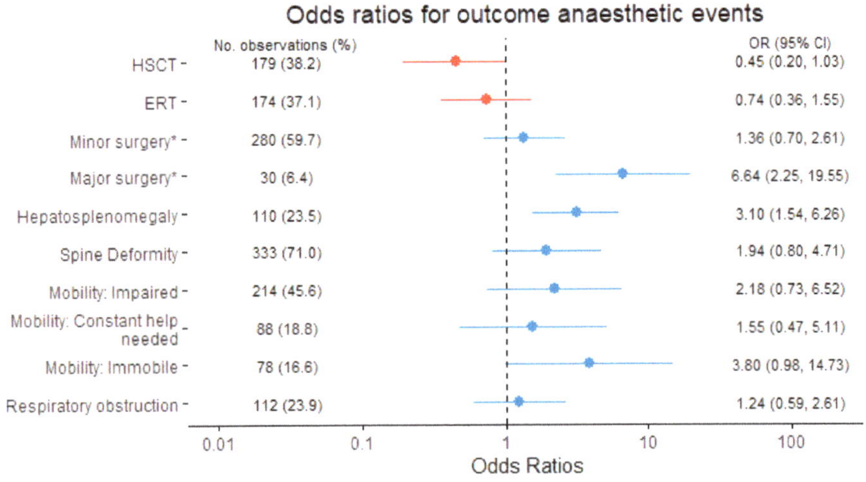

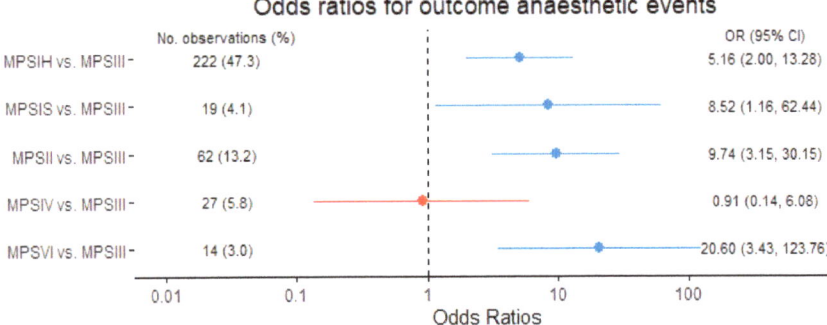

Figure 3. Estimated odds ratios and 95% confidence intervals (CI) for anaesthesia-related complications from a multivariable model based on automatic variable selection via lasso regression. Variables are presented in blue color (increased risk) or red color (decreased risk), respectively. * Reference: diagnostics and interventions. Abbreviations: CI, confidence interval; ERT, enzyme replacement therapy; HSCT, haematopoietic stem cell transplantation.

Figure 4. Estimated odds ratios and 95% confidence intervals (CI) for anaesthesia-related complications from a multivariable model based on disease subtypes. Variables are presented in blue color (increased risk) or red color (decreased risk), respectively. Abbreviations: CI, confidence interval; MPS, mucopolysaccharidosis.

4. Discussion

With 99 patients, the present study is one of the largest case series performed so far describing multi-organ manifestations in children and adults with the orphan disease MPS [17–19]. Moreover, with 484 anaesthetic cases in the study patients it is the largest study published as yet on anaesthetic risk in MPS and the first one to assess preoperative risk factors responsible for high peri- and postoperative morbidity [5]. In this study, almost a quarter of all cases experienced anaesthesia-related complications. According to the great phenotypical variability even within one MPS type, the best predictability power is not attributed to the underlying subtype, but to a prediction model based on the clinical manifestations and indication for anaesthesia. Precisely, this study suggests that the most relevant predictors for anaesthetic complications are hepatosplenomegaly, immobility, and planned major surgery.

By systematic chart review, this study specifies various disease manifestations in the different MPS types with a slight focus on symptoms relevant for anaesthesia planning. The natural history of MPSIII has so far only been described concerning neurocognition and behavioural patterns [20,21]. Hence, this is the first study on peripheral symptoms in MPSIII. Considering that no approved therapy exists for MPSIII, information on the natural disease course is essential to assess effects of evoking therapies. This is also one of the first studies to comprehend peripheral symptoms in a large transplanted MPSI patient cohort. Furthermore, specifics on spine disease have never been published for different disease types [22].

The prevalent MPS types vary globally. In Germany, most MPS patients suffer from MPSIII (44%), followed by MPSI (20%), MPSII (18%), MPSIV (11%) and MPSVI (7%) [12]. This order matches with the distribution pattern of this study with a shift towards MPSI as the division of paediatric stem cell transplantation of our institution is specialised in metabolic diseases. Concerning disease manifestations, it is noteworthy that airway-related symptoms such as macroglossia, sleep apnoea and airway obstruction were present throughout all MPS types, confirming the risk of difficult airway and the need for adequate precautions and postoperative monitoring potentially for all MPS patients. This is in line with a report by Berger et al. [2], who highlighted the frequency of respiratory problems in MPS, which are among the first symptoms. Patients with MPSIVA (Morquio A syndrome) can furthermore suffer from tracheal narrowing or tortuous appearance of the trachea or bronchi [23,24]. Considering the burden of spine disease in MPS [22], correct preoperative positioning is indispensable. In our study, despite precautions, two patients experienced temporary neurological deficits or even tetraplegia. Patients with MPSIVA are at particular risk for myelopathy during anaesthesia considering their skeletal phenotype with manifestations such as spinal deformities, cord compressions, adontoid hypoplasia and atlantoaxial instability, accompanied by ligamentous laxity [23,25,26]. This is supported by our data as 83% of the MPSIVA patients presented with cervical spine pathologies. Overall, 24% of the MPS patients manifested cervical spine instability and 62% cervical spine stenosis, which pose contraindications for extension of the head during intubation [5].

The overall event rate (22.7%) is consistent with the previous study performed by our centre (25.6%) [11]. The event rates vary between the different MPS types, with the highest burden in MPSII (38.7%), followed by MPSVI (31.8%) and MPSI (27.4%). For MPSIII, the event rate (7.2%) was only slightly higher than in the healthy population: 0.14–5.2% [27,28]. The overall 30-day in-hospital mortality of 0.4% is increased compared to the healthy paediatric population (0.1%) [27]. A high postoperative mortality has been described before by Arn et al., who reported on 32 of 196 deceased MPS patients, who had undergone surgery within one month of death [9].

Notably, during the study period over almost 17 years, the event rate has decreased substantially. The anaesthesia management of MPS patients hence became safer. As the ICLD is a specialised metabolic centre for MPS, a high MPS patient turnover also affects the anaesthesiologists to gain experience with this otherwise rare patient group. Actually, the necessity for an anaesthesia team experienced with MPS-specific challenges has already been deliberately emphasised on [5,25]. Nonetheless, the event rate over time should be interpreted with caution as the patient population may have changed with improved clinical management, including disease detection, specific therapies and multidisciplinary follow-up programs.

The multivariable regression models show that MPSII prones most for anaesthetic complications, followed by MPSVI and MPSI, respectively. However, additional patient-based information such as individual disease manifestations improve overall risk prediction. The model based on clinical aspects selected by the lasso regression has the best performance. In the final model, hepatosplenomegaly, immobility, and planned major surgery are the most important preoperative risk factors. Interestingly, not only the age and gender, but also the disease subtypes were dismissed as predictors in the automated parameter selection process of the clinical model. This suggests a substitution of the disease subtypes as a relevant predictor by clinical surrogate parameters. The manifestations hepatosplenomegaly and immobility imply a progressed disease stage or a poorly treated condition. Patients capable to perform lung function testing form a preselected patient group concerning age, disease type and progression (mental capacity). In case of sleep apnoea with the need for non-invasive ventilation, precautions such as postoperative transfer to the intensive care unit were taken. Therefore, respiratory manifestations might have been underestimated as predictors. As this study has an explorative design, the results of the multivariable models cannot be generalized or applied to other cohorts and hence are not designated for the clinical use. A score, by which the preoperative disease status can be translated into a predicted individual risk for anaesthetic complications requires an external validation. For this purpose, a prospective validation study is needed.

The clinical prediction model showed that disease-specific therapies might have a protective effect against anaesthesia-related complications. In the clinical multivariable model, HSCT is associated with a relevant risk reduction. Other studies strengthen our finding that HSCT decreases the overall event incidence [8,29]. Whether ERT actually has a protective effect remains unclear looking at the small effect size and large confidence interval. Other studies indicate that ERT alone does not improve difficult airway management in MPS Types I, II and VI [8,29]. Interestingly, the risk for anaesthesia-related complications was increased both in MPSIH and MPSIS to a similar extend. Thus, all individuals with MPSI are at high-risk.

In MPS patients with an expected difficult airway or cervical spine disease, intubation is typically facilitated by videolaryngoscopy or by use of a flexible bronchoscope with or without guidance via a supraglottic conduit. This approach produces the lowest conversion rate [5,11]. Our previous study suggested that the application of advanced techniques would be especially important for patients with MPS I, II, IV and VI [11,23]. Well noted, in this study, we aimed to analyse preoperative risk factors. Hence, the risk factor analysis of this study did not incorporate perioperative management factors (e.g., airway management, duration of anaesthesia). Thus, we cannot draw any concrete anaesthesia management recommendations from our findings. We previously found that airway management is the most important technical factor associated with anaesthetic events [11].

This study has few limitations. As the primary endpoint is a composite, we cannot differentiate which influencing factors exactly account for which type of adverse event. It is a retrospective study, so the documentation, also of the adverse events, may have been incomplete. Due to the high risk for anaesthetic complications in MPS, the indication for anaesthesia has to be carefully verified. For the purpose of primary endpoints, we could only include and describe patients, who actually underwent anaesthesia. The strict indication for anaesthesia and the centre experience may produce selection biases. For a better understanding and prediction of the actual risk, one would have to conduct a multi-centred, retrospective analysis of anaesthesias performed in unawareness of the risk.

5. Conclusions

The present study gives full particulars of the multi-morbidity of 99 MPS patients undergoing anaesthesia and is with 484 anaesthetic cases the largest cohort published so far. The rate of anaesthesia-related complications was as high as 22.7%. This study suggests that the most relevant predictors are planned major surgery, hepatosplenomegaly, and immobility, surrogate parameters for a generally advanced disease stage or an insufficiently or untreated condition. Disease-specific therapies such as HSCT and ERT produce an overall protective effect. Nonetheless, multidisciplinary preoperative diagnostics are indispensable in all patients. The burden of cardiorespiratory manifestations and spine disease call for carefully planned patient positioning and postoperative monitoring, if applicable at the intensive care unit. A better prediction of the anaesthetic risk might enable more patient-based and feasible precautionary measures. For this purpose, a prospective validation study is needed, to generate a score, by which the preoperative disease status can be translated into an individual risk assessment for anaesthetic complications.

Supplementary Materials: The following are available online at https://www.mdpi.com/2077-0383/10/16/3518/s1, Table S1: cervical spine disease in MPS. Table S2: characteristics or anaesthetic cases. Figure S1: variable selection path for the model based on the lasso method.

Author Contributions: Conceptualization, M.P., N.M.M., L.S.A. and T.D.; formal analysis, L.S.A., T.D., A.L., M.P. and N.M.M.; data acquisition, A.L., L.S.A., T.D. and S.R.B.; statistical analysis, A.-K.O. and T.D.; writing—original draft preparation, L.S.A. and T.D.; writing—review and editing, L.S.A., T.D., M.P., N.M.M. and A.-K.O.; visualization and editing, L.S.A. and T.D.; supervision, M.P. and N.M.M.; All authors have read and agreed to the published version of the manuscript.

Funding: This research received no external funding.

Institutional Review Board Statement: The study was conducted according to the guidelines of the Declaration of Helsinki, and approved by the ethical committee of the medical board Hamburg, Germany (ethical code number WF-056/18, 30 October 2018).

Informed Consent Statement: Patient consent was waived as this is a retrospective chart analysis of anonymized data acquired during clinical routine visits.

Data Availability Statement: The data that support the findings of this study are available from the corresponding author, upon reasonable request. The data are not publicly available to ensure, that the privacy of the study patients with rare diseases is not compromised.

Conflicts of Interest: The authors declare no conflict of interest.

References

1. Galimberti, C.; Madeo, A.; Di Rocco, M.; Fiumara, A. Mucopolysaccharidoses: Early diagnostic signs in infants and children. *Ital. J. Pediatr.* **2018**, *44*, 133. [CrossRef]
2. Berger, K.I.; Fagondes, S.C.; Giugliani, R.; Hardy, K.A.; Lee, K.S.; McArdle, C.; Scarpa, M.; Tobin, M.J.; Ward, S.A.; Rapoport, D.M. Respiratory and sleep disorders in mucopolysaccharidosis. *J. Inherit. Metab. Dis.* **2013**, *36*, 201–210. [CrossRef]
3. De Ru, M.H.; Boelens, J.J.; Das, A.M.; Jones, S.A.; van der Lee, J.H.; Mahlaoui, N.; Mengel, E.; Offringa, M.; O'Meara, A.; Parini, R.; et al. Enzyme replacement therapy and/or hematopoietic stem cell transplantation at diagnosis in patients with mucopolysaccharidosis type I: Results of a European consensus procedure. *Orphanet J. Rare Dis.* **2011**, *6*, 55. [CrossRef]
4. Arn, P.; Wraith, J.E.; Underhill, L. Characterization of surgical procedures in patients with mucopolysaccharidosis type I: Findings from the MPS I Registry. *J. Pediatr.* **2009**, *154*, 859–864. [CrossRef] [PubMed]
5. Moretto, A.; Bosatra, M.G.; Marchesini, L.; Tesoro, S. Anesthesiological risks in mucopolysaccharidoses. *Ital. J. Pediatr.* **2018**, *44*, 116. [CrossRef]
6. Walker, R.; Belani, K.G.; Braunlin, E.A.; Bruce, I.A.; Hack, H.; Harmatz, P.R.; Jones, S.; Rowe, R.; Solanki, G.A.; Valdemarsson, B. Anaesthesia and airway management in mucopolysaccharidosis. *J. Inherit. Metab. Dis.* **2013**, *36*, 211–219. [CrossRef] [PubMed]
7. Scaravilli, V.; Zanella, A.; Ciceri, V.; Bosatra, M.; Flandoli, C.; La Bruna, A.; Sosio, S.; Parini, R.; Gasperini, S.; Pesenti, A.; et al. Safety of anesthesia for children with mucopolysaccharidoses: A retrospective analysis of 54 patients. *Paediatr. Anaesth.* **2018**, *28*, 436–442. [CrossRef]
8. Kirkpatrick, K.; Ellwood, J.; Walker, R.W. Mucopolysaccharidosis type I (*Hurler syndrome*) and anesthesia: The impact of bone marrow transplantation, enzyme replacement therapy, and fiberoptic intubation on airway management. *Paediatr. Anaesth.* **2012**, *22*, 745–751. [CrossRef] [PubMed]
9. Arn, P.; Whitley, C.; Wraith, J.E.; Webb, H.W.; Underhill, L.; Rangachari, L.; Cox, G.F. High rate of postoperative mortality in patients with mucopolysaccharidosis I: Findings from the MPS I Registry. *J. Pediatr. Surg.* **2012**, *47*, 477–484. [CrossRef] [PubMed]
10. Jöhr, M.; Berger, T.M. Fiberoptic intubation through the laryngeal mask airway (LMA) as a standardized procedure. *Paediatr. Anaesth.* **2004**, *14*, 614. [CrossRef] [PubMed]
11. Dohrmann, T.; Muschol, N.M.; Sehner, S.; Punke, M.A.; Haas, S.A.; Roeher, K.; Breyer, S.; Koehn, A.F.; Ullrich, K.; Zöllner, C.; et al. Airway management and perioperative adverse events in children with mucopolysaccharidoses and mucolipidoses: A retrospective cohort study. *Paediatr. Anaesth.* **2020**, *30*, 181–190. [CrossRef]
12. Zhou, J.; Lin, J.; Leung, W.T.; Wang, L. A basic understanding of mucopolysaccharidosis: Incidence, clinical features, diagnosis, and management. *Intractable Rare Dis. Res.* **2020**, *9*, 1–9. [CrossRef]
13. Madoff, L.U.; Kordun, A.; Cravero, J.P. Airway management in patients with mucopolysaccharidoses: The progression toward difficult intubation. *Paediatr. Anaesth.* **2019**, *29*, 620–627. [CrossRef]
14. Meyer, A.; Kossow, K.; Gal, A.; Mühlhausen, C.; Ullrich, K.; Braulke, T.; Muschol, N. Scoring evaluation of the natural course of mucopolysaccharidosis type IIIA (*Sanfilippo syndrome* type A). *Pediatrics* **2007**, *120*, e1255–e1261. [CrossRef] [PubMed]

15. Groll, A.; Trutz, G. Variable selection for generalized linear mixed models by L1-penalized estimation. *Stat. Comput.* **2014**, *24*, 137–154. [CrossRef]
16. Bates, D.; Maechler, M.; Bolker, B.; Walker, S. Fitting Linear Mixed-Effects Models Using lme4. *J. Stat. Softw.* **2015**, *67*, 1–48. [CrossRef]
17. Arn, P.; Bruce, I.A.; Wraith, J.E.; Travers, H.; Fallet, S. Airway-related symptoms and surgeries in patients with mucopolysaccharidosis I. *Ann. Otol. Rhinol. Laryngol.* **2015**, *124*, 198–205. [CrossRef] [PubMed]
18. Beck, M.; Arn, P.; Giugliani, R.; Muenzer, J.; Okuyama, T.; Taylor, J.; Fallet, S. The natural history of MPS I: Global perspectives from the MPS I Registry. *Genet. Med. Off. J. Am. Coll. Med. Genet.* **2014**, *16*, 759–765. [CrossRef] [PubMed]
19. Montaño, A.M.; Tomatsu, S.; Gottesman, G.S.; Smith, M.; Orii, T. International Morquio A Registry: Clinical manifestation and natural course of Morquio A disease. *J. Inherit. Metab. Dis.* **2007**, *30*, 165–174. [CrossRef] [PubMed]
20. Shapiro, E.G.; Jones, S.A.; Escolar, M.L. Developmental and behavioral aspects of mucopolysaccharidoses with brain manifestations—Neurological signs and symptoms. *Mol. Genet. Metab.* **2017**, *122*, 1–7. [CrossRef] [PubMed]
21. Shapiro, E.G.; Escolar, M.L.; Delaney, K.A.; Mitchell, J.J. Assessments of neurocognitive and behavioral function in the mucopolysaccharidoses. *Mol. Genet. Metab.* **2017**, *122*, 8–16. [CrossRef] [PubMed]
22. Remondino, R.G.; Tello, C.A.; Noel, M.; Wilson, A.F.; Galaretto, E.; Bersusky, E.; Piantoni, L. Clinical Manifestations and Surgical Management of Spinal Lesions in Patients With Mucopolysaccharidosis: A Report of 52 Cases. *Spine Deform.* **2019**, *7*, 298–303. [CrossRef] [PubMed]
23. Theroux, M.C.; Nerker, T.; Ditro, C.; Mackenzie, W.G. Anesthetic care and perioperative complications of children with Morquio syndrome. *Paediatr. Anaesth.* **2012**, *22*, 901–907. [CrossRef]
24. Averill, L.W.; Kecskemethy, H.H.; Theroux, M.C.; Mackenzie, W.G.; Pizarro, C.; Bober, M.B.; Ditro, C.P.; Tomatsu, S. Tracheal narrowing in children and adults with mucopolysaccharidosis type IVA: Evaluation with computed tomography angiography. *Pediatr. Radiol.* **2021**, *51*, 1202–1213. [CrossRef] [PubMed]
25. Charrow, J.; Alden, T.D.; Breathnach, C.A.; Frawley, G.P.; Hendriksz, C.J.; Link, B.; Mackenzie, W.G.; Manara, R.; Offiah, A.C.; Solano, M.L.; et al. Diagnostic evaluation, monitoring, and perioperative management of spinal cord compression in patients with Morquio syndrome. *Mol. Genet. Metab.* **2015**, *114*, 11–18. [CrossRef]
26. Tomatsu, S.; Mackenzie, W.G.; Theroux, M.C.; Mason, R.W.; Thacker, M.M.; Shaffer, T.H.; Montaño, A.M.; Rowan, D.; Sly, W.; Alméciga-Díaz, C.J.; et al. Current and emerging treatments and surgical interventions for Morquio A syndrome: A review. *Res. Rep. Endocr. Disord.* **2012**, *2012*, 65–77. [CrossRef] [PubMed]
27. Habre, W.; Disma, N.; Virag, K.; Becke, K.; Hansen, T.G.; Jöhr, M.; Leva, B.; Morton, N.S.; Vermeulen, P.M.; Zielinska, M.; et al. Incidence of severe critical events in paediatric anaesthesia (APRICOT): A prospective multicentre observational study in 261 hospitals in Europe. *Lancet Respir. Med.* **2017**, *5*, 412–425. [CrossRef]
28. Kurth, C.D.; Tyler, D.; Heitmiller, E.; Tosone, S.R.; Martin, L.; Deshpande, J.K. National pediatric anesthesia safety quality improvement program in the United States. *Anesth. Analg.* **2014**, *119*, 112–121. [CrossRef] [PubMed]
29. Frawley, G.; Fuenzalida, D.; Donath, S.; Yaplito-Lee, J.; Peters, H. A retrospective audit of anesthetic techniques and complications in children with mucopolysaccharidoses. *Paediatr. Anaesth.* **2012**, *22*, 737–744. [CrossRef]

Article

Molecular Diagnosis of Pompe Disease in the Genomic Era: Correlation with Acid Alpha-Glucosidase Activity in Dried Blood Spots

Fanny Thuriot [1,2], Elaine Gravel [1,2], Katherine Hodson [3], Jorge Ganopolsky [3], Bojana Rakic [4], Paula J. Waters [1], Serge Gravel [1,2] and Sébastien Lévesque [1,2,*]

1. Department of Pediatrics, Université de Sherbrooke, Sherbrooke, QC J1H 5H3, Canada; Fanny.Thuriot@USherbrooke.ca (F.T.); Elaine.Gravel@USherbrooke.ca (E.G.); Paula.J.Waters@USherbrooke.ca (P.J.W.); Serge.Gravel@USherbrooke.ca (S.G.)
2. Sherbrooke Genomic Medicine, Sherbrooke, QC J1H 5H3, Canada
3. Dynacare, Laval, QC H7L 4S3, Canada; hodsonk@dynacare.ca (K.H.); ganopolskyj@dynacare.ca (J.G.)
4. BC Children's Hospital, Vancouver, BC V6H 3N1, Canada; bojana.rakic@cw.bc.ca
* Correspondence: Sebastien.A.Levesque@USherbrooke.ca

Abstract: Measurement of alpha-glucosidase activity on dried blood spots has been the main method to screen for Pompe disease, but a paradigm shift has been observed in recent years with the incorporation of gene panels and exome sequencing in molecular diagnostic laboratories. An 89-gene panel has been available to Canadian physicians since 2017 and was analyzed in 2030 patients with a suspected muscle disease. Acid alpha-glucosidase activity was measured in parallel in dried blood spots from 1430 patients. Pompe disease was diagnosed in 14 patients, representing 0.69% of our cohort. In 7 other patients, low enzyme activities overlapping those of Pompe disease cases were attributable to the presence of pseudodeficiency alleles. Only two other patients had enzymatic activity in the Pompe disease range, and a single heterozygous pathogenic variant was identified. It is possible that a second variant could have been missed; we suggest that RNA analysis should be considered in such cases. With gene panel testing increasingly being performed as a first-tier analysis of patients with suspected muscle disorders, our study supports the relevance of performing reflex enzymatic activity assay in selected patients, such as those with a single *GAA* variant identified and those in whom the observed genotype is of uncertain clinical significance.

Keywords: Pompe disease; gene panel sequencing; alpha-glucosidase; GAA; dried-blood spots

1. Introduction

Pompe disease is an autosomal recessive disorder caused by pathogenic variants in the *GAA* gene, which encodes an acid alpha-glucosidase enzyme [1]. This lysosomal glycogen storage disorder has a prevalence of 1:40,000 in individuals in the United States, with increased incidence in African Americans [2,3]. It may present at any age, from infancy to late adulthood [4]. Patients with infantile onset Pompe disease (IOPD) often present with hypotonia, respiratory insufficiency, and cardiomyopathy, resulting in death in the first year of life if untreated. Patients with late onset Pompe disease (LOPD) present with a slowly progressive phenotype, including muscle weakness, mainly limb-girdle, and respiratory failure [5]. Most adult patients share the common c.-32-13T>G leaky splicing variant [6]. Because of the variable severity of this disease, its rarity, and the extensive differential diagnoses, diagnosis is typically made years after the onset of symptoms [7,8]. In 2006, enzyme replacement therapy was first approved to treat patients with Pompe disease [9]. To be effective, the treatment must be administered as soon as possible, as delay may cause irreversible damage [10]. In that context, newborn screening was proposed to enable early diagnosis. Several pilot studies subsequently demonstrated its favorable impact on patient outcomes, leading to the introduction of population newborn screening for Pompe disease in some jurisdictions [11,12]. To provide a low-cost and rapid screening test, dried blood spots (DBS) are used to measure acid alpha-glucosidase enzymatic activity, by fluorometric assays or by tandem mass spectrometry [11,13]. However, pseudodeficiency alleles can generate false-positive results, as these benign hypomorphic variants cause a decrease in the observed enzymatic activity, but without causing Pompe disease. To confirm diagnosis, sequencing analysis of the *GAA* gene must be performed [14,15].

With decreasing cost of sequencing technologies, targeted and whole-exome sequencing have increasingly been used to diagnose patients with Pompe disease, especially in adults with suggestive symptoms or in populations where newborn screening is not yet available. These methods have been shown to have a high diagnostic yield in contexts where differential diagnoses, such as other limb-girdle muscular dystrophies (LGMD), cannot be discounted [16–18].

Here we present data supporting the use of acid alpha-glucosidase enzymatic assay on dried blood spot as a reflex test following molecular analysis, for the confirmation of diagnosis of Pompe disease in symptomatic patients.

2. Materials and Methods

Clinical molecular testing was performed on a total of 2030 pediatric and adult patients with a suspected muscle disorder who were followed in outpatient clinics across Canada (general neurology, specialized neuromuscular, clinical genetics). To be eligible for testing, the patient had to have no reported diagnosis explaining their phenotype and to present weakness (any pattern) or symptom(s) suggestive of muscle involvement (i.e., myalgia, rhabdomyolysis, exercise intolerance, or unexplained respiratory insufficiency). Most patients (93.5%) also presented at least one abnormal laboratory finding suggestive of muscle involvement (plasma creatine kinase (CK), EMG, muscle biopsy, or MRI). Demographics and clinical information were obtained from the laboratory requisition [18]. Genetic counselling and follow up tests were recommended, when appropriate, to the referring physician. Patients were referred to different specialized genetic services across the country, and additional genetic counselling support was available at Dynacare (Laval, QC, Canada) by phone or virtual consultation when needed.

2.1. Acid Alpha-Glucosidase Enzymatic Activity Assays

Dried blood spots (DBS) were collected for measurement of acid alpha-glucosidase activity at either Dynacare laboratory (Laval, QC, Canada) or the BC Children's Hospital (Vancouver, BC, Canada). Both laboratories used similar fluorometric assays, based on a previously published methodology [13] with minor modifications. These assays rely upon enzymatic cleavage of the alpha-glucosidase substrate 4-methylumbelliferyl-alpha-D-glucopyranoside (4-MUG) at acidic pH in the presence of acarbose, which inhibits potentially interfering isoenzymes, such as maltose-glycoamylase. After stopping the enzymatic reaction by addition of a strongly alkaline buffer, fluorescence of the free 4-methylumbelliferone (4-MU) reaction product is measured, and its concentration calculated using a 4-MU calibration curve. Both laboratories also assayed at least one other enzyme in parallel (data not shown), which provided a control for specimen quality. Further information on assay procedures specific to each laboratory are summarised as follows.

At Dynacare, an extract containing the enzyme was eluted from a 3 mm DBS punch with 40 mM sodium acetate buffer (pH 3.8) for 1 h at 4 °C, then incubated with 4-MUG for 20 h at 37 °C in the presence of acarbose. Fluorescence was read with a fluorometer with excitation at 355 nm and emission at 460 nm, within one hour after stopping the enzymatic reaction with 150 mM EDTA, pH 11.3–12. Acid alpha-glucosidase enzymatic activity was expressed in pmol/hour/punch. Cut-off values were 4.49 and 5.39 pmol/hour/punch for "reduced" and "borderline" enzymatic activities, respectively. Values above 5.39 pmol/hour/punch were considered normal.

At BC Children's Hospital, two 3 mm DBS punches from each specimen were extracted with 400 µL of deionized water in a 1.5 mL microcentrifuge tube. Each sample was vortexed for 10 s followed by gentle mixing at room temperature for 1 h on a rocking platform. After 1 h the tubes were spun in a refrigerated centrifuge (11,600 rpm, 5 min). The working substrate solution was 2.8 mM 4-MUG in 40 mM sodium acetate buffer, pH 3.8, with 15 µM acarbose. Enzyme reactions consisted of 32 µL DBS extract and 48 µL substrate solution. The reactions were incubated overnight for 20 h at 37 °C in a PCR machine. DBS extracts for blanks were also incubated. After 20 h the reaction was stopped by adding 160 µL of 10 mM NaOH stop buffer, pH 10.5, to all tubes including blanks. Fluorescence was measured in a 96-well plate (Synergy 2 microplate reader). Results for acid alpha-glucosidase activity were reported with a normal reference range of 2.0–9.4 pmol/h/µL).

Since enzymatic activity assays for patients in this study were performed by two different laboratories, we normalized each reported value relative to the corresponding lower limit of the normal reference range. We do not have DBS values for all patients who underwent gene panel testing because parallel enzymatic testing was not supported at the beginning of the program. Enzyme activity results were available for 1430 patients (1314 measured at Dynacare; 108 measured at BC Children's Hospital), representing 70.4% of the study cohort.

2.2. Gene Panel and Next Generation Sequencing Method

Blood samples were collected to extract genomic DNA using a MagnaPure instrument (Roche, MA). A clinical gene panel test was performed at the Sherbrooke Genomic Medicine laboratory (a not-for-profit organization), and the cost of the test was covered by a special program with financial support from Sanofi Genzyme Canada. This gene panel included the *GAA* gene for Pompe disease, and genes with muscle-associated disorders, mainly limb-girdle muscular dystrophies, but also congenital muscular dystrophies, congenital myasthenic syndromes, nemaline myopathy, myofibrillar myopathy, centronuclear myopathy, collagen VI–related myopathies, inclusion myopathies, metabolic myopathies, rigid spine syndromes, and scapuloperoneal syndromes [18]. DNA libraries were prepared according to standard protocol (Kapa Biosystems, Roche, MA), following targeted capture (xGen Predesigned Gene Capture Pools, Integrated DNA Technologies, Kanata, ON, Canada, and sequencing on a NextSeq 550 (Illumina, CA, USA) sequencer with a 150-bp paired-end protocol.

2.3. Splicing Analysis

Blood sample was collected in Tempus Blood RNA Tubes and RNA was extracted using MagMAX™ for Stabilized Blood Tubes RNA Isolation Kit, according to standard protocol (ThermoFisher, Waltham, MA, USA). RNA integrity was assessed with an Agilent 2100 Bioanalyzer (Agilent Technologies, Saint-Laurent, QC, Canada). Reverse transcription was performed on 750 ng total RNA with Transcriptor reverse transcriptase, random hexamers, dNTPs (Roche Diagnostics, Laval, QC, Canada), and 10 units of RNAse OUT (Invitrogen, Waltham, MA, USA) following the manufacturer's protocol in a total volume of 10 µL. All forward and reverse primers were individually resuspended to 20–100 µM stock solution in Tris-EDTA buffer (IDT) and diluted as a primer pair to 1.2 µM in RNase DNase-free water (IDT). End-point PCR reactions were done on 10 ng cDNA in 10 µL final volume containing 0.2 mmol/L each dNTP, 0.6 µmol/L each primer, and 0.2 units of TransStart FastPfu Fly DNA Polymerase (Trans). An initial incubation of 2 min at 95 °C was followed by 35 cycles at 95 °C 20 s, 55 °C 20 s, and 72 °C 60 s. The amplification was completed by a 5-min incubation at 72 °C. PCR reactions are carried on thermocyclers C1000 Touch Thermal cycler (Bio-Rad), and the amplified products were analyzed by automated chip-based microcapillary electrophoresis on Labchip GX Touch HT instruments (Perkin Elmer, Woodbridge, ON, Canada). Amplicon sizing and relative quantitation was performed by the manufacturer's software, before being uploaded to the LIMS database.

2.4. Bioinformatics

We analyzed the sequencing data using a Linux-based bioinformatics pipeline based on the one developed by the McGill University and Genome Quebec Innovation Centre (bitbucket.org/mugqic/mugqic_pipelines (accessed on 14 June 2021)) as previously described [18]. Filtered variant lists obtained from the bioinformatics pipeline were then interpreted with an inhouse script and manual revision. Deletion and duplication analysis were performed using the CoNVaDING software [19] and manual review of binary alignment map files before quantitative PCR confirmation using Taqman Copy Number Assay (ThermoFisher Scientific, Montreal, QC, Canada). The recurrent *GAA* exon 18 deletion could be detected with both visual inspection of the sequencing reads and the CoNVaDING software, using a previously known positive control [17]. Variants were revised manually and were reported according to the American College of Medical Genetics and Genomics guidelines [20].

2.5. Statistical Analysis

Statistical analysis was performed using GraphPad Prism version 8.2.0 for Windows, GraphPad Software, San Diego, CA, USA, www.graphpad.com (accessed on 21 June 2021).

3. Results

3.1. Patients with Pompe Disease

A molecular diagnosis was identified in 272 of the 2030 patients. Of these, 14 patients were diagnosed with Pompe disease, representing 5.1% of all diagnoses, 1.15% of our LGMD patients, and 0.69% of our entire cohort. All 14 Pompe disease patients were found to be compound heterozygous for two variants, each considered pathogenic or likely pathogenic [20], in the *GAA* gene.

Among these patients with Pompe disease, 3 had IOPD, ranging from 1 month-old to 2 years-old. The 11 remaining patients had LOPD, ranging from 33 to 68 years-old (mean, 50 years-old). All patients with LOPD carried the c.-32-13T>G variant in a compound heterozygous state, whereas only one infantile onset patient carried the c.-32-13T>G variant. Most variants were identified in only one patient. All reported causal variants found in these patients are listed in Table 1. The c.1805C>T (p.Thr602Ile) variant was not previously known to be disease-causing, but was reclassified as likely pathogenic based on the very low acid alpha-glucosidase activity and the presence of a second pathogenic variant in a patient with phenotype consistent with IOPD. Later, the two variants were shown to be *in trans* following parental study.

Table 1. Pathogenic and likely pathogenic variants found in the *GAA* gene in patients with Pompe disease. All variants were observed only in the compound heterozygous state. Occurrence denotes the number of times each variant was observed in this group (14 patients; 28 alleles).

Pathogenic/Likely Pathogenic Variants	Occurrence
c.32-13T>G	12
c.655G>A (p.Gly219Arg)	2
c.1115A>T (p.His372Leu)	2
c.1-?_2859+?del (p.Met1_Cys952del)	1
c.258dupC (p.Asn87fs)	1
c.525delT (p.Glu176fs)	1
c.706delG (p.Val236fs)	1
c.896T>C (p.Leu299Pro)	1
c.1396dupG (p.Val466fs)	1
c.1551+1G>C	1
c.1805C>T (p.Thr602Ile)	1
c.1912G>T (p.Gly638Trp)	1
c.1927G>A (p.Gly643Arg)	1
c.2242dupG (p.Glu748fs)	1
c.2577G>A (p.Trp859*)	1

Patients with IOPD presented with hypotonia or limb-girdle weakness. One among the three IOPD cases did not show cardiomyopathy at the time of diagnosis.

All but one LOPD patient presented with limb-girdle weakness, and 5 of them presented with respiratory insufficiency as well. A single LOPD patient presented only with unexplained respiratory insufficiency and showed normal CK levels and EMG.

Among all patients with available CK data (12), only one patient (LOPD) had normal CK at the time of diagnosis.

3.2. Enzymatic Activity and Genotype

Among our cohort of 2030 patients, results of acid alpha-glucosidase activity were available for 1430 patients. Overall, 58 of the 1430 patients (4.1%) had a decreased enzymatic activity (Figure 1). Of those, only 14 (24.1%) had two pathogenic or likely pathogenic variants confirming the diagnosis of Pompe disease. Fourteen (24.1%) patients did not harbor any variant which could explain this decreased enzymatic activity. Conversely, all Pompe disease patients identified through the gene panel had a low enzymatic activity, as expected.

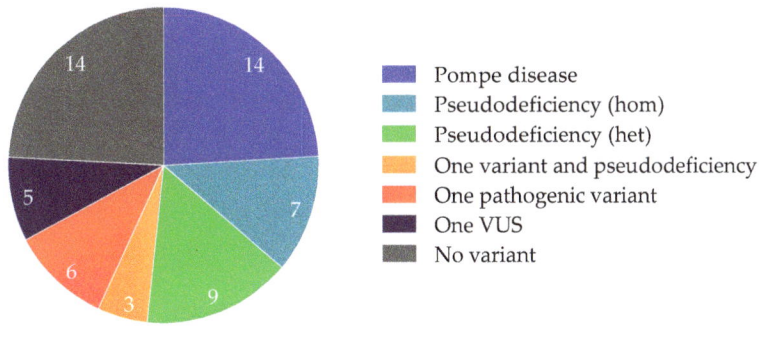

Figure 1. Genotype-based categories of patients with decreased acid alpha-glucosidase activity. Pompe disease—2 pathogenic or likely pathogenic *GAA* variants identified. Pseudodeficiency (hom)—One known pseudodeficiency allele was identified in a homozygous state, in the absence of any other identified variant. Pseudodeficiency (het)—One known pseudodeficiency allele was identified in a heterozygous state, in the absence of any other identified variant. One variant + pseudodeficiency—A single variant (pathogenic or of uncertain significance was identified in a heterozygous state, together with at least one known pseudodeficiency allele. One pathogenic variant—A single pathogenic or likely pathogenic variant was identified. One VUS—A single heterozygous variant of uncertain significance was identified. No variant—No variant of any kind was identified in the *GAA* gene.

Enzymatic activities, grouped according to the patients' *GAA* genotype categories, and the corresponding statistical comparisons using a Mann–Whitney test, are illustrated in Figure 2. The decreasing order of median values for enzymatic activities was as follows: no variant (2.35) > one VUS (1.96) > pseudodeficiency het (1.72) > one pathogenic variant (1.21) > one variant + pseudodeficiency (0.81) > pseudodeficiency hom (0.61) > Pompe disease (0.31). Enzymatic activity of patients with Pompe disease were statistically different from all other classes of genotype, including pseudodeficiency. Pompe disease patients had an enzymatic activity of less than 0.65 normalized activity, meaning less than 65% of activity of the lower reference limit.

Notably, 9 other patients had an enzymatic activity lower than 0.65, including 7 patients with pseudodeficiency alleles and 2 patients with a single pathogenic variant (c.-32-13T>G) identified. Of the 7 patients with pseudodeficiency alleles, 6 harboured these variants in the homozygous state and one in the heterozygous state. Enzymatic activity measurement was repeated for one of the patients with a single pathogenic variant, on a new specimen, giving a similar result. To exclude a possible second variant not detected by DNA sequencing of coding sequences, RNA studies were suggested to check for potential splicing defects (reflecting a deep intronic splicing variant) for the patient with repeated low enzymatic activity. However, the suggestion was declined by the referring physician, who considered that the patient's evolution was not suggestive of Pompe disease. Splicing studies could be performed on the second patient with a single pathogenic variant but no splicing defect was detected. Ultimately, none of these two patients received a diagnosis of Pompe disease nor did they have access to enzyme replacement therapy. Detailed clinical description of these patients was not available to us, therefore we could not exclude the possibility of Pompe disease. For comparison, we note that 8 other patients found to be heterozygous carriers of the c.-32-13T>G variant had normal enzymatic activity (>1.00), while 2 others showed "borderline" enzyme results (normalized activities between 0.65 and 1.00).

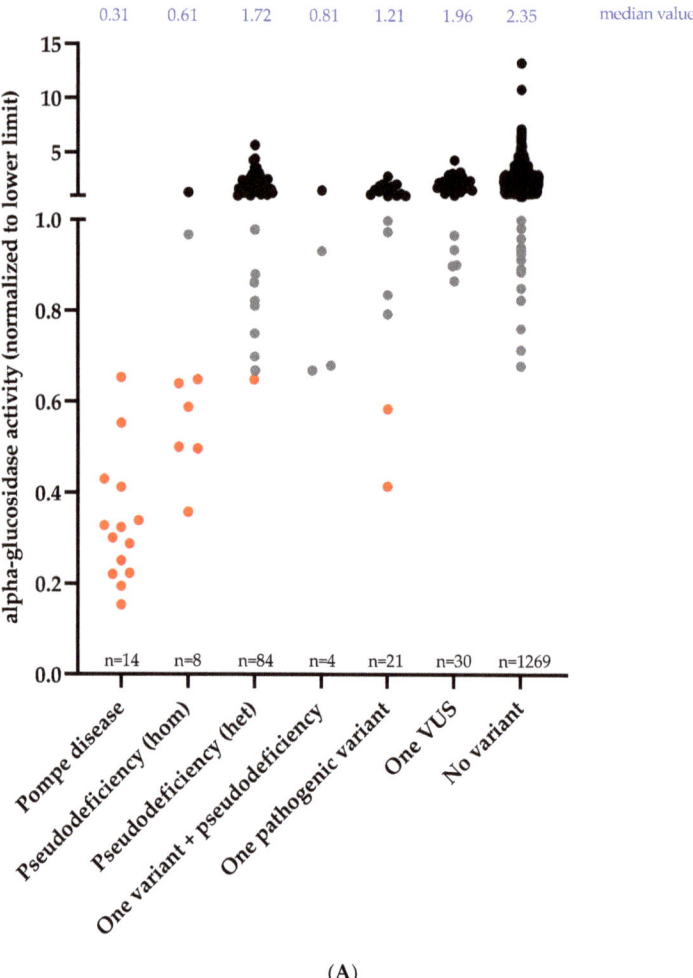

Figure 2. Cont.

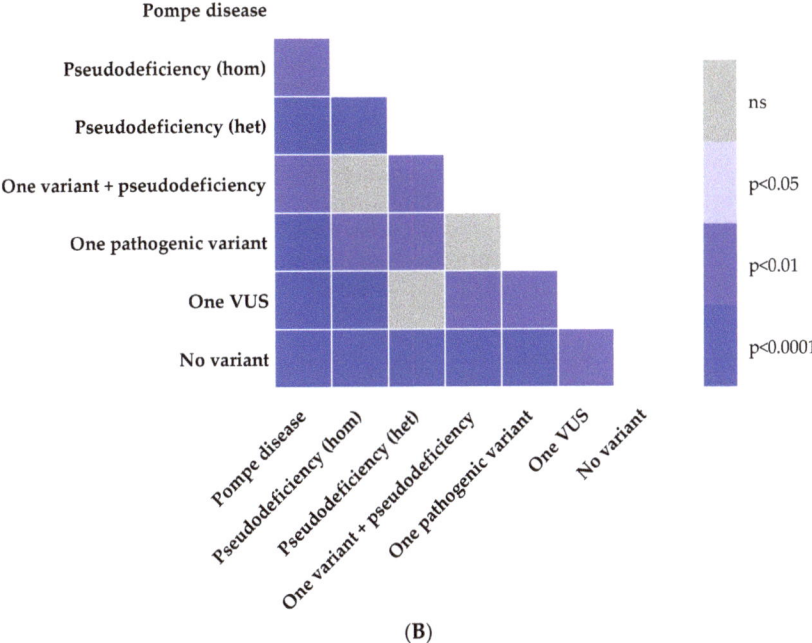

(B)

Figure 2. Acid alpha-glucosidase activity and genotypes of our cohort (n = 1430). Since enzymatic activity was assayed in two different centres, activity is reported normalized to the lower limit of the normal reference range according to the corresponding laboratory. (**A**) Black: normal enzymatic activity (>1.00); grey: borderline enzymatic activity (0.65–1.00); red: decreased enzymatic activity corresponding to the levels observed in Pompe disease (<0.65). The median value of each subgroup is reported in blue. (**B**) p values calculated using Mann–Whitney test. ns = not significant.

4. Discussion

Measurement of acid alpha-glucosidase activity on dried blood spots is used for newborn screening and has also been used widely in "high-risk" populations to screen for Pompe disease [11,12,21]. Although it is an efficient and low-cost approach to identify potential cases of Pompe disease, putative positive cases require confirmation by mutation analysis and exclusion of pseudodeficiency alleles [22]. The increased availability of gene panel and whole-exome sequencing is changing clinical practice, as these methods can address the wide differential diagnoses that are facing clinicians during their investigations of patients with muscle weakness. Measurement of acid alpha-glucosidase activity as a first-tier test in this context is therefore being questioned. In this study, we show the relevance of combining sequencing and enzymatic assays to avoid missing a diagnosis of Pompe disease or to clarify the implications of an observed variant of uncertain significance.

In our cohort, Pompe disease showed a prevalence of 0.69%, and accounted for 1.15% of patients with limb-girdle weakness. The clinical presentation of the 14 patients identified with Pompe disease is similar to historical cohorts and, not surprisingly, all LOPD cases carried the common c.-32-13T>G variant [23,24]. Table 2 provides a review of recent sequencing studies (2015–2021) which included more than 50 patients with muscle disorders. These studies cover wider genetic approaches such as whole-exome sequencing (WES) as well as targeted sequencing of gene panels [25–33]. The proportion of Pompe disease patients identified in our study is similar to previous studies, although it is slightly lower than the mean value of 1.27%. Variability in prevalence between studies is likely to be explained by differences in recruitment criteria. Indeed, some cohorts included only patients with limb-girdle muscular weakness, which is known to be the main type of weakness in patients with Pompe disease [34]. Since our cohort included other types of weakness, such as predominant distal weakness, it tended to incorporate patients with a broader spectrum of muscular disorders and thus dilute the proportion of Pompe patients. The higher proportion of 1.15% of Pompe disease within the group of patients with limb-girdle weakness supports this hypothesis. Finally, it is interesting to note that the rate of Pompe disease identified by these sequencing studies and our in patients presenting with limb-girdle weakness is similar to previous studies screening with measurement of acid alpha-glucosidase activity [15,35,36]. This suggests that if cases are missed by first-tier sequencing approaches (thus presumed to be heterozygous carriers), it is likely to represent a small proportion a priori.

Table 2. Literature review of cohorts including patients with Pompe disease.

Reference	Genetic Approach	Cohort	Number of Patients	Proportion of Pompe Patients	Recruitment
Ghaoui et al., 2015 PMID: 26436962 [30]	WES	LGMD	100	1.00%	Australia, retrospective research, muscle biopsies
Reddy et al., 2017 PMID: 27708273 [26]	WES	LGMD	55	1.82%	United States, research protocol
Chakravorty et al., 2020 PMID: 33250842 [27]	WES	Myopathy	201	1.00%	India, tertiary care hospital
Mean proportion of Pompe disease patients (whole-exome sequencing)				1.27%	
Töpf et al., 2020 PMID: 32528171 [31]	WES (429 genes analyzed)	LGMD and/or elevated CK	1001	1.00%	Europe and Middle East, 43 neuromuscular referral centers
Johnson et al., 2017 PMID: 29149851 [25]	WES (169 genes analyzed)	LGMD and/or elevated CK	606	1.98%	England, referred by clinicians
Nallamilli et al., 2018 PMID: 30564623 [28]	Targeted sequencing (35 genes)	LGMD	4656	0.82%	United States, Emory Genetics Laboratory
Savarese et al., 2018 PMID: 29880332 [32]	Targeted sequencing (93 genes)	LGMD, myopathies and/or isolated hyperCKemia	504	3.17%	Italy, tertiary centers for neuromuscular disorders
Bevilacqua et al., 2020 PMID: 31931849 [29]	Targeted sequencing (10 genes)	LGMD	2103	0.43%	Latin America, 20 institutions
Winder et al., 2020 PMID: 32337338 [33]	Targeted sequencing (266 genes)	Cardiomyopathy/skeletal muscle, muscular dystrophy, neuromuscular disorders, LGMD	6493	0.25%	United States, Invitae Laboratory
Mean proportion of Pompe disease patients (targeted sequencing)				1.28%	
This study	Targeted sequencing (89 genes)	Suspected muscle disorders	2030	0.69% (entire cohort) 1.15% (LGMD)	Canada, outpatient clinics

Our study provides a direct comparison between results of sequencing and enzymatic activity measurement. Acid alpha-glucosidase activity was assayed using dried blood spots and results were available for 1430 patients, representing 70.4% of our entire cohort. A total of 58 patients had decreased acid alpha-glucosidase activity, with Pompe disease accounting for a quarter of the patients with decreased enzymatic activity (<1.00 normalized activity). Another quarter was explained by pseudodeficiency. In a third quarter, only a single heterozygous *GAA* variant (pathogenic or of uncertain significance, together with a co-existing pseudodeficiency allele in some cases) was found. Finally, the last quarter was composed of patients without any detected *GAA* variant. However, by setting the threshold at 0.65 normalized activity, we showed that only 23 patients had enzymatic values falling within the range corresponding to Pompe disease. Fourteen were explained by molecularly confirmed Pompe disease, while seven were explained by the presence of one or more pseudodeficiency alleles, which are known to reduce enzymatic activity without causing clinical disease [15]. This and data from Figure 2 illustrate well the difficulty in differentiating homozygous pseudodeficiency alleles from Pompe disease cases based on enzyme activity alone. The two remaining low values represented two patients with only one pathogenic variant (c.-32-13T>G) identified; one whose enzymatic activity was confirmed to be low on a second specimen. In both cases, we were not able to confirm a diagnosis of Pompe disease. Either we did not have the opportunity to perform RNA studies to exclude the possibility that a second causal variant could have been missed, or the results of these studies did not suggest the presence of second variant. An example of such a deep intronic variant has been reported in a Pompe disease patient previously [37]. Although whole-genome sequencing has the potential to identify deep intronic variants, RNA studies and enzymatic activity measurement are likely to be required as reflex testing to confirm bioinformatic predictions of splicing events. The scarce availability of whole-genome sequencing and RNA sequencing in clinical laboratories probably explain why deep intronic variants are currently absent from the Pompe disease variants database [38]. Other factors such as promoter hypermethylation could be considered, and muscle biopsy remains helpful in absence of a second variant to support a diagnosis of Pompe disease by showing the pathogenic accumulation of glycogen.

Enzymatic activity measurement as a reflex test can also be used to reclassify variants of uncertain significance in certain circumstances. In particular, as illustrated by our patient carrying a pathogenic variant and the variant of uncertain significance c.1805C>T (p.Thr602Ile), a low enzyme activity consistent with Pompe disease may contribute to reclassify the latter as likely pathogenic, according to ACMG guidelines [20]. Indeed, ClinGen's expert panel has been working on a modified version of the ACMG guidelines for improvement of classification of variants in the *GAA* gene, and includes acid alpha-glucosidase activity in their interpretation in a variety of scenarios [39]; [https://clinicalgenome.org/site/assets/files/3969/clingen_lsd_acmg_specifications_v1.pdf (accessed on 22 June 2021)].

We conclude that a combined approach, using DNA sequencing followed by dried blood spot acid alpha-glucosidase activity assay as a reflex test when indicated, can be recommended as best practice to identify Pompe disease patients in the molecular era. Although the rate of diagnosis of Pompe disease is similar in LGMD patients using gene panels or WES compared to enzymatic screening, reflex enzymatic testing potentially decreases the risk of missing a diagnosis when only one pathogenic variant is detected by DNA sequencing, and may also be used to confirm or rule out a diagnosis of Pompe disease following the observation of a genotype of uncertain clinical significance.

Author Contributions: Conceptualization, S.G. and S.L.; methodology, F.T., E.G., K.H., J.G. and B.R.; software, F.T.; validation S.G. and S.L.; formal analysis, F.T., E.G., S.G. and S.L.; investigation, S.G and S.L.; resources, S.L.; data curation, F.T.; writing—original draft preparation, F.T and S.L.; writing—review and editing, E.G., K.H., J.G., B.R., P.J.W. and S.G.; visualization, F.T.; supervision, S.L.; project administration, S.L.; funding acquisition, S.L. All authors have read and agreed to the published version of the manuscript.

Funding: The cost of the test was covered by a special program with financial support from Sanofi Genzyme Canada.

Institutional Review Board Statement: The study was conducted according to the guidelines of the Declaration of Helsinki, and approved by the Institutional Ethics Review Board of Université de Sherbrooke (project ##MP-31-2013-533, 12-208, approved on 10 March 2015).

Informed Consent Statement: Informed consent was obtained from all subjects involved in the study.

Data Availability Statement: Anonymized data will be shared by request from any qualified investigator. When not possible, given the risk to identify rare patients, additional aggregate data in table form will be produced to address specific questions.

Acknowledgments: The authors are thankful to Elvy Lapointe and Mathieu Durand at the RNomics Platform (Université de Sherbrooke, QC, Canada) for her contribution to gene panel sequencing and his contribution for splicing analysis, Philippe Thibault and Safa Jammali for their help in bioinformatics, Dynacare for their contribution in samples' logistics and genetic counselling, Calcul Quebec and Compute Canada for providing part of the computing infrastructure used to analyze the data. They are also grateful to the patients and their families, neurologists, neuromuscular specialists, genetics counsellor, and clinical geneticists across Canada for their participation in this study. F. Thuriot is supported by doctoral scholarship from the Fonds de recherche du Quebec–Santé (FRQS).

Conflicts of Interest: S.G. and S.L. received speaker honoraria from Sanofi Genzyme. All other authors declare no conflicts of interest. The funders had no role in the design of the study, in the collection, analyses, or interpretation of data, in the writing of the manuscript, or in the decision to publish the results.

References

1. Dasouki, M.; Jawdat, O.; Almadhoun, O.; Pasnoor, M.; McVey, A.L.; Abuzinadah, A.R.; Herbelin, L.; Barohn, R.J.; Dimachkie, M.M. Pompe Disease. *Neurol. Clin.* **2014**, *32*, 751–776. [CrossRef]
2. Martiniuk, F.; Chen, A.; Mack, A.; Arvanitopoulos, E.; Chen, Y.; Rom, W.; Codd, W.J.; Hanna, B.; Alcabes, P.; Raben, N.; et al. Carrier frequency for glycogen storage disease type II in New York and estimates of affected individuals born with the disease. *Am. J. Med. Genet.* **1998**, *79*, 69–72. [CrossRef]
3. Chien, Y.-H.; Hwu, W.-L.; Lee, N.-C. Pompe Disease: Early Diagnosis and Early Treatment Make a Difference. *Pediatr. Neonatol.* **2013**, *54*, 219–227. [CrossRef] [PubMed]
4. van der Ploeg, A.T.; Reuser, A.J. Pompe's disease. *Lancet* **2008**, *372*, 1342–1353. [CrossRef]
5. Manganelli, F.; Ruggiero, L. Clinical features of Pompe disease. *Acta Myol.* **2013**, *32*, 82–84. [PubMed]
6. Dardis, A.; Zanin, I.; Zampieri, S.; Stuani, C.; Pianta, A.; Romanello, M.; Baralle, F.E.; Bembi, B.; Buratti, E. Functional characterization of the common c.-32-13T>G mutation of GAA gene: Identification of potential therapeutic agents. *Nucleic Acids Res.* **2014**, *42*, 1291–1302. [CrossRef]
7. Byrne, B.J.; Kishnani, P.S.; Case, L.; Merlini, L.; Müller-Felber, W.; Prasad, S.; van der Ploeg, A. Pompe disease: Design, methodology, and early findings from the Pompe Registry. *Mol. Genet. Metab.* **2011**, *103*, 1–11. [CrossRef]
8. Regnery, C.; Kornblum, C.; Hanisch, F.; Vielhaber, S.; Strigl-Pill, N.; Grunert, B.; Müller-Felber, W.; Glocker, F.X.; Spranger, M.; Deschauer, M.; et al. 36 months observational clinical study of 38 adult Pompe disease patients under alglucosidase alfa enzyme replacement therapy. *J. Inherit. Metab. Dis.* **2012**, *35*, 837–845. [CrossRef] [PubMed]
9. Van Der Ploeg, A.T.; Clemens, P.R.; Corzo, D.; Escolar, D.M.; Florence, J.; Groeneveld, G.J.; Herson, S.; Kishnani, P.S.; Laforet, P.; Lake, S.L.; et al. A Randomized Study of Alglucosidase Alfa in Late-Onset Pompe's Disease. *N. Engl. J. Med.* **2010**, *362*, 1396–1406. [CrossRef]
10. Prater, S.N.; Banugaria, S.G.; DeArmey, S.M.; Botha, E.G.; Stege, E.M.; Case, L.; Jones, H.N.; Phornphutkul, C.; Wang, R.; Young, S.P.; et al. The emerging phenotype of long-term survivors with infantile Pompe disease. *Genet. Med.* **2012**, *14*, 800–810. [CrossRef]
11. Bodamer, O.A.; Scott, C.R.; Giugliani, R. Pompe Disease Newborn Screening Working Group; on behalf of the Pompe Disease Newborn Screening Working Group Newborn Screening for Pompe Disease. *Pediatrics* **2017**, *140*, S4–S13. [CrossRef]
12. Sawada, T.; Kido, J.; Nakamura, K. Newborn Screening for Pompe Disease. *Int. J. Neonatal Screen.* **2020**, *6*, 31. [CrossRef] [PubMed]
13. Kallwass, H.; Carr, C.; Gerrein, J.; Titlow, M.; Pomponio, R.; Bali, D.; Dai, J.; Kishnani, P.; Skrinar, A.; Corzo, D.; et al. Rapid diagnosis of late-onset Pompe disease by fluorometric assay of α-glucosidase activities in dried blood spots. *Mol. Genet. Metab.* **2007**, *90*, 449–452. [CrossRef] [PubMed]
14. Peruzzo, P.; Pavan, E.; Dardis, A. Molecular genetics of Pompe disease: A comprehensive overview. *Ann. Transl. Med.* **2019**, *7*, 278. [CrossRef] [PubMed]
15. Niño, M.Y.; Wijgerde, M.; de Faria, D.O.S.; Hoogeveen-Westerveld, M.; Bergsma, A.J.; Broeders, M.; van der Beek, N.A.M.E.; Hout, H.J.M.V.D.; van der Ploeg, A.T.; Verheijen, F.W.; et al. Enzymatic diagnosis of Pompe disease: Lessons from 28 years of experience. *Eur. J. Hum. Genet.* **2021**, *29*, 434–446. [CrossRef]
16. Mori, M.; Haskell, G.; Kazi, Z.; Zhu, X.; DeArmey, S.M.; Goldstein, J.L.; Bali, D.; Rehder, C.; Cirulli, E.T.; Kishnani, P.S. Sensitivity of whole exome sequencing in detecting infantile- and late-onset Pompe disease. *Mol. Genet. Metab.* **2017**, *122*, 189–197. [CrossRef] [PubMed]
17. Lévesque, S.; Auray-Blais, C.; Gravel, E.; Boutin, M.; Dempsey-Nunez, L.; Jacques, P.-E.; Chenier, S.; LaRue, S.; Rioux, M.-F.; Al-Hertani, W.; et al. Diagnosis of late-onset Pompe disease and other muscle disorders by next-generation sequencing. *Orphanet J. Rare Dis.* **2016**, *11*, 8. [CrossRef]
18. Thuriot, F.; Gravel, E.; Buote, C.; Doyon, M.; Lapointe, E.; Marcoux, L.; Larue, S.; Nadeau, A.; Chénier, S.; Waters, P.J.; et al. Molecular diagnosis of muscular diseases in outpatient clinics. *Neurol. Genet.* **2020**, *6*, e408. [CrossRef]
19. Johansson, L.F.; Van Dijk, F.; De Boer, E.N.; Van Dijk-Bos, K.K.; Jongbloed, J.D.; Van Der Hout, A.H.; Westers, H.; Sinke, R.J.; Swertz, M.A.; Sijmons, R.H.; et al. CoNVaDING: Single Exon Variation Detection in Targeted NGS Data. *Hum. Mutat.* **2016**, *37*, 457–464. [CrossRef]
20. Richards, S.; Aziz, N.; Bale, S.; Bick, D.; Das, S.; Gastier-Foster, J.; Grody, W.W.; Hegde, M.; Lyon, E.; Spector, E.; et al. Standards and guidelines for the interpretation of sequence variants: A joint consensus recommendation of the American College of Medical Genetics and Genomics and the Association for Molecular Pathology. *Genet. Med.* **2015**, *17*, 405–423. [CrossRef]
21. Almeida, V.; Conceição, I.; Fineza, I.; Coelho, T.; Silveira, F.; Santos, M.; Valverde, A.; Geraldo, A.; Maré, R.; Aguiar, T.C.; et al. Screening for Pompe disease in a Portuguese high risk population. *Neuromuscul. Disord.* **2017**, *27*, 777–781. [CrossRef]
22. Jastrzębska, A.; Potulska-Chromik, A.; Łusakowska, A.; Jastrzębski, M.; Lipowska, M.; Kierdaszuk, B.; Kamińska, A.; Kostera-Pruszczyk, A. Screening for late-onset Pompe disease in Poland. *Acta Neurol. Scand.* **2019**, *140*, 239–243. [CrossRef]

23. Herbert, M.; Case, L.E.; Rairikar, M.; Cope, H.; Bailey, L.; Austin, S.L.; Kishnani, P.S. Early-onset of symptoms and clinical course of Pompe disease associated with the c.-32–13 T > G variant. *Mol. Genet. Metab.* **2019**, *126*, 106–116. [CrossRef] [PubMed]
24. Vanherpe, P.; Fieuws, S.; D'Hondt, A.; Bleyenheuft, C.; Demaerel, P.; De Bleecker, J.; Bergh, P.V.D.; Baets, J.; Remiche, G.; Verhoeven, K.; et al. Late-onset Pompe disease (LOPD) in Belgium: Clinical characteristics and outcome measures. *Orphanet J. Rare Dis.* **2020**, *15*, 83. [CrossRef]
25. Johnson, K.; Töpf, A.; Bertoli, M.; Phillips, L.; Claeys, K.; Stojanovic, V.R.; Perić, S.; Hahn, A.; Maddison, P.; Akay, E.; et al. Identification of GAA variants through whole exome sequencing targeted to a cohort of 606 patients with unexplained limb-girdle muscle weakness. *Orphanet J. Rare Dis.* **2017**, *12*, 173. [CrossRef]
26. Reddy, H.; Cho, K.-A.; Lek, M.; Estrella, E.; Valkanas, E.; Jones, M.D.; Mitsuhashi, S.; Darras, B.; Amato, A.A.; Lidov, H.G.; et al. The sensitivity of exome sequencing in identifying pathogenic mutations for LGMD in the United States. *J. Hum. Genet.* **2017**, *62*, 243–252. [CrossRef] [PubMed]
27. Chakravorty, S.; Nallamilli, B.R.R.; Khadilkar, S.V.; Singla, M.B.; Bhutada, A.; Dastur, R.; Gaitonde, P.S.; Rufibach, L.E.; Gloster, L.; Hegde, M. Clinical and Genomic Evaluation of 207 Genetic Myopathies in the Indian Subcontinent. *Front. Neurol.* **2020**, *11*, 559327. [CrossRef]
28. Nallamilli, B.R.R.; Chakravorty, S.; Kesari, A.; Tanner, A.; Ankala, A.; Schneider, T.; Da Silva, C.; Beadling, R.; Alexander, J.J.; Askree, S.H.; et al. Genetic landscape and novel disease mechanisms from a large LGMD cohort of 4656 patients. *Ann. Clin. Transl. Neurol.* **2018**, *5*, 1574–1587. [CrossRef] [PubMed]
29. Bevilacqua, J.A.; Ehuletche, M.D.R.G.; Perna, A.; Dubrovsky, A.; Franca, M.C.; Vargas, S.; Hegde, M.; Claeys, K.G.; Straub, V.; Daba, N.; et al. The Latin American experience with a next generation sequencing genetic panel for recessive limb-girdle muscular weakness and Pompe disease. *Orphanet J. Rare Dis.* **2020**, *15*, 1–11. [CrossRef] [PubMed]
30. Ghaoui, R.; Cooper, S.; Lek, M.; Jones, K.; Corbett, A.; Reddel, S.W.; Needham, M.; Liang, C.; Waddell, L.B.; Nicholson, G.; et al. Use of Whole-Exome Sequencing for Diagnosis of Limb-Girdle Muscular Dystrophy. *JAMA Neurol.* **2015**, *72*, 1424–1432. [CrossRef] [PubMed]
31. Töpf, A.; Johnson, K.; Bates, A.; Phillips, L.; Chao, K.R.; England, E.M.; Laricchia, K.M.; Mullen, T.; Valkanas, E.; Xu, L.; et al. Sequential targeted exome sequencing of 1001 patients affected by unexplained limb-girdle weakness. *Genet. Med.* **2020**, *22*, 1478–1488. [CrossRef] [PubMed]
32. Savarese, M.; Torella, A.; Musumeci, O.; Angelini, C.; Astrea, G.; Bello, L.; Bruno, C.; Comi, G.P.; Di Fruscio, G.; Piluso, G.; et al. Targeted gene panel screening is an effective tool to identify undiagnosed late onset Pompe disease. *Neuromuscul. Disord.* **2018**, *28*, 586–591. [CrossRef]
33. Winder, T.L.; Tan, C.A.; Klemm, S.; White, H.; Westbrook, J.M.; Wang, J.Z.; Entezam, A.; Truty, R.; Nussbaum, R.L.; McNally, E.M.; et al. Clinical utility of multigene analysis in over 25,000 patients with neuromuscular disorders. *Neurol. Genet.* **2020**, *6*, e412. [CrossRef] [PubMed]
34. Chan, J.; Desai, A.K.; Kazi, Z.; Corey, K.; Austin, S.; Hobson-Webb, L.D.; Case, L.E.; Jones, H.N.; Kishnani, P.S. The emerging phenotype of late-onset Pompe disease: A systematic literature review. *Mol. Genet. Metab.* **2017**, *120*, 163–172. [CrossRef] [PubMed]
35. Preisler, N.; Lukacs, Z.; Vinge, L.; Madsen, K.L.; Husu, E.; Hansen, R.S.; Duno, M.; Andersen, H.; Laub, M.; Vissing, J. Late-onset Pompe disease is prevalent in unclassified limb-girdle muscular dystrophies. *Mol. Genet. Metab.* **2013**, *110*, 287–289. [CrossRef]
36. Gutiérrez-Rivas, E.; Bautista, J.; Vílchez, J.; Muelas, N.; Diaz-Manera, J.; Illa, I.; Martínez-Arroyo, A.; Olive, M.; Sanz, I.; Arpa, J.; et al. Targeted screening for the detection of Pompe disease in patients with unclassified limb-girdle muscular dystrophy or asymptomatic hyperCKemia using dried blood: A Spanish cohort. *Neuromuscul. Disord.* **2015**, *25*, 548–553. [CrossRef]
37. Bergsma, A.J.; Groen, S.L.I.T.; Verheijen, F.W.; Van Der Ploeg, A.T.; Pijnappel, W.W.M.P. From Cryptic Toward Canonical Pre-mRNA Splicing in Pompe Disease: A Pipeline for the Development of Antisense Oligonucleotides. *Mol. Ther. Nucleic Acids* **2016**, *5*, e361. [CrossRef]
38. Reuser, A.J.J.; Van Der Ploeg, A.T.; Chien, Y.; Llerena, J.; Abbott, M.; Clemens, P.R.; Kimonis, V.E.; Leslie, N.; Maruti, S.S.; Sanson, B.; et al. GAA variants and phenotypes among 1,079 patients with Pompe disease: Data from the Pompe Registry. *Hum. Mutat.* **2019**, *40*, 2146–2164. [CrossRef]
39. Rivera-Muñoz, E.A.; Milko, L.V.; Harrison, S.M.; Azzariti, D.R.; Kurtz, C.L.; Lee, K.; Mester, J.L.; Weaver, M.A.; Currey, E.; Craigen, W.; et al. ClinGen Variant Curation Expert Panel experiences and standardized processes for disease and gene-level specification of the ACMG/AMP guidelines for sequence variant interpretation. *Hum. Mutat.* **2018**, *39*, 1614–1622. [CrossRef] [PubMed]

Review

Management of Corneal Clouding in Patients with Mucopolysaccharidosis

Orlaith McGrath *, Leon Au and Jane Ashworth

Manchester Royal Eye Hospital, Central Manchester University Hospitals NHS Foundation Trust, Oxford Road, Manchester M13 9WL, UK; leon.au@mft.nhs.uk (L.A.); jane.ashworth@mft.nhs.uk (J.A.)
* Correspondence: orlaith.mcgrath@mft.nhs.uk; Tel.: +44-0161-701-4841

Abstract: Mucopolysaccharidoses (MPS) are a rare group of lysosomal storage disorders characterized by the accumulation of incompletely degraded glycosaminoglycans (GAGs) in multiple organ systems including the eye. Visual loss occurs in MPS predominantly due to corneal clouding and retinopathy, but the sclera, trabecular meshwork and optic nerve may all be affected. Despite the success of therapies such as enzyme replacement therapy (ERT) and hematopoietic stem-cell transplantation (HSCT) in improving many of the systemic manifestations of MPS, their effect on corneal clouding is minimal. The only current definitive treatment for corneal clouding is corneal transplantation, usually in the form of a penetrating keratoplasty or a deep anterior lamellar keratoplasty. This article aims to provide an overview of corneal clouding, its current clinical and surgical management, and significant research progress.

Keywords: Mucopolysaccharidosis; corneal clouding; penetrating keratoplasty; deep anterior lamellar keratoplasty

1. Introduction

Corneal clouding resulting in photophobia and compromised vision is frequently observed in mucopolysaccharidoses (MPS) subtypes, including MPS I, MPS IV, MPS VI, and MPS VII [1]. While enzyme replacement therapy (ERT) and Hematopoietic stem-cell transplantation (HSCT), improve many of the systemic manifestations of MPS, vision loss remains a significant complication which may adversely affect quality of life. The MPS I registry quantified that over 80% of 302 patients had corneal clouding [2]. Ashworth et al. [1] showed that approximately 80% of 50 patients with MPS type I had visual acuity worse than 6/12 (Snellen) in their better eye and 11% had profound visual impairment (<3/60) in their better eye.

Visual deterioration in MPS occurs due to corneal clouding, retinopathy, glaucoma, and optic neuropathy [1]. (See Table 1 for a summary of the ocular manifestations of MPS). Patients developing retinopathy may complain of a decrease in their peripheral vision and nyctalopia [3]. However, this can be detracted from clinically by visual loss secondary to corneal clouding. Ultimately, the patient develops central visual field loss. Signs on fundus examination may include narrowing of arterioles, foveal external limiting membrane pigmentation/deposition, RPE atrophy, bulls eye maculopathy, and later, bone-spicules [1]. Widespread rod–cone dystrophy can occur [1].

Glycosaminoglycan (GAG) accumulation and consequential corneal thickening can lead to trabecular outflow obstruction and narrowing of the anterior chamber angle. Raised IOP can lead to damage to the optic nerve and glaucoma. In a multicenter case note review study involving four tertiary referral centers, the prevalence of glaucoma ranged from 2.1% to 12.5% in patients with MPS [4]. Peripheral corneal vascularization can develop in patients with MPS, due to blepharitis, exposure, or persistent corneal oedema secondary to raised IOP [5].

Table 1. Ocular findings in patients with mucopolysaccharidoses. Data from Ashworth et al. [1].

Disease	Corneal Opacity	Retinopathy	Optic Nerve Abnormalities	Glaucoma
MPS IH Hurler	Very common, mild to severe	Moderate, thickened ELM, parafoveal thinning, parafoveal retinal folds, bulls eye retinopathy	Common, mild to moderate	Uncommon, mild
MPS IH/S Hurler–Scheie	Very common, mild to severe	Moderate, retinal pigment epithelial degeneration	Common, mild to moderate	Uncommon, mild
MPS IS Scheie	Very common, mild to severe	Moderate	Quite common	Uncommon, mild
MPS II Hunter	Rare	Moderate, Pigmented retinopathy	Moderate	Uncommon
MPS III Sanfilippo A-D	Not usually significant	Moderate to severe, with pigmentary retinal degeneration	Rare	Rare
MPS IV Morquio	Some cases, usually mild	Pigmentary retinopathy	Some cases reported	Some cases reported
MPS VI Maroteau x-Lamy	Very common, often severe	Very rare, pigmented retinopathy, parafoveal retinal folds	Common	Unknown frequency
MPS VII Sly	Mild to moderate, can be severe	Unknown frequency	Quite common	Unknown frequency
MPS IX Natowicz	Unknown frequency	Unknown frequency	Unknown frequency	Unknown frequency

Shallow orbits that cause progressive pseudo-exophthalmos, hypertelorism, strabismus, hypermetropia, and astigmatism are common [1]. Non-ocular causes, such as cortical visual impairment, could also result in visual impairment [6]. Graft-versus-host disease is a rare complication following HSCT which could lead to conjunctivitis, keratoconjunctivitis sicca, corneal epithelial defects, and pseudo membrane formation [7]. Diagnosing ocular pathologies in patients with MPS can be a challenging task because of physical or mental disabilities which can reduce patient cooperation and tolerance of the exam. If dense, corneal clouding can interfere with accurate ophthalmological examination of the lens, vitreous, and retina [1,5,8–10]. Photophobia due to corneal clouding can lead to difficulty tolerating the slit lamp light beam [5].

In patients who have MPS, the frequency of ophthalmic involvement and related visual deterioration requires careful clinical examination, optimal glasses prescription, management of raised IOP and the corneal surface, and, when corneal clouding is the cause of the visual loss, corneal transplantation.

Corneal clouding treatment remains an unmet need in ophthalmology despite considerable advances in the systemic therapy of MPS. This review article aims to provide an overview of corneal clouding, its current clinical and surgical management, and noteworthy research progress.

2. Corneal Clouding in MPS

While corneal clouding is seen most commonly in MPS I, it is usually most severe in patients with MPS VI (see Figure 1, which demonstrates corneal opacification in MPS I) [1]. It is also seen to some extent in MPS IV, VI, and VII (See Table 1). Corneal clouding is a slowly progressive symptom, therefore visual acuity may be surprisingly good in the early stages of corneal clouding, but subsequently the patient may suffer from photophobia and a slowly progressive loss of visual acuity [6]. It is often present from early childhood [6]. Photochromatic glasses can help to ease symptoms in photophobic patients [11].

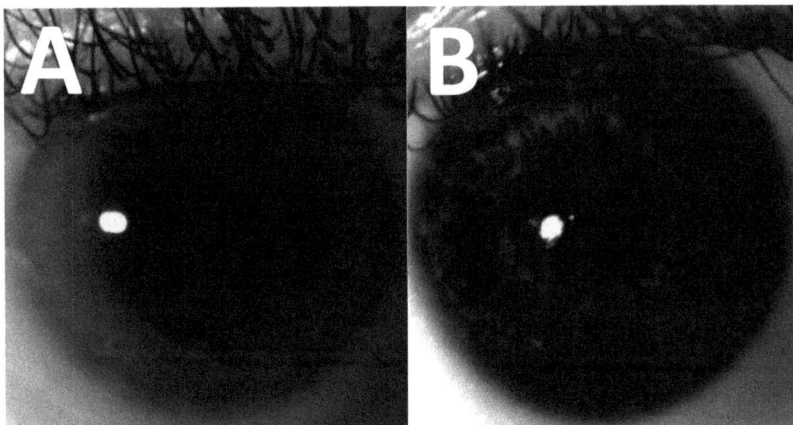

Figure 1. (**A**) Corneal image of a patient with MPS I Hurler demonstrating significant corneal clouding. (**B**) Corneal image of a patient without corneal clouding. Images were taken using IrisGuard AD100, MREH.

Corneal transparency is the outcome of the regular spacing of collagen fibers which have an extraordinarily regular diameter and maintain a consistent interfibrillar space [12,13]. Corneal opacification in MPS is caused by the accumulation of GAGs (see Table 2 which depicts the GAGs that accumulate in the various MPS types), particularly keratan sulphate, in all corneal layers, but particularly within the corneal stroma. The GAG accumulation induces significant light scattering, as the regular arrangement of collagen fibrils that maintain corneal transparency are lost [14,15]. In vivo confocal microscopy typically shows bright intercellular spaces in the corneal layers, extracellular stromal matrix microdeposits, and keratocytes that also have microdeposits and are morphologically modified [15,16]. Corneal clouding affects the entire cornea and it has a characteristic 'ground glass' appearance [14].

Thickest at the central cornea, the stromal layer is organized predominantly by type I collagens and proteoglycans (a protein core, with GAG side chains composed of either keratin (KS) or dermatan sulphate (DS)) [12]. Keratin proteoglycans manage collagen fibril diameter and dermatan proteoglycans regulate interfibrillar positioning and collagen adhesion [12]. Patients with MPS II are generally spared from corneal clouding [1,6,9,15] (see Table 1.) The deficient enzyme in MPS II (Iduronate-2-sulfatase) results in the build-up of DS containing an additional sulfate group as compared to MPS I and VI. It is thought that the additional sulfate group on the DS in MPS II exhibits a protective effect in the prevention of corneal clouding [17].

GAG deposition in the lysosomes of the keratocytes effects hysteresis, increasing corneal thickness and reducing corneal elasticity, therefore affecting IOP measurements, which rely on normal corneal rigidity for accuracy [4]. Therefore, IOP measurements may be falsely raised in patients with MPS and corneal clouding, potentially leading to difficulty in deciphering whether a raised IOP is secondary to corneal clouding or if it is an indication of potential glaucoma [18,19]. Ashworth et al. found a statistically significant relationship between IOP and the extent of corneal opacification in patients with MPS I and MPS VI [1,6].

Table 2. Enzyme defect, glycosaminoglycan deposited and inheritance pattern of the mucopolysaccharidoses. Data from Ashworth et al. [1].

MPS Type	Enzyme Defect	Glycosaminoglycan	Inheritance
MPS IH Hurler	α-L-Iduronidase	Dermatan sulphate, Heparin sulphate	AR
MPS IH/S Hurler–Scheie	α-L-Iduronidase	Dermatan sulphate, Heparin sulphate	AR
MPS IS Scheie	α-L-Iduronidase	Dermatan sulphate, Heparin sulphate	AR
MPS II Hunter	Iduronate-2-sulfatase	Dermatan sulphate, Heparin sulphate	X-linked
MPS IIIA Sanfilippo A	Heparan sulfamidase	Heparin sulphate	AR
MPS IIIB Sanfilippo B	N-Acetyl-α-D-glucosaminidase	Heparin sulphate	AR
MPS IIIC Sanfilippo C	Acetyl-CoA:αglucosaminidase N-acetyltransferase	Heparin sulphate	AR
MPS IIID Sanfilippo D	N-Acetylglucosamine-6-sulfatase	Heparin sulphate	AR
MPS IV Morquio	N-Acetylgalactosamine-6-sulfatase	Keratin sulphate	AR
MPS VI Maroteaux-Lamy	N-acetylgalactosamine-4-sulfatase	Dermatan sulphate,	AR
MPS VII Sly	β-D-Glucuronidase	Dermatan sulphate, Heparin sulphate, Chondroitin sulphate	AR
MPS IX Natowicz	Hyaluronidase	Chondroitin sulphate	AR

AR = autosomal recessive.

3. Systemic Therapies and Their Effect on Corneal Clouding

Improvements in quality of life and lifespan due to early systemic treatment have meant that the management of ocular complications and the preservation of vision has increased importance for patients with MPS [1,8]. While systemic treatments significantly improve disease manifestations and prolong life, a considerable burden of disease remains in areas which are not affected by systemic treatments, for example, corneal clouding [17,20].

Early diagnosis of MPS is important, since HSCT is indicated before two years of age and early treatment is associated with better outcomes [21–24]. Diagnosis is often made after irreversible damage of various tissues has already occurred. Beginning treatment at the asymptomatic stage of the disease has been proven effective at reducing urinary GAGs and organomegaly [23,25]. However, the efficacy of improving functions of the brain and avascular regions, such as the cornea, remains an unmet problem. A key component of more favorable outcomes seems to be starting therapy as early as possible, at diagnosis, before 16 months of age [16,26,27].

There are several sibling studies demonstrating the effectiveness of early treatment on the ocular manifestations of MPS [28]. A 2016 study by Laraway et al. [24,29] studied the outcomes of treatment with ERT in 35 patients with MPS I over a mean study period of 6.5 years. Corneal clouding remained stable in 78% of patients, visual acuity remained stable in 33%, and visual acuity improved in 42%. Younger patients (<10 years at treatment initiation) maintained disease measures closer to norms for age compared with patients aged ≥10 years at treatment initiation [29].

3.1. Enzyme Replacement Therapy (ERT)

ERT provides an impact on most visceral organs, although there is uneven organ biodistribution. ERT has a very limited effect on cornea, bone, central nervous system (CNS), and heart valves, due to the blood–brain barrier. The avascular nature of the cornea means that large proteins are prevented from passing through the blood–cornea or the blood–brain barrier. Despite lowering lysosomal GAG storage amounts to the normal level [30], reports suggest ERT does not seem to prevent progression of corneal or optic disc pathology and, thus, the related worsening of visual function [31]. Photophobia and conjunctival irritation diminish, but corneal clouding and other ocular complications do not usually improve [31–33].

There is a paucity of literature about the effect of ERT on corneal clouding specifically. Some studies report an overall stabilizing effect [15,34]; however, other studies describe a worsening of corneal clouding despite treatment [35].

The first ERT clinical trial in 2001 involved 10 patients with MPS I, treated over 52 weeks with weekly intravenous infusions of 0.58 mg/kg laronidase. The extent of corneal clouding did not change in any of the eight patients with corneal clouding. Several patients reported decreased photophobia or conjunctival irritation. Visual acuity improved from 20/1000 to 20/200 (in one eye) in one patient and slightly improved in two others [33].

No changes in corneal opacity were observed by Kakkis and coworkers [33] in 10 patients with MPS I undergoing ERT for one year. Some patients treated with ERT noted an improvement in photosensitivity and corneal clouding, but this was not seen in most [15,29,31,32] Where there are improvements, they are partial and possibly vary among individuals.

In a study by Pitz et al. [31], eight patients with MPS I were followed up for four years while undergoing ERT. One patient had a worsening of VA related to increasing corneal opacity and had subsequent corneal transplantation. Despite repeat immunogenic graft rejections, this patient's VA improved significantly, from logMAR 0.50 to 0.10, in both eyes.

A case report by Sarfraz et al. [35] described a patient who was diagnosed with MPS VI at age six. He suffered progressive visual loss and corneal clouding despite being treated with ERT from age 10. His follow up period was over 18 years.

Corneal clouding is difficult to quantify, as it is currently based on the subjective judgement of the clinician. There are also examination difficulties in assessing young children. VA can be more difficult to assess due to comorbid ocular conditions which may be present including glaucoma, optic nerve oedema, optic atrophy, and retinal degeneration [5]. There have recently been studies that demonstrate that corneal densitometry or iris recognition cameras can provide a reliable and objective determination of opacification [19,36–38]. These will be useful to determine the effectiveness of treatments in research settings and in clinical practice. ERT's effect on corneal clouding is limited and variable [20,39].

3.2. Hematopoietic Stem-Cell Transplantation (HSCT)

The ocular risks of HSCT include the development of cataracts, epithelial punctate keratopathy, and dry eye syndrome [40,41].

Recent studies detected large numbers of myofibroblasts in the cornea of an MPS I patient after HSCT, indicating that corneal clouding may be caused by the transformation of keratocytes into myofibroblasts, which would not be affected by HSCT [20].

A 2015 international multi-center study reported on 217 MPS I Hurler patients. Approximately 98% of the patients had corneal clouding before starting HSCT. After treatment, approximately 74% had either stabilized or had shown a decrease in the degree of their corneal clouding [21].

A 2021 study by Guffon et al. [42] analyzed more than 30 years' worth of data regarding 25 patients with MPS I (Hurler Syndrome) who were treated with HSCT. All 25 patients demonstrated some degree of corneal clouding. In 84%, corneal clouding was diagnosed at a median age of 13 months, before HSCT had begun. Despite HSCT, corneal clouding progressed in all patients and approximately half underwent corneal transplant at a median age of 17.8 years [42].

In a retrospective case series, Gullingsrud et al. [43] showed that six patients (30% of a study group of 25 patients with various types of MPS), showed improvements in their corneal clouding, whereas five patients (25%) had worse corneal clouding during follow-up ranging from 7 to 24 months following BMT. No correlation could be made to age at BMT. No eyes with corneal clouding showed complete clouding resolution over the follow up period. One patient required bilateral keratoplasty.

Vellodi and colleagues [44] reported upon two patients with MPS I (Hurler syndrome) who showed complete resolution of corneal clouding after BMT.

Javed et al. carried out a study of nine patients with MPS I (Hurler) or VI (Maroteaux-Lamy) and found that 5/17 (29%) had a significant deterioration in corneal clouding despite ERT or HSCT. One patient whose corneal clouding improved had been treated with ERT from the age of 12 months, before starting HSCT [38].

Corneal clouding may progress despite systemic therapy [5]. In a 2018 study by Fahnehjelm et al. [45], which studied eight patients with MPS I Hurler Syndrome, corneal opacities were present in all patients before or shortly after beginning therapy with HSCT. The clouding increased during follow up, despite HSCT, in 5/8 patients. This analysis of ocular disease in a cohort of children with MPS I after HSCT revealed ongoing corneal clouding, as seen in other studies [46]. These studies highlight the need for new MPS treatments that will prevent and reverse corneal clouding.

Sometimes, despite having had systemic therapy from an early age, corneal clouding progresses, impacting on visual acuity and quality of life. A more direct approach is needed to treat ocular pathologies in MPS patients, rather than just ERT and HSCT [46].

4. Surgical Treatment for Corneal Clouding

The only current definitive treatment for corneal clouding is corneal transplantation. When the cornea becomes so opacified that vision and quality of life is affected, the patient's suitability for keratoplasty must be considered. The decision to proceed with a corneal transplant depends on the following factors:

1. The effect of visual impairment on the patient's daily activities and quality of life, and the wishes of the patient to improve their vision;
2. The exclusion of other ocular factors (retinopathy or optic neuropathy) as a cause of visual impairment;
3. The condition of the ocular surface; dryness or vascularization of the cornea;
4. The general health of the patient and their suitability for anesthesia.

4.1. Pre-Operative Planning for Keratoplasty

The decision to undergo a corneal transplant is a joint one between the patient, their family, their ophthalmologist(s), and their metabolic team, based on whether surgical treatment of corneal clouding is in the patient's best interests. The possibility of graft re-opacification and the risk of only temporary improvements in vision must be thoroughly discussed. Improvements in visual function and quality of life that corneal transplantation can offer to patients with MPS must be weighed against their usually heightened anesthetic risk [9]. Many MPS patients will have concomitant cardiovascular disease, cervical spine instability, short neck, and intubation difficulties. Although local anesthesia may be possible for some types of corneal transplants, very young patients and patients with mental disabilities or behavioral problems may not tolerate surgery without a general anesthetic. This should only be carried out at a specialized center for MPS by an experienced anesthesiologist. Other concomitant eye pathologies must also be taken into careful consideration.

If there is concomitant retinopathy, optic nerve pathology, or glaucoma, visual improvement may be limited, as other factors also affect vision. A corneal transplant might resolve such patients' corneal opacification, but it will not resolve other ocular issues [47].

Patients should undergo additional tests if possible, such as visual fields, optical coherence tomography (OCT) of the retina and optic nerve, electroretinography (to assess retinal function), and visual evoked potentials (to assess optic nerve function) [5]. If corneal clouding is the principal factor affecting vision, then a corneal transplant can be considered.

Corneal transplantation demands scrupulous preparation to maximise success. This includes optimisation of the ocular surface condition by use of actions to minimize the harmful effects of ocular surface diseases [48]. Blepharitis, dry eyes, and corneal vascularization may need treatment to reduce the risk of infection and rejection [49]. Preoperative control of glaucoma is also crucial to ensure a successful surgery. Simultaneous cataract surgery along with keratoplasty is something for the surgeon to consider. Glaucoma following keratoplasty is relatively common, it can appear at any period in the evolution of the graft, it can be difficult to diagnose and to monitor and its treatment can hinder the progress of the transplant [50]. Simultaneous cataract surgery and keratoplasty could reduce the risk of anterior chamber angle compromise over time as well as in the immediate post-operative period [51,52].

The surgeon must also acknowledge the patient's postoperative management. Is the patient driven, motivated and suitable for the surgery? The assessment and operation should be carried out in a specialized center for MPS [48].

A slit lamp examination (with photographs to help rate the degree of corneal opacification over time) permits the detection of corneal opacities, atypical epithelial corneal changes, or vascularization. It also allows evaluation of the anterior chamber depth to assess for narrow-angle glaucoma. Most studies that evaluate corneal clouding are limited by the subjective results. That is why precise and objective cornea photography methods using the iris camera and Pentacam are useful [36,37]. Corneal topography is of use too [38].

Anterior segment optical coherence tomography is useful to measure the corneal thickness and to study the layers of the cornea. It can provide detailed morphological information for the anterior segment in patients with severe corneal clouding [53]. Additionally, in vivo confocal microscopy facilitates thorough examination of corneal cellular changes, assisting in the distinction between stromal and endothelial disease [37].

Tonometry (to measure intra-ocular pressure) and corneal pachymetry (to assess corneal thickness) are important, bearing in mind that intraocular pressure may be falsely raised in patients with MPS [15]. Corneal thickness can be measured using a pachymeter or anterior segment optical coherence tomography (OCT) [54].

Dilated fundus examination could show typical MPS findings such as atrophic optic nerve heads, swollen discs, pathological optic disc cupping, attenuated arterioles, or retinal pigmentary epithelial changes [15]. However, it is important to note that dilation in a phakic patient could result in an attack of acute angle closure. This is because patients with MPS often have occludable angles due to a thickened peripheral cornea and iris [55,56]. A study by Zhang et al. [57] used anterior segment swept-source OCT to analyse anterior chamber angles and found that 5 of 6 patients with MPS I had narrow to closed angles. Even in cases of severe corneal clouding, fundal photographs are recommended as it may be possible to visualise the retina and optic nerve even when this is very difficult via ophthalmoscopy [5,17]. In some cases, examination is hindered by the patient's photophobia. OCT is important as it could demonstrate cystoid macular oedema, or atrophy of the nerve fibre layer or atrophy of the photoreceptor layer sometimes found in patients with MPS [5].

In patients who have supposed damage to the optic nerve, pattern visual evoked potentials (VEPs) can be useful. Progressive optic nerve swelling and consequent axonal atrophy can lead to trace amplitude reduction [6]. Peak latency increase can result from fiber demyelination caused by the optic nerve compression [15].

Electroretinography (ERG) is recommended in cases of clinical suspicion of retinopathy [1]. ERG recordings in patients with MPS I, II, and III have revealed retinal dysfunctions ranging from none to severe [58]. The ERG abnormalities in patients with MPS show a pattern typical for rod–cone degeneration [1].

There are two main types of corneal transplant, Penetrating Keratoplasty (PK) and Deep Anterior Lamellar Keratoplasty (DALK).

4.2. Penetrating Keratoplasty (PK)

PK is the most widely used surgical treatment for corneal opacification. In PK, all five corneal layers are transplanted. Penetrating keratoplasty has been evolving with the use of technology such as femtosecond lasers to generate PKP incisions [59]. An international study of 32 penetrating keratoplasties, performed in patients with MPS and published in 2016, had a graft success rate of 96% [60]. Literature reporting on the PK graft survival rate in patients without MPS indicates a graft survival range of 62% to 86% [61,62]. It is postulated that this higher graft survival rate is because patients with MPS are more receptive to corneal grafts [60].

An international 2017 study [60] involving 48 eyes from 32 patients with MPS I, IV, or VI was reported upon. Mean follow-up was 70 months (range: 5–186). PK was performed in 45 eyes and DALK in three eyes. At the last follow-up, a successful visual outcome for PK was found in 63%. Rejection episodes occurred in 23% of grafts; however, a clear graft was recorded at last follow-up in 94% [60]. This study demonstrated that clear corneal grafts can be obtained for patients with corneal clouding due to MPS with improvement in visual acuity in the majority [60]. According to Bothun et al. [47], MPS VI may be associated with a higher graft rejection risk.

Case reports denote that the donor cornea may re-opacify because GAGs can accumulate in donor keratocytes [60,63]. This likely relates to the severity of the MPS and could be due to host keratocyte anterior–posterior spread. There can be gradual replacement of the donor epithelial cells by the host epithelium [9,63]. Käsmann-Kellner et al. [63] suggest that PK may have better outcomes in the MPS types that have dermatan sulphate accumulation (MPS VI, MPS VII) than in the MPS types that have with keratan sulphate accumulation (MPS IV). Dermatan sulphate is present in healed corneal wounds, rejected grafts, and post-viral opacification [63].

Various case reports on MPS patients following PK denote that a clear donor cornea was retained from three months up to five years, without systemic treatment [47,64,65]. A literature review by Bothun et al. described 23 reports that recorded 40 initial and 3 repeat cases of PK in patients with MPS. Thirty-one initial and two repeat corneal grafts were reported as clear, varying from 3 months to 12 years of follow up [47]. A patient with MPS VII had a PK for corneal clouding and this remained clear two years post-transplant [64]. Naumann et al. [65] performed PKs successfully in three children with MPS VI-A (severe type) at the age of 7–11 years. The transplants remained clear during the follow-up over 2.5–5 years and the long-term visual acuity was encouraging. Intriguingly, two of the three patients displayed some clearing of the host cornea adjacent to the transplant. This phenomenon was presumed to have been caused by diffusion of the normal enzyme from the graft to the recipient avascular cornea, to correct the enzyme defect and restore transparency. However, this result has not been reported in any other type of MPS and it could not be duplicated in a study involving a cat model of MPS VI [66].

PK, being an open globe procedure, requires general anesthesia. During corneal transplant surgery, there is often a significant mismatch of corneal thickness between the graft (normal) and the host (abnormally thick). Care should be taken when suturing to allow a smooth anterior corneal surface. This is easier in PK surgery where one can offset the posterior surface but harder to achieve in DALK surgery due to the intact Descemet membrane and the fixed posterior surface [67]. PK is sometimes associated with the loosening of sutures, suture infiltrates, and suture-produced astigmatism [68]. Astigmatism post PK can cause a clear graft to have vision that is not as good as expected [69]. Another important cause of vision poorer than predicted is postopretive glaucoma. Numerous factors can contribute to an increase in the incidence of glaucoma, such as post-operative glaucoma, increased intra-operative manipulation, and severe post-operative inflammation [70]. Rarely, PK can be associated with disastrous problems such as expulsive choroidal hemorrhage [69].

4.3. Deep Anterior Lamellar Keratoplasty (DALK)

DALK is a partial-thickness cornea transplant that involves the selective transplantation of the epithelium and the stroma, leaving the patient's native Descemet membrane and endothelium in place. These outer two layers are replaced with a donor epithelium and stroma. In patients with MPS, DALK is often preferred, since corneal clouding is due to GAGs accumulating in the corneal stroma, sometimes sparing Descemet's membrane and the corneal endothelium. Endothelial involvement occurs only in late stages of MPS, and an intact Descemet's membrane can act as a barrier to prevent stromal recurrence of MPS in the graft [10]. DALK is contraindicated in patients who have clouding of the endothelium or Descemet's membrane [60]. DALK may be carried out under local anesthetic in cooperative patients [60]. However, one must take into consideration that conversion to PK may need to happen and good anesthesia and blood pressure control is still very important to avoid complications such as suprachoroidal hemorrhage [71].

A report by the American Academy of Ophthalmology by Reinhart et al. found that there is no advantage to DALK over PK for refractive error outcomes [72]. However, DALK is superior to PK for preservation of endothelial cell density. DALK has an associated lower risk of infection, bleeding, and decreased rates of rejection [69]. Studies comparing the PK procedure to the DALK procedure have demonstrated that DALK can have lower complication rates [73,74]. Because DALK is not a full-thickness procedure, the resultant wound is stronger than that of a PK so the sutures can be removed sooner [72]. Leaving the host endothelium intact considerably reduces the risk of endothelial rejection [75,76]. As DALK is a closed-system operation, there is also decreased risk of immune rejection [76]. Another major DALK advantage is that late corneal failure due to endothelial cell loss, which can be quite common after penetrating keratoplasty, cannot occur after DALK [72]. This is associated with easier postoperative management. Reduced concentration, duration and frequency of topical steroids reduces the risk of steroid-induced glaucoma and cataract [77]. DALK is currently favored over conventional PK in MPS patients due to its similar effectiveness and lower risks [9]. Initially, DALK was performed using manual corneal dissection. Now, DALK can also be performed using a femtosecond laser [67]. Good visual outcomes have been described in patients with conditions such as keratoconus who underwent femtosecond laser-assisted DALK [78].

Phacoemulsification can also be safely performed along with DALK [79]. In patients with MPS, simultaneous keratoplasty and cataract surgery could reduce the risk of postoperative glaucoma [79]. Glaucoma following PK has a relatively high frequency; it can appear early, as well as late, in the evolution of the transplant, it is very hard to diagnose and also to follow-up and the medical or surgical treatment can interfere negatively with the evolution of the corneal graft Over time, there is a risk of anterior chamber angle compromise following DALK. Simultaneous cataract surgery could negate this risk.

Complications are associated with the fundamental difficulty in parting Descemet's membrane from the stroma [48]. DALK is a more difficult surgery to perform than PK [80]. In patients with MPS, the stroma is more rigid to handle due to GAG deposition which makes the surgical technique of dissection more of a challenge. The poor view due to corneal clouding can pose difficulties for surgeons who prefer a manual dissection technique in DALK surgery. Big bubble technique can be successfully applied but the cloudiness still poses a challenge in gauging the right depth to insert the air needle for big bubble formation [80]. DALK is usually more difficult to perform in younger patients because Descemet's membrane does not separate as easily [67]. Intra-operative complications include micro perforations and macro perforations of Descemet's membrane (in which conversion to PK is usually necessary) [48,81]. Post-operative complications include the formation of a double (pseudo-) anterior chamber [67,82]. This is where the donor epithelium separates from the host Descemet's membrane. It is usually seen in the immediate postoperative period. Risk factors include instances where there was Descemet's Membrane perforation during surgery [80,83]. To rectify this complication, air is injected surgically into the anterior chamber to tamponade the detached Descemet's membrane.

Epithelial, stromal, and mixed epithelial and stromal graft rejection occur at a rate of approximately 8 to 10% [84]. Rejection can present any time after three months postoperatively [85]. Graft dehiscence may occur following early suture removal. An interface haze may be apparent in the late post-operative follow-up phase. Haze can occur in cases where stromal fibers have been retained and Descemet's membrane folds can form as a result [86]. Interface keratitis could occur in the interface, or empty space, that is left. Air or gas in the anterior chamber could lead to pupillary block.

4.4. Postoperative Management

Topical antibiotics and steroid drops should be used during the first post-op month, followed by steroid and lubricant drops for the next six months. After this time period, steroid drop duration is determined by the surgeon's judgement. Check-ups should be given twice during the first post-operative month, every three months throughout the first post-operative year, and biannually henceforth, until suture removal [15].

Intra- and post-surgical complications are the same as those connected to keratoplasty in any patient. Late complications such as rejection can occur, and it is of paramount importance to assess any case of possible inflammation (red eye and/or visual acuity loss) so that therapy can be administered as early as possible [15]. The eye should be kept completely clean, especially during the first month, and potentially treacherous activities should be prevented to avoid trauma that could cause graft dehiscence. An eye shield can be worn [15].

Re-opacification as early as one-year post graft can occur due to GAG deposition in donor keratocytes [9]. Effectiveness is dependent on the type of GAG deposited and the severity of the disease [63]. Sutures should remain in place for at least one year post-transplantation and following consideration of astigmatism and of the suture condition [5,87]. Suture removal can be done at the slit lamp but may require anesthesia in an uncooperative patient.

5. Future Corneal Clouding Treatment Options

5.1. Gene Therapy

Gene therapy is currently under development as an MPS treatment option. Gene therapy seems to have the most promise as an effective and permanent solution if it proves to be as safe and effective as seen in animal models. A study published in June 2020 by Miyadera et al. [88] showed that intrastromal gene therapy prevents and reverses advanced corneal clouding in a canine model of MPS I. The eyes with advanced disease demonstrated resolution of corneal clouding as early as one week post-injection, followed by sustained corneal transparency until the experimental endpoint of 25 weeks [88]. This study showed the potential ability of gene therapy to reverse, as well as prevent, corneal clouding. Kamata et al. [89] injected an adenovirus expressing human beta-glucuronidase into the anterior chamber or intrastromal region the cornea of mice who had MPS VII. It successfully treated corneal clouding. Adenovirus-mediated transduction was found throughout the mouse cornea, but it peaked after a few days and then declined after one week.

Vance et al. [90] explored adeno-associated virus gene therapy for alpha-L-iduronidase (IUDA) enzyme delivery by intrastromal injection as a viable remedy for MPS I-related corneal clouding. Seven days after intrastromal injection into human corneas, the enzyme was overproduced in the corneal stroma with extensive dispersal in numerous cell types. There was also a 10-fold escalation in enzyme activity without toxicity.

5.2. Substrate Reduction Therapy

Substrate reduction therapy is expected to affect "difficult-to-treat" tissues such as the cornea and the central nervous system [91]. Small chemical inhibitors are expected to cross the blood–brain barrier as well as the blood–cornea barrier, reaching tissues not accessible to the large recombinant lysosomal enzymes of ERT. Rhodamine B was shown to reduce GAG synthesis in MPS IIIA and VI in vitro studies and in studies of mice with MPS IIIA [91]. Clinical trials are needed to assess the effect on corneal clouding.

In 2006, genistein, a compound that can be purified from soya beans and acts as a tyrosine kinase inhibitor, was identified as showing in vivo reduction of GAG production in MPS I, II, III, VI, and VII fibroblast cells [92]. This drug acts via the epidermal growth factor-dependent pathway to prevent the synthesis of GAGs [93].

Further research needs consistent and repeatable techniques which involve assessing corneal clouding as part of clinical trials to improve current MPS treatment strategies.

6. Conclusions

Management of the ocular manifestations of MPS requires a multi-disciplinary approach, with early diagnosis, early initiation of systemic treatment, and careful ocular assessment. Severe corneal clouding may require corneal transplantation. However, novel therapies aim to prevent corneal opacification before the need for surgery arises. Clinical trials need to consistently evaluate the effect of new MPS treatments on corneal clouding to ultimately improve patient outcomes.

Author Contributions: Conceptualization, O.M. and J.A.; methodology, O.M. and J.A.; writing—original draft preparation, O.M.; writing—review and editing, J.A. and L.A.; visualization, O.M. and L.A. and J.A.; supervision, L.A. and J.A.; project administration, J.A. All authors have read and agreed to the published version of the manuscript.

Funding: This research received no external funding.

Institutional Review Board Statement: Not applicable.

Informed Consent Statement: Not applicable.

Conflicts of Interest: The authors declare no conflict of interest.

References

1. Ashworth, J.L.; Biswas, S.; Wraith, E.; Lloyd, I.C. Mucopolysaccharidoses and the Eye. *Surv. Ophthalmol.* **2006**, *51*, 1–17. [CrossRef]
2. Pastores, G.M.; Arn, P.; Beck, M.; Clarke, J.T.; Guffon, N.; Kaplan, P.; Muenzer, J.; Norato, D.Y.; Shapiro, E.; Thomas, J.; et al. The MPS I registry: Design, methodology, and early findings of a global disease registry for monitoring patients with Mucopolysaccharidosis Type I. *Mol. Genet. Metab.* **2007**, *91*, 37–47. [CrossRef] [PubMed]
3. Summers, C.G.; Ashworth, J.L. Ocular manifestations as key features for diagnosing mucopolysaccharidoses. *Rheumatology* **2011**, *50*, v34–v40. [CrossRef]
4. Ashworth, J.; Flaherty, M.; Pitz, S.; Ramlee, A. Assessment and diagnosis of suspected glaucoma in patients with mucopolysaccharidosis. *Acta Ophthalmol.* **2015**, *93*, 111–117. [CrossRef] [PubMed]
5. Del Longo, A.; Piozzi, E.; Schweizer, F. Ocular features in mucopolysaccharidosis: Diagnosis and treatment. *Ital. J. Pediatr.* **2018**, *44*, 125. [CrossRef]
6. Ashworth, J.L.; Kruse, F.E.; Bachmann, B.; Tormene, A.P.; Suppiej, A.; Parini, R.; Guffon, N. Ocular manifestations in the mucopolysaccharidoses—A review. *Clin. Exp. Ophthalmol.* **2010**, *38*, 12–22. [CrossRef]
7. Nassar, A.; Tabbara, K.F.; Aljurf, M. Ocular manifestations of graft-versus-host disease. *Saudi. J. Ophthalmol.* **2013**, *27*, 215–222. [CrossRef] [PubMed]
8. Fenzl, C.; Teramoto, K.; Moshirfar, M. Ocular manifestations and management recommendations of lysosomal storage disorders I: Mucopolysaccharidoses. *Clin. Ophthalmol.* **2015**, *9*, 1633–1644. [CrossRef] [PubMed]
9. Ferrari, S.; Ponzin, D.; Ashworth, J.L.; Fahnehjelm, K.T.; Summers, C.G.; Harmatz, P.R.; Scarpa, M. Diagnosis and management of ophthalmological features in patients with mucopolysaccharidosis. *Br. J. Ophthalmol.* **2011**, *95*, 613–619. [CrossRef]
10. Ganesh, A.; Bruwer, Z.; Al-Thihli, K. An update on ocular involvement in mucopolysaccharidoses. *Curr. Opin. Ophthalmol.* **2013**, *24*, 379–388. [CrossRef]
11. Fahnehjelm, K.T.; Malm, G.; Winiarski, J.; Törnquist, A.-L. Ocular findings in four children with mucopolysaccharidosis I-Hurler (MPS I-H) treated early with haematopoietic stem cell transplantation. *Acta Ophthalmol. Scand.* **2006**, *84*, 781–785. [CrossRef]
12. Michelacci, Y.M. Collagens and proteoglycans of the corneal extracellular matrix. *Braz. J. Med. Biol. Res.* **2003**, *36*, 1037–1046. [CrossRef] [PubMed]
13. Meek, K.M.; Knupp, C. Corneal structure and transparency. *Prog. Retin. Eye Res.* **2015**, *49*, 1–16. [CrossRef]

14. Müller, L.J.; Pels, E.; Schurmans, L.R.; Vrensen, G.F. A new three-dimensional model of the organization of proteoglycans and collagen fibrils in the human corneal stroma. *Exp. Eye Res.* **2004**, *78*, 493–501. [CrossRef]
15. Fahnehjelm, K.T.; Ashworth, J.L.; Pitz, S.; Olsson, M.; Törnquist, A.L.; Lindahl, P.; Summers, C.G. Clinical guidelines for diagnosing and managing ocular manifestations in children with mucopolysaccharidosis. *Acta Ophthalmol.* **2012**, *90*, 595–602. [CrossRef] [PubMed]
16. Grupcheva, C.; Craig, J.P.; McGhee, C.N. In Vivo Microstructural Analysis of the Cornea in Scheie's Syndrome. *Cornea* **2003**, *22*, 76–79. [CrossRef]
17. Tomatsu, S.; Pitz, S.; Hampel, U. Ophthalmological Findings in Mucopolysaccharidoses. *J. Clin. Med.* **2019**, *8*, 1467. [CrossRef]
18. Fahnehjelm, K.T.; Chen, E.; Winiarski, J. Corneal hysteresis in mucopolysaccharidosis I and VI. *Acta Ophthalmol.* **2012**, *90*, 445–448. [CrossRef]
19. Elflein, H.M.; Hofherr, T.; Berisha-Ramadani, F.; Weyer, V.; Lampe, C.; Beck, M.; Pitz, S. Measuring corneal clouding in patients suffering from mucopolysaccharidosis with the Pentacam densitometry programme. *Br. J. Ophthalmol.* **2013**, *97*, 829–833. [CrossRef]
20. Hampe, C.; Wesley, J.; Lund, T.; Orchard, P.; Polgreen, L.; Eisengart, J.; McLoon, L.; Cureoglu, S.; Schachern, P.; McIvor, R. Mucopolysaccharidosis Type I: Current Treatments, Limitations and Prospects for Improvement. *Biomolecules* **2021**, *11*, 189. [CrossRef] [PubMed]
21. Aldenhoven, M.; Wynn, R.F.; Orchard, P.J.; O'Meara, A.; Veys, P.; Fischer, A.; Valayannopoulos, V.; Neven, B.; Rovelli, A.; Prasad, V.K.; et al. Long-term outcome of Hurler syndrome patients after hematopoietic cell transplantation: An international multicenter study. *Blood* **2015**, *125*, 2164–2172. [CrossRef] [PubMed]
22. Poe, M.D.; Chagnon, S.L.; Escolar, M.L. Early treatment is associated with improved cognition in Hurler syndrome. *Ann. Neurol.* **2014**, *76*, 747–753. [CrossRef] [PubMed]
23. Muenzer, J. Early initiation of enzyme replacement therapy for the mucopolysaccharidoses. *Mol. Genet. Metab.* **2014**, *111*, 63–72. [CrossRef]
24. Laraway, S.; Breen, C.; Mercer, J.; Jones, S.; Wraith, J.E. Does early use of enzyme replacement therapy alter the natural history of mucopolysaccharidosis I? Experience in three siblings. *Mol. Genet. Metab.* **2013**, *109*, 315–316. [CrossRef]
25. Clarke, L.A.; Wraith, J.E.; Beck, M.; Kolodny, E.H.; Pastores, G.M.; Muenzer, J.; Rapoport, D.; Berger, K.; Sidman, M.; Kakkis, E.D.; et al. Long-term Efficacy and Safety of Laronidase in the Treatment of Mucopolysaccharidosis I. *Pediatrics* **2009**, *123*, 229–240. [CrossRef]
26. Giugliani, R.; Muschol, N.; Keenan, H.A.; Dant, M.; Muenzer, J. Improvement in time to treatment, but not time to diagnosis, in patients with mucopolysaccharidosis type I. *Arch. Dis. Child.* **2021**, *106*, 674–679. [CrossRef]
27. De Ru, M.H.; Boelens, J.J.; Das, A.M.; Jones, S.A.; Van Der Lee, J.H.; Mahlaoui, N.; Mengel, E.; Offringa, M.; O'Meara, A.; Parini, R.; et al. Enzyme Replacement Therapy and/or Hematopoietic Stem Cell Transplantation at diagnosis in patients with Mucopolysaccharidosis type I: Results of a European consensus procedure. *Orphanet. J. Rare Dis.* **2011**, *6*, 55. [CrossRef]
28. McGill, J.J.; Inwood, A.C.; Coman, D.; Lipke, M.L.; De Lore, D.; Swiedler, S.J.; Hopwood, J.J. Enzyme replacement therapy for mucopolysaccharidosis VI from 8 weeks of age-a sibling control study. *Clin. Genet.* **2010**, *77*, 492–498. [CrossRef] [PubMed]
29. Laraway, S.; Mercer, J.; Jameson, E.; Ashworth, J.; Hensman, P.; Jones, S. Outcomes of Long-Term Treatment with Laronidase in Patients with Mucopolysaccharidosis Type I. *J. Pediatr.* **2016**, *178*, 219–226. [CrossRef]
30. Gaffke, L.; Pierzynowska, K.; Podlacha, M.; Brokowska, J.; Węgrzyn, G. Changes in cellular processes occurring in mucopolysaccharidoses as underestimated pathomechanisms of these diseases. *Cell Biol. Int.* **2021**, *45*, 498–506. [CrossRef]
31. Pitz, S.; Ogun, O.; Bajbouj, M.; Arash, L.; Schulze-Frenking, G.; Beck, M. Ocular Changes in Patients With Mucopolysaccharidosis I Receiving Enzyme Replacement Therapy. *Arch. Ophthalmol.* **2007**, *125*, 1353–1356. [CrossRef] [PubMed]
32. Wraith, J.E. The first 5 years of clinical experience with laronidase enzyme replacement therapy for mucopolysaccharidosis I. *Expert Opin. Pharmacother.* **2005**, *6*, 489–506. [CrossRef]
33. Kakkis, E.D.; Muenzer, J.; Tiller, G.E.; Waber, L.; Belmont, J.; Passage, M.; Izykowski, B.; Phillips, J.; Doroshow, R.; Walot, I.; et al. Enzyme-Replacement Therapy in Mucopolysaccharidosis I. *N. Engl. J. Med.* **2001**, *344*, 182–188. [CrossRef]
34. Pitz, S.; Ogun, O.; Arash, L.; Miebach, E.; Beck, M. Does enzyme replacement therapy influence the ocular changes in type VI mucopolysaccharidosis? *Graefe's Arch. Clin. Exp. Ophthalmol.* **2009**, *247*, 975–980. [CrossRef]
35. Sarfraz, M.W.; Smith, M.; Jones, S.; Ashworth, J. Progression of eye disease over 15 years in a patient with mucopolysaccharidosis type VI on enzyme replacement therapy. *BMJ Case Rep.* **2021**, *14*, e238544. [CrossRef]
36. Aslam, T.; Shakir, S.; Wong, J.; Au, L.; Ashworth, J. Use of iris recognition camera technology for the quantification of corneal opacification in mucopolysaccharidoses. *Br. J. Ophthalmol.* **2012**, *96*, 1466–1468. [CrossRef] [PubMed]
37. Javed, A.; Aslam, T.; Ashworth, J. Use of new imaging in detecting and monitoring ocular manifestations of the mucopolysaccharidoses. *Acta Ophthalmol.* **2016**, *94*, e676–e682. [CrossRef] [PubMed]
38. Javed, A.; Aslam, T.; Jones, S.; Ashworth, J. Objective Quantification of Changes in Corneal Clouding Over Time in Patients With Mucopolysaccharidosis. *Investig. Ophthalmol. Vis. Sci.* **2017**, *58*, 954–958. [CrossRef]
39. Summers, C.G.; Fahnehjelm, K.T.; Pitz, S.; Guffon, N.; Koseoglu, S.T.; Harmatz, P.; Scarpa, M. Systemic therapies for mucopolysaccharidosis: Ocular changes following haematopoietic stem cell transplantation or enzyme replacement therapy—A review. *Clin. Exp. Ophthalmol.* **2010**, *38*, 34–42. [CrossRef]

40. Fahnehjelm, K.T.; Törnquist, A.-L.; Olsson, M.; Winiarski, J. Visual outcome and cataract development after allogeneic stem-cell transplantation in children. *Acta Ophthalmol. Scand.* **2007**, *85*, 724–733. [CrossRef]
41. Fahnehjelm, K.T.; Winiarski, J.; Törnquist, A.-L. Dry-eye syndrome after allogeneic stem-cell transplantation in children. *Acta Ophthalmol.* **2008**, *86*, 253–258. [CrossRef]
42. Guffon, N.; Pettazzoni, M.; Pangaud, N.; Garin, C.; Lina-Granade, G.; Plault, C.; Mottolese, C.; Froissart, R.; Fouilhoux, A. Long term disease burden post-transplantation: Three decades of observations in 25 Hurler patients successfully treated with hematopoietic stem cell transplantation (HSCT). *Orphanet. J. Rare Dis.* **2021**, *16*, 1–20. [CrossRef] [PubMed]
43. Gullingsrud, E.O. Ocular abnormalities in the mucopolysaccharidoses after bone marrow transplantation Longer follow-up. *Ophthalmology* **1998**, *105*, 1099–1105. [CrossRef]
44. Vellodi, A.; Young, E.P.; Cooper, A.; Wraith, J.E.; Winchester, B.; Meaney, C.; Ramaswami, U.; Will, A. Bone marrow transplantation for mucopolysaccharidosis type I: Experience of two British centres. *Arch. Dis. Child.* **1997**, *76*, 92–99. [CrossRef]
45. Fahnehjelm, K.T.; Olsson, M.; Chen, E.; Hengstler, J.; Naess, K.; Winiarski, J. Children with mucopolysaccharidosis risk progressive visual dysfunction despite haematopoietic stem cell transplants. *Acta Paediatr.* **2018**, *107*, 1995–2003. [CrossRef]
46. Broek, B.T.V.D.; van Egmond-Ebbeling, M.B.; Achterberg, J.A.; Boelens, J.J.; Vlessert, I.C.; Prinsen, H.C.; van Doorn, J.; van Hasselt, P.M. Longitudinal Analysis of Ocular Disease in Children with Mucopolysaccharidosis I after Hematopoietic Cell Transplantation. *Biol. Blood Marrow Transplant.* **2020**, *26*, 928–935. [CrossRef]
47. Bothun, E.D.; Decanini, A.; Summers, C.G.; Orchard, P.J.; Tolar, J. Outcome of Penetrating Keratoplasty for Mucopolysaccharidoses. *Arch. Ophthalmol.* **2011**, *129*, 138–144. [CrossRef]
48. Tan, D.T.; Dart, J.K.; Holland, E.J.; Kinoshita, S. Corneal transplantation. *Lancet* **2012**, *379*, 1749–1761. [CrossRef]
49. Pinello, L.; Busin, M.; Fontana, L.; Dua, H.S. Application of (lamellar) keratoplasty and limbal stem cell transplantation for corneal clouding in the mucopolysaccharidoses—A review. *Clin. Exp. Ophthalmol.* **2010**, *38*, 52–62. [CrossRef]
50. Ayyala, R.S. Penetrating Keratoplasty and Glaucoma. *Surv. Ophthalmol.* **2000**, *45*, 91–105. [CrossRef]
51. Chaurasia, S.; Price, F.W.; Gunderson, L.; Price, M. Descemet's Membrane Endothelial Keratoplasty. *Ophthalmology* **2014**, *121*, 454–458. [CrossRef]
52. Jones, S.M.; Fajgenbaum, M.A.; Hollick, E.J. Endothelial cell loss and complication rates with combined Descemets stripping endothelial keratoplasty and cataract surgery in a UK centre. *Eye* **2015**, *29*, 675–680. [CrossRef]
53. Matoba, A.; Oie, Y.; Tanibuchi, H.; Winegarner, A.; Nishida, K. Anterior segment optical coherence tomography and in vivo confocal microscopy in cases of mucopolysaccharidosis. *Am. J. Ophthalmol. Case Rep.* **2020**, *19*, 100728. [CrossRef]
54. Ramesh, P.V.; Jha, K.N.; Srikanth, K. Comparison of Central Corneal Thickness using Anterior Segment Optical Coherence Tomography Versus Ultrasound Pachymetry. *J. Clin. Diagn. Res.* **2017**, *11*, NC08–NC11. [CrossRef] [PubMed]
55. Mullaney, P.; Awad, A.H.; Millar, L. Glaucoma in mucopolysaccharidosis 1-H/S. *J. Pediatr. Ophthalmol. Strabismus* **1996**, *33*, 127–131. [CrossRef]
56. Quigley, H.A.; Maumenee, A.E.; Stark, W.J. Acute glaucoma in systemic mucopolysaccharidosis I-S. *Am. J. Ophthalmol.* **1975**, *80*, 70–72. [CrossRef]
57. Zhang, J.R.; Wang, J.H.; Lin, H.Z.; Lee, Y.C. Anterior Chamber Angles in Different Types of Mucopolysaccharidoses. *Am. J. Ophthalmol.* **2020**, *212*, 175–184. [CrossRef]
58. Caruso, R.C.; Kaiser-Kupfer, M.I.; Muenzer, J.; Ludwig, I.H.; Zasloff, M.A.; Mercer, P.A. Electroretinographic Findings in the Mucopolysaccharidoses. *Ophthalmology* **1986**, *93*, 1612–1616. [CrossRef]
59. Price, F.W.; Price, M.; Grandin, J.C.; Kwon, R. Deep anterior lamellar keratoplasty with femtosecond-laser zigzag incisions. *J. Cataract. Refract. Surg.* **2009**, *35*, 804–808. [CrossRef] [PubMed]
60. Ohden, K.L.; Pitz, S.; Ashworth, J.; Magalhães, A.; Marinho, D.R.; Lindahl, P.; Fahnehjelm, K.T.; Summers, C.G. Outcomes of keratoplasty in the mucopolysaccharidoses: An international perspective. *Br. J. Ophthalmol.* **2017**, *101*, 909–912. [CrossRef]
61. Williams, K.A.; Esterman, A.J.; Bartlett, C.; Holland, H.; Hornsby, N.B.; Coster, D.J. How effective is penetrating corneal transplantation? Factors influencing long-term outcome in multivariate analysis. *Transplantation* **2006**, *81*, 896–901. [CrossRef]
62. Borderie, V.M.; Boëlle, P.Y.; Touzeau, O.; Allouch, C.; Boutboul, S.; Laroche, L. Predicted long-term outcome of corneal transplantation. *Ophthalmology* **2009**, *116*, 2354–2360. [CrossRef] [PubMed]
63. Käsmann-Kellner, B.; Weindler, J.; Pfau, B.; Ruprecht, K. Ocular Changes in Mucopolysaccharidosis IV A (Morquio A Syndrome) and Long-Term Results of Perforating Keratoplasty. *Ophthalmology* **1999**, *213*, 200–205. [CrossRef]
64. Bergwerk, K.; Falk, R.E.; Glasgow, B.J.; Rabinowitz, Y.S. Corneal transplantation in a patient with mucopolysaccharidosis type VII (Sly disease). *Ophthalmic Genet.* **2000**, *21*, 17–20. [CrossRef]
65. Naumann, G.O.; Rummelt, V. Clearing of the para-transplant host cornea after perforating keratoplasty in Maroteaux-Lamy syndrome (type VI-A mucopolysaccharidosis). *Klin. Mon. Fur. Augenheilkd.* **1993**, *203*, 351–360. [CrossRef] [PubMed]
66. Aguirre, G.; Raber, I.; Yanoff, M.; Haskins, M. Reciprocal corneal transplantation fails to correct mucopolysaccharidosis VI corneal storage. *Investig. Ophthalmol. Vis. Sci.* **1992**, *33*, 2702–2713.
67. Nanavaty, M.A.; Vijjan, K.S.; Yvon, C. Deep anterior lamellar keratoplasty: A surgeon's guide. *J. Curr. Ophthalmol.* **2018**, *30*, 297–310. [CrossRef]
68. Christo, C.G.; Van Rooij, J.; Geerards, A.J.; Remeijer, L.; Beekhuis, W.H. Suture-related Complications Following Keratoplasty. *Cornea* **2001**, *20*, 816–819. [CrossRef]

69. Tandon, R.; Singh, R.; Gupta, N.; Vanathi, M. Corneal transplantation in the modern era. *Indian J. Med Res.* **2019**, *150*, 7–22. [CrossRef]
70. Al-Mahmood, A.M.; Al-Swailem, S.A.; Edward, D. Glaucoma and Corneal Transplant Procedures. *J. Ophthalmol.* **2012**, *2012*, 1–9. [CrossRef]
71. Chua, A.; Chua, M.J.; Kam, P. Recent advances and anaesthetic considerations in corneal transplantation. *Anaesth. Intensive Care* **2018**, *46*, 162–170. [CrossRef]
72. Reinhart, W.J.; Musch, D.; Jacobs, D.; Lee, W.B.; Kaufman, S.C.; Shtein, R. Deep Anterior Lamellar Keratoplasty as an Alternative to Penetrating Keratoplasty: A Report by the American Academy of Ophthalmology. *Ophthalmology* **2011**, *118*, 209–218. [CrossRef]
73. Abdelaal, A.M.; Alqassimi, A.H.; Malak, M.; Hijazi, H.T.; Hadrawi, M.; Khan, M.A. Indications of Keratoplasty and Outcomes of Deep Anterior Lamellar Keratoplasty Compared to Penetrating Keratoplasty. *Cureus* **2021**, *13*, e13825. [CrossRef] [PubMed]
74. Janiszewska-Bil, D.; Czarnota-Nowakowska, B.; Krysik, K.; Lyssek-Boroń, A.; Dobrowolski, D.; Grabarek, B.; Wylęgała, E. Comparison of Long-Term Outcomes of the Lamellar and Penetrating Keratoplasty Approaches in Patients with Keratoconus. *J. Clin. Med.* **2021**, *10*, 2421. [CrossRef] [PubMed]
75. Espandar, L.; Carlson, A.N. Lamellar Keratoplasty: A Literature Review. *J. Ophthalmol.* **2013**, *2013*, 1–8. [CrossRef]
76. Hos, D.; Matthaei, M.; Bock, F.; Maruyama, K.; Notara, M.; Clahsen, T.; Hou, Y.; Le, V.N.H.; Salabarria, A.-C.; Horstmann, J.; et al. Immune reactions after modern lamellar (DALK, DSAEK, DMEK) versus conventional penetrating corneal transplantation. *Prog. Retin. Eye Res.* **2019**, *73*, 100768. [CrossRef] [PubMed]
77. Sharma, R.A.; Bursztyn, L.L.; Golesic, E.; Mather, R.; Tingey, D.P. Comparison of intraocular pressure post penetrating keratoplasty vs Descemet's stripping endothelial keratoplasty. *Can. J. Ophthalmol.* **2016**, *51*, 19–24. [CrossRef] [PubMed]
78. De Macedo, J.P.; de Oliveira, L.A.; Hirai, F.; De Sousa, L.B. Femtosecond laser-assisted deep anterior lamellar keratoplasty in phototherapeutic keratectomy versus the big-bubble technique in keratoconus. *Int. J. Ophthalmol.* **2018**, *11*, 807–812. [CrossRef] [PubMed]
79. Zaki, A.A.; Elalfy, M.S.; Said, D.G.; Dua, H.S. Deep anterior lamellar keratoplasty—Triple procedure: A useful clinical application of the pre-Descemet's layer (Dua's layer). *Eye* **2015**, *29*, 323–326. [CrossRef]
80. Ricardo, J.R.D.S.; Medhi, J.; Pineda, R. Indications for and Outcomes of Deep Anterior Lamellar Keratoplasty in Mucopolysaccharidoses. *J. Pediatr. Ophthalmol. Strabismus* **2013**, *50*, 376–381. [CrossRef]
81. Jhanji, V.; Sharma, N.; Vajpayee, R.B. Intraoperative perforation of Descemet's membrane during "big bubble" deep anterior lamellar keratoplasty. *Int. Ophthalmol.* **2010**, *30*, 291–295. [CrossRef]
82. Karimian, F.; Feizi, S. Deep Anterior Lamellar Keratoplasty: Indications, Surgical Techniques and Complications. *Middle East Afr. J. Ophthalmol.* **2010**, *17*, 28–37. [CrossRef]
83. Basak, S.K.; Basak, S. Complications and management in Descemet's stripping endothelial keratoplasty: Analysis of consecutive 430 cases. *Indian J. Ophthalmol.* **2014**, *62*, 209–218. [CrossRef] [PubMed]
84. Watson, S.L.; Tuft, S.J.; Dart, J.K. Patterns of Rejection after Deep Lamellar Keratoplasty. *Ophthalmology* **2006**, *113*, 556–560. [CrossRef]
85. Perera, C.; Jhanji, V.; Lamoureux, E.; Pollock, G.; Favilla, I.; Vajpayee, R.B. Clinical presentation, risk factors and treatment outcomes of first allograft rejection after penetrating keratoplasty in early and late postoperative period. *Eye* **2012**, *26*, 711–717. [CrossRef]
86. Tan, D.; Ang, M.; Arundhati, A.; Khor, W.-B. Development of Selective Lamellar Keratoplasty within an Asian Corneal Transplant Program: The Singapore Corneal Transplant Study (An American Ophthalmological Society Thesis). *Trans. Am. Ophthalmol. Soc.* **2015**, *113*.
87. Feizi, S.; Zare, M. Current Approaches for Management of Postpenetrating Keratoplasty Astigmatism. *J. Ophthalmol.* **2011**, *2011*, 1–8. [CrossRef] [PubMed]
88. Miyadera, K.; Conatser, L.; Llanga, T.A.; Carlin, K.; O'Donnell, P.; Bagel, J.; Song, L.; Kurtzberg, J.; Samulski, R.J.; Gilger, B.; et al. Intrastromal Gene Therapy Prevents and Reverses Advanced Corneal Clouding in a Canine Model of Mucopolysaccharidosis I. *Mol. Ther.* **2020**, *28*, 1455–1463. [CrossRef] [PubMed]
89. Kamata, Y.; Okuyama, T.; Kosuga, M.; O'Hira, A.; Kanaji, A.; Sasaki, K.; Yamada, M.; Azuma, N. Adenovirus-Mediated Gene Therapy for Corneal Clouding in Mice with Mucopolysaccharidosis Type VII. *Mol. Ther.* **2001**, *4*, 307–312. [CrossRef]
90. Vance, M.; Llanga, T.; Bennett, W.; Woodard, K.; Murlidharan, G.; Chungfat, N.; Asokan, A.; Gilger, B.; Kurtzberg, J.; Samulski, R.J.; et al. AAV Gene Therapy for MPS1-associated Corneal Blindness. *Sci. Rep.* **2016**, *6*, 22131. [CrossRef] [PubMed]
91. Roberts, A.L.K.; Thomas, B.J.; Wilkinson, A.S.; Fletcher, J.M.; Byers, S. Inhibition of Glycosaminoglycan Synthesis Using Rhodamine B in a Mouse Model of Mucopolysaccharidosis Type IIIA. *Pediatr. Res.* **2006**, *60*, 309–314. [CrossRef] [PubMed]
92. Vadalà, M.; Castellucci, M.; Guarrasi, G.; Terrasi, M.; La Blasca, T.; Mulè, G. Retinal and choroidal vasculature changes associated with chronic kidney disease. *Graefe's Arch. Clin. Exp. Ophthalmol.* **2019**, *257*, 1687–1698. [CrossRef] [PubMed]
93. Jakóbkiewicz-Banecka, J.; Piotrowska, E.; Narajczyk, M.; Barańska, S.; Węgrzyn, G. Genistein-mediated inhibition of glycosaminoglycan synthesis, which corrects storage in cells of patients suffering from mucopolysaccharidoses, acts by influencing an epidermal growth factor-dependent pathway. *J. Biomed. Sci.* **2009**, *16*, 26. [CrossRef] [PubMed]

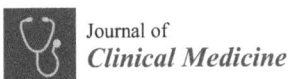

Article

Gastrointestinal Manifestations in Mucopolysaccharidosis Type III: Review of Death Certificates and the Literature

Sophie Thomas [1,*], Uma Ramaswami [2], Maureen Cleary [3], Medeah Yaqub [4] and Eva M. Raebel [4,*]

[1] The Society for Mucopolysaccharide and Related Diseases, MPS House, Amersham HP7 9LP, UK
[2] Lysosomal Disorders Unit, Royal Free London NHS Foundation Trust, London NW3 2QG, UK; uma.ramaswami@nhs.net
[3] Great Ormond Street Hospital for Children NHS Foundation Trust, Great Ormond St., London WC1N 3JH, UK; Maureen.Cleary@gosh.nhs.uk
[4] Rare Disease Research Partners, MPS House, Amersham HP7 9LP, UK; m.yaqub@rd-rp.com
* Correspondence: s.thomas@mpssociety.org.uk (S.T.); e.raebel@rd-rp.com (E.M.R.); Tel.: +44-345-389-9901 (S.T. & E.M.R.)

Abstract: Background: Mucopolysaccharidosis type III (MPS III, Sanfilippo disease) is a life-limiting recessive lysosomal storage disorder caused by a deficiency in the enzymes involved in degrading glycosaminoglycan heparan sulfate. MPS III is characterized by progressive deterioration of the central nervous system. Respiratory tract infections have been reported as frequent and as the most common cause of death, but gastrointestinal (GI) manifestations have not been acknowledged as a cause of concern. The aim of this study was to determine the incidence of GI problems as a primary cause of death and to review GI symptoms reported in published studies. Methods: Causes of death from 221 UK death certificates (1957–2020) were reviewed and the literature was searched to ascertain reported GI symptoms. Results: GI manifestations were listed in 5.9% (n = 13) of death certificates. Median (IQR) age at death was 16.7 (5.3) years. Causes of death included GI failure, GI bleed, haemorrhagic pancreatitis, perforation due to gastrostomies, paralytic ileus and emaciation. Twenty-one GI conditions were reported in 30 studies, mostly related to functional GI disorders, including diarrhoea, dysphagia, constipation, faecal incontinence, abdominal pain/distension and cachexia. Conclusions: GI manifestations may be an under-recognized but important clinical feature of MPS III. Early recognition of GI symptoms and timely interventions is an important part of the management of MPS III patients.

Keywords: mucopolysaccharidosis; Sanfilippo syndrome; mortality; gastrointestinal

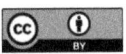

1. Introduction

Mucopolysaccharidosis type III (MPS III, Sanfilippo disease) is a rare autosomal recessive lysosomal storage disorder (LSD) caused by the accumulation of glycosaminoglycan (GAG) heparan sulfate due to the deficiency of specific enzymes responsible for its degradation [1]. Four distinct MPS III subtypes have been recognized, depending on the enzyme deficiency: MPS III type A (heparan N-sulphatase, sulfamidase; MIM #252900), type B (α-N-acetylglucosaminidase; MIM #252920), type C (acetyl-CoA α-glucosaminide N-acetyltransferase; MIM #252930), and type D (N-acetylglucosamine 6-sulfatase; MIM #252940) [1,2]. Overall prevalence is estimated at 1–9 births per one-million population, with subtypes varying geographically and incidence of subtypes A and B being the most diagnosed in Europe [1,3]. UK prevalence has been estimated at approximately 1.21 per 100,000 live births [4].

MPSIII is a life-limiting condition prevalently characterized by a progressive severe deterioration of the central nervous system (CNS), including neurocognitive and behavioural decline [5]. Following an initial normal birth and development, the disease tends to progress through three main phases: the first phase usually begins at 1–3 years of age and is characterized by delayed cognitive development, specially speech delay; the second phase starts between 3–4 years of age and it is marked by the beginning of cognitive decline with challenging behaviour, including aggression, hyperactivity and sleep disturbance; the third stage, usually from 10 years of age onwards, is quieter as behavioural difficulties disappear but there is a rapid loss of cognitive processes and motor functions, including walking, swallowing and the development of seizures and pyramidal symptoms [1,2,6–8]. Patients in this last phase tend to be immobile, fed by enteral tube and incontinent, becoming fully dependent on care. MPS III also presents with somatic symptoms, but those are relatively less severe if compared to other MPS disorders [5,9,10]. Associated somatic signs and symptoms can include mild facial dysmorphology, hirsutism, recurrent ear, nose and throat (ENT) infections, frequent upper respiratory infections, umbilical and inguinal hernias, coarse hair, hepatomegaly, splenomegaly, recurrent diarrhoea, constipation, hearing loss, scoliosis, odontoid hypoplasia, femoral head osteonecrosis, cardiac disease and abnormal dentition [5–7,9,11–16].

Life expectancy for individuals with MPS III varies greatly but death usually occurs between the second and third decades of life, even though survival into later decades has been reported, depending on the disorder's subtype and the phenotype (severe and attenuated forms) [11,17,18]. Pneumonia and respiratory tract infections have been reported as the most common causes of death (>50%) in MPS III individuals with types A, B [11,17–19] and C [20].

The large differences in disease onset, clinical manifestations and life span between individuals are the result of genetic heterogeneity producing inter- and intra- type variability [21]. Due to the rarity of MPS III and the non-specificity of early-symptoms, early diagnosis of MPS III remains a challenge and median diagnostic delay between initial symptoms and diagnosis can range from 2 years in MPS IIIA [6] to 28 years in MPS IIIB individuals with the attenuated phenotype [18]. Currently, there is no approved disease-modifying therapy for MPS III, with treatment being limited to the management of clinical symptoms and palliative care [2].

The UK Society for Mucopolysaccharide and Related Diseases (MPS Society) is a patient support group providing advocacy and support to individuals and families diagnosed with a MPS or related conditions. Through its work with clinicians, patients, and their families, the MPS Society was made aware of gastro-intestinal (GI) problems presenting in patients with MPS III. Personal communication [ST] with patients and LSD medical specialists from UK metabolic centres revealed GI symptoms and signs are frequently reported, including constipation, diarrhoea, intolerance to feeds, recto-vaginal fistulas, malabsorption of feeds, bowel volvulus, bowel stasis, ulcerative colitis, GI bleeding and pseudo-obstruction, with some individuals having had a diagnosis of irritable bowel syndrome or Crohn's disease.

To date, GI symptoms have not been acknowledged in previous studies as a primary cause of concern in the MPS III population, however, parents have identified digestive, toileting and feeding issues as an unmet treatment need in MPS III, causing significant concerns and challenges on the child's family [22]. Determining their incidence and severity is paramount to understand MPS III natural history and disease progression, and to improve the future clinical management of these patients. The aim of this study is to review death certificates of individuals with MPS III to determine the incidence of GI manifestations as a leading or contributing cause of death, and to review GI symptoms and signs reported in published studies of live or deceased individuals with MPS III.

2. Materials and Methods

2.1. GI Manifestations as a Cause of Death in UK Patients with MPS III

The MPS Society UK holds details of 416 individuals with MPS III in their database. According to the UK Data Protection Act 2018, the General Data Protection Regulation (GDPR) only applies in the UK to living individuals (https://www.legislation.gov.uk/ukpga/2018/12/section/3/enacted (accessed on 20 July 2021)). Data on deceased patients with MPS III were retrospectively extracted, including: name, date of birth, date of death, gender, and type of MPS III, where available. To ascertain the cause of death, death certificates, were obtained.

In the UK, a death certificate includes an exact copy of the cause of death given by a medic on the Medical Certificate of Cause of Death (MCCD) [23]. The cause of death section of UK death certificates is divided into two parts. Part I starts on line (a) with the immediate, direct cause of death, and it is followed on subsequent lines (b and/or c) by the sequence of events or conditions that led to death, until reaching the underlaying cause of death which is the condition that started the fatal sequence. Part II includes other significant conditions that contributed to death but were not related to the disease or condition causing it [23]. Under UK legislation, death certificates are considered public records and duplicate certificates can be requested by anyone if the full name of the deceased individual and date of death is available, to obtain the General Register Office (GRO) index reference number (Births and Deaths Registration Act 1953; (https://www.legislation.gov.uk/ukpga/Eliz2/1-2/20/section/30 (accessed on 20 July 2021)). If the date of death is not available, this can be found in the register if the birth year is available. For individuals ≤ 16 years of age, the full name of both parents is required, together with the latest registered address. This was available for some members on the database. The MPS Society held copies of death certificates registered from January 1957–March 2006, including some from a previous mortality study [17]. Death certificates from April 2006–October 2020 were obtained, with the last request made on 21 May 2021. Death certificates were reviewed for listed GI manifestations recorded as cause of death. Causes of death for one individual could include different conditions leading to death (e.g., respiratory and gastrointestinal conditions). Data was anonymised and all patients were deceased, hence ethical approval was not required.

2.2. GI Manifestations in the Literature

A literature search was conducted in PubMed to ascertain GI symptoms and signs in MPS III patients reported in published studies. The pre-determined search terms 'Sanfilippo syndrome' and 'Mucopolysaccharidosis type III' were combined using the Boolean 'OR' operator. Studies were retrieved if the title/abstract/keyword contained at least one of the terms. The Boolean term 'NOT' was used to exclude animal studies. Searches were completed on 20 April 2021. The Rayyan Web app [24] was used to screen titles, abstracts and keywords by two researchers (ER, MY) to identify potential studies for inclusion. Further animal studies were excluded. Full texts of relevant papers were subjected to further scrutiny with final papers being selected based on the inclusion criteria in Table 1. GI symptoms and sigs mentioned within the studies were recorded (ER, MY). GI manifestations affecting the liver, or the mouth, were excluded (e.g., hepatomegaly, abnormal dentition). This literature review only aimed to identify the number of studies reporting GI symptoms.

Table 1. Inclusion and exclusion criteria of studies.

Inclusion Criteria	Exclusion Criteria
Article in English	Full-text paper not available
Patients with a diagnosis of MPS III	In-vitro, embryonic, pre-natal and molecular level studies
Case studies, retrospective, or prospective studies	
Mention of a GI symptom/sign	

3. Results

3.1. GI Manifestations as Cause of Death in Patients with MPS III: Death Certificates

3.1.1. Death Certificates

Records of 240 deceased members with MPS III were found on the MPS Society database. Three records did not include the full names of the individuals and seven were of children ≤16 years old for whom the name of both parents was not available. For three individuals, the date of death was not recorded and alternative searches within the government website did not yield any results. Death records for six individuals were not available from the General Register Office even though full name and date of death were provided. A total of 221 death certificates from deceased individuals were included in this study: 113 death certificates were available from Lavery et al. [17], 24 from the MPS Society UK, and 84 new certificates with full records were obtained.

3.1.2. Demographics of Deceased Patients

Median (IQR) age at death of the 221 individuals was 16.0 (6.4) years (mean 17.7 (±7.4), range 3.2–47.8) and 110 (49.8%) of deceased individuals were female. Type of MPS III and decade at death are shown in Table 2. Dates of birth ranged from April 1946 to August 2004, with dates of death between January 1957 to September 2020. Age at death increased over time from a mean age of 16.5 years (±4.3, $n = 51$) in 1990–1999 to 21.8 years (±9.9, $n = 50$) in 2010–2020. A total of 72.4% ($n = 160$) of deaths occurred during the patient's second decade of life (i.e., between 10–19 years of age) (Table 2).

Table 2. Characteristics of deceased individuals with MPSIII on death certificates ($n = 221$) and of individuals with GI conditions listed on their death certificate ($n = 13$).

	Deceased Individuals			GI Condition on Death Certificate		
N	221			13		
Gender						
Males	111			8		
Females	110			5		
MPS III subtype	*n* (%)			*n* (%)		
A	148	(67.0)		10	(76.9)	
B	34	(15.4)		2	(15.4)	
C	9	(4.1)		—		
Unknown	30	(13.6)		1	(7.7)	
Age at death (years)						
Mean age (±SD)	17.7 (±7.4)			18.1 (±7.3)		
Median (IQR)	16.0 (6.4)			16.7 (5.3)		
Range	3.2–47.8			11.2–39.7		
Range (years)	*n* (%)			*n* (%)		
0–9	9	(4.1)		—		
10–19	160	(72.4)		10	(76.9)	
20–29	36	(16.3)		2	(15.4)	
30–39	12	(5.4)		1	(7.7)	
40–49	4	(1.8)		—		
Decade at death	*n* (%)		Mean age (±SD)	*n* (%)		Mean age (±SD)
1950–1959	1	(0.5)	10.7 (—)	—		—
1960–1969	—		—	—		—
1970–1979	4	(1.8)	10.7 (±3.1)	—		—
1980–1989	36	(16.3)	13.4 (±3.6)	2	(16.7)	12.2 (±1.5)
1990–1999	51	(23.1)	16.5 (±4.3)	3	(25.0)	19.1 (±2.7)
2000–2009	78	(35.3)	18.2 (±7.1)	4	(33.3)	21.0 (±12.7)
2010–2020	51	(23.1)	21.8 (±9.9)	4	(33.3)	17.4 (±3.7)

3.1.3. GI Manifestations Leading or Contributing to Death on Death Certificates

A total of 5.9% ($n = 13$) of deceased individuals had GI conditions listed on their death certificates: 12 (5.4%) certificates had GI conditions recorded as leading to death (Table 3, Part I) and one as significantly contributing to death (Table 3, Part II). Three deaths were associated with complications of percutaneous endoscopic gastrostomies (PEG) (Table 3). Median (IQR) age at death of these individuals was 16.7 (5.3) years (mean 18.1 (±7.3), range

11.2–39.7) and 38.5% (*n* = 5) were female. Type of MPS III and decade at death are shown in Table 2. Dates of birth ranged from January 1966 to March 2002, with dates of death between January 1981 to August 2018. Nine deaths (76.9%) occurred during the patient's second decade of life (i.e., between 10–19 years of age). Two patients died in their third decade of life and one in their fourth (Table 2).

Table 3. GI-related conditions (*in italics*) leading or contributing to death on death certificates (*n* = 13). Causes of death recorded on death certificates follow the Medical Certificate of Cause of Death (MCCD) classification [23].

	Cause of Death Listed on Death Certificates			
	Part I: Disease or Condition Leading to Death			**Part II:** Other Significant Conditions Contributing to Death but not Related to the Disease or Condition Causing It
Patient	I(a) Disease or Condition Leading Directly to Death	I (b) Other Disease or Condition, if Any, Leading to I(a)	I (c) Other Disease or Condition, if Any, Leading to I(b)	
1	*Acute haemorrhagic pancreatitis*	—	—	—
2	Respiratory and *gastrointestinal failure*	MPS IIIB	—	Von Willebrand's Disease
3	*Gut failure*	MPS III	—	ESBL colonisation of chest
4	*Perforation of the bowel*	*Migrated PEG*	MPS III	—
5	*Gastroenteritis*	MPS III	—	Coma
6	*Gastrointestinal bleed*	MPS III	—	—
7	MPS IIIA treated by *palliative gastrostomy with complications*	—	—	—
8	*Aspiration of gastric contents*	MPS III	—	—
9	*Vomiting and aspiration*	MPS III	—	—
10	Sepsis	*Perforated PEG*	—	—
11	*Peritonitis*	*Abdominal abscess*	—	MPS III
12	*Dehydration*	*Paralytic ileus*	MPS III	—
13	Bronchopneumonia	MPS IIIA	—	*Extreme emaciation*

ESBL: extended spectrum beta-lactamase; PEG: percutaneous endoscopic gastrostomy.

3.2. GI Manifestations Reported in the Literature

A total of 837 papers were identified in the PubMed search and were subjected to abstract review; of these, 731 were excluded, based on the pre-determined inclusion/exclusion criteria (Table 1). Full-text review was performed on 53 papers, from which 30 reported GI manifestations, both as individual case studies, a case series, or as aggregated data within retrospective/prospective studies.

Twenty-one GI signs and symptoms were reported in the literature, mostly related to functional GI disorders (Table 4). Diarrhoea and dysphagia were commonest (*n* = 16 and 12 studies, respectively), followed by constipation (*n* = 5) and loss of bowel control/faecal incontinence (*n* = 4). Nine studies reported patients needing a gastrostomy and four studies mention nasogastric/feeding tube.

Table 4. GI manifestations in MPS III reported in the literature.

GI Manifestations	No. of Studies	Studies
Upper GI tract		
Gastroesophageal reflux	1	[25]
Gastroenteritis	1	[26]
Pyloric stenosis	1	[27]
Swallowing difficulties (Dysphagia)	12	[19,21,27–36]
Nasopharyngeal/feeding tube—management	4	[11,18,21,27]
PEG *—management	9	[19,29,32–34,36–39]
Vomiting	1	[34]
Abdominal distention/ protuberant abdomen	3	[28,29,40]
Abdominal pain	2	[30,41]

Table 4. Cont.

GI Manifestations	No. of Studies	Studies
Lower GI tract		
Constipation	5	[10,11,18,33,34]
Diarrhoea	16	[7,10,11,18–21,26,28,33–35,37,41–43]
Faecal impaction	1	[31]
Intestinal fistula due to stenosis of pyloric ring	1	[27]
Intestinal lymphangiectasia	1	[41]
Loss of bowel control/faecal incontinence	4	[6,29,41,44]
General/Others		
Cachexia	1	[21,33]
Emaciation	1	[28]
Erratic appetite	1	[45]
Excessive weight	1	[10]
Weight loss	1	[31]
Food allergy—multiple	1	[26]

* PEG: percutaneous endoscopic gastrostomy.

4. Discussion

This is the first retrospective study of individuals with MPS III presenting with significant GI manifestations leading or contributing to death. Our results showed that gastrointestinal complications led or contributed to 5.9% of deaths in this population. Lavery et al. [17] showed that some conditions can be relatively high within the non-pulmonary related deaths. Although pulmonary conditions in our study were listed in 50.7% of death certificates, cardiac arrest led or contributed to 2.3% of deaths, aspiration pneumonia to 3.6%, congestive/cardiac failure to 4.5%, respiratory failure to 5% and epilepsy/seizures to 6.8%, while other conditions had a prevalence of <1% (e.g., renal failure, sepsis). Our results could not be directly compared to those in Lavery et al.'s publication as it was not possible to ascertain how the causes of death had been classified in the study.

Most degenerative disorders can present with feeding problems because of functional decline. By the time MPS III children reach their second decade of life, dysphagia and an increased need for aspiration usually result in the requirement of a nasogastric tube or gastrostomy feeding to avoid chocking and severe debility [19,26]. Indeed, extreme emaciation contributed to the cause of death in one of the individuals in our study and three deaths were a consequence of PEG-related complications. A Dutch study on adult phenotype and natural history of patients with MPS IIIB reported six deaths, including a 51 old male who died from complications after gastrostomy replacement and a 68 year old female who died of cachexia a year after developing difficulties with swallowing [33]. Review of the death certificates indicated that, besides deaths related to feeding problems, other GI conditions play a role in MPS III mortality, including GI failure, GI bleed, gastroenteritis and paralytic ileus. Information on causes of death in MPS III patients is limited in the literature with numerous studies stating the number of deceased individuals but not their cause of death, suggesting that GI manifestations as a cause of mortality may be underreported.

Death certificates showed that the trend for increased survival reported by Lavery et al. [17] continued in 2010 to 2020. Improved medical care (e.g., enteral feeding such as gastrostomies), supportive and multidisciplinary care, better awareness of the disease in the community leading to earlier diagnosis and detection of attenuated cases, and referral of patients to specialist centres, are possible reasons for this increase in life expectancy [17,37].

Inflammation may be a contributor to neurodegeneration in LSDs and problems related to inflammatory bowel disease (IBD) in some LSDs have been reported. In Fabry Disease, IBD-like symptoms can include unspecified functional bowel disorder, functional abdominal bloating/distension, irritable bowel syndrome (IBS), diarrhoea, constipation, abdominal pain and early satiety [46,47]. GI signs and symptoms are common in Fabry

Disease, possibly due to the accumulation of Gb3 (globotriaosylceramide) substrate in neuronal and muscle intestinal cells, although the physiological processes are not fully understood [47]. GI manifestations in Fabry Disease do not result in mortality. In Niemann Pick C, severe GI symptoms resembling carbohydrate malabsorption leading to extreme weight loss [48] and perianal fistulas indicative of Chron's disease [49,50] have also been reported. In MPS III, it is speculated that GAGs may infiltrate into the human GI tract, as evaluation of the GI tract in MPS IIIA mice has demonstrated lysosomal GAG accumulation in the lamina propria of the villi of the duodenum, jejunum and ileum, and an increased lysosomal storage in the submucosa throughout the GI system [51]. Autopsy examination of a deceased MPS III patient reported in the literature revealed GAG accumulation and vacuolization in the pyloric ring and the extrinsic nerves of the Auerbach nerve plexuses [27]. Although much focus has been placed on MPS III pathology in the CNS, mouse models have demonstrated lesions in the peripheral nervous system (PNS), with lysosomal storage damage in the myenteric plexus and submucosal plexus, which involve enteric neurons in the GI tract [52]. This effect on the PNS may explain the autonomic abnormality of GI peristalsis in MPS III patients and some of the GI manifestations reported in this study.

Despite GI symptoms not being a well-recognised clinical finding in MPS disorders, non-specific GI symptoms were reported for MPS III individuals in the literature, including abdominal pain and distension, recurrent diarrhoea, reflux, weight loss and vomiting. A mini-review of MPS III [1] described diarrhoea as episodic, with other studies showing recurrent diarrhoea can affect 50–92% of patients with MPS IIIA, B & C [11,18,19,21,34], interspersed with bouts of constipation, frequently present as patients get older [11,18]. Diarrhoea has been well recognized in MPS II children [53]. Loss of bowel control and faecal incontinence was reported in four studies from our review. Although adaptive behaviours in MPS III individuals persist for longer than cognitive functions, loss of bowel control is one of the adaptive behaviours most affected by disease progression [6]. Since these symptoms are non-specific and functional, thus not explainable by structural or biochemical abnormalities, the exact cause of these GI symptoms is still unclear.

It is not currently known if GI manifestations are disease related, or if there are other contributing factors, such as comorbidities or the consequence of side-effects and interactions between the numerous medications prescribed to these patients. For example, intestinal dysmotility caused by neuronal dysfunction and immobility as disease progresses may contribute to the development of fistulas. However, enemas administered to treat constipation can also contribute to the development of fistulas and rectal perforations [54] and the regular use of laxatives to treat constipation has been associated with increased constipation and faecal impaction [55]. Similarly, imodium-based antidiarrheals (e.g., loperamide hydrochloride) are widely and chronically used in these patients to treat diarrhoea and fistulas [56], but GI-related side-effects include constipation, nausea, vomiting, abdominal pain and, in rare circumstances, paralytic ileus [57]. MPS III patients have also been found to be particularly susceptible to extrapyramidal side effects (e.g., dystonia, ataxia) of certain behaviour management treatments (i.e., risperidone, olanzapine, or lamotrigine) [58]. There may be a burden of medication in MPS III patients due to the need to ameliorate symptoms of multiple conditions and polypharmacy, defined as taking more than five medications at any one time, has been identified as a risk factor for developing GI conditions and GI motility delays [59]. A study assessing sleep disturbance in MPS III children lists two participants as taking 5–10 concurrent medications to manage sleep, epilepsy, seizures, pain, GI symptoms and other conditions [60]. The implications of polypharmacy on GI manifestations in MPS III patients have not been studied and warrant further investigation.

A limitation of this study is the use of death certificates, which in 22.6% ($n = 50$) of cases only reported 'MPS III', 'Sanfilippo syndrome' or 'MPS' as the cause of death. In addition, GI conditions contributing to death may not be reflected in death certificates. For example, one death certificate listed aspiration pneumonitis and seven aspiration pneumonia as the cause of death, which may have been initiated by gastroesophageal reflux or by the inhalation of food, drink, vomit or saliva as a consequence of dysphagia. Limitations and advantages on the use of death certificates to determine cause of death in MPS III individuals have been reviewed in Lavery et al. [17]. A further limitation with the use of death certificates and reported cases in the literature is the lack of clinical data and information on the disease journey of these patients, which may have helped with elucidating at what age GI symptoms first presented, how long these symptoms were managed with medication, how long PEGs were required for, and whether symptoms were the consequence of disease progression, the result of long-term medication and surgeries, or an outcome of patients now living longer. Furthermore, only a compilation of GI manifestations mentioned in these studies is included here, further analysis, including the number of cases within case series and GI symptoms reported as aggregated data will be presented elsewhere.

To be able to support MPS III patients and their families with achieving the best quality of life throughout their disease journey, and to be able to characterise these results further, a prospective study using clinical data is warranted to ascertain the prevalence, morbidity and mortality associated with GI manifestations in individuals with MPS III.

5. Conclusions

This retrospective study has identified significant GI pathology leading or contributing to the cause of death in individuals with MPS III. GI manifestations may be an under-recognized, but important clinical feature of LSDs, including MPS III. Early recognition of GI symptoms and signs, and timely interventions, are an important part of the management of MPS III patients.

Author Contributions: Conceptualization, S.T. and E.M.R.; methodology, S.T. and E.M.R.; formal analysis, E.M.R.; data curation, E.M.R. and M.Y.; writing—original draft preparation, E.M.R.; writing—review and editing, E.M.R., S.T., U.R. and M.C. All authors have read and agreed to the published version of the manuscript.

Funding: This research received no external funding.

Institutional Review Board Statement: Not applicable as subjects were deceased.

Informed Consent Statement: Not applicable.

Data Availability Statement: Death certificates are publicly available at the following location: https://www.gov.uk/order-copy-birth-death-marriage-certificate (accessed on 20 July 2021).

Acknowledgments: The authors would like to thank Christian Hendriksz, Anupam Chakrapani and Ana Amado Fondo for their input in early clinical discussions.

Conflicts of Interest: The authors declare no conflict of interest related to this manuscript.

References

1. Valstar, M.J.; Ruijter, G.J.; van Diggelen, O.P.; Poorthuis, B.J.; Wijburg, F.A. Sanfilippo syndrome: A mini-review. *J. Inherit. Metab. Dis.* **2008**, *31*, 240–252. [CrossRef]
2. Fedele, A.O. Sanfilippo syndrome: Causes, consequences, and treatments. *Appl. Clin. Genet.* **2015**, *8*, 269–281. [CrossRef]
3. Orphanet. Mucopolysaccharidosis Type 3. Available online: https://www.orpha.net/consor/cgi-bin/OC_Exp.php?Expert=581 (accessed on 1 June 2021).
4. Héron, B.; Mikaeloff, Y.; Froissart, R.; Caridade, G.; Maire, I.; Caillaud, C.; Levade, T.; Chabrol, B.; Feillet, F.; Ogier, H.; et al. Incidence and natural history of mucopolysaccharidosis type III in France and comparison with United Kingdom and Greece. *Am. J. Med. Genet. A* **2011**, *155*, 58–68. [CrossRef]
5. Neufeld, E.F.; Muenzer, J. The Mucopolysaccharidoses. In *The Online Metabolic and Molecular Bases of Inherited Disease*; Valle, D.L., Antonarakis, S., Ballabio, A., Beaudet, A.L., Mitchell, G.A., Eds.; McGraw-Hill Education: New York, NY, USA, 2001; pp. 3421–3452.
6. Buhrman, D.; Thakkar, K.; Poe, M.; Escolar, M.L. Natural history of Sanfilippo syndrome type A. *J. Inherit. Metab. Dis.* **2014**, *37*, 431–437. [CrossRef]
7. Meyer, A.; Kossow, K.; Gal, A.; Mühlhausen, C.; Ullrich, K.; Braulke, T.; Muschol, N. Scoring evaluation of the natural course of mucopolysaccharidosis type IIIA (Sanfilippo syndrome type A). *Pediatrics* **2007**, *120*, e1255–e1261. [CrossRef]

8. Fraser, J.; Wraith, J.E.; Delatycki, M.B. Sleep disturbance in Mucopolysaccharidosis type III (Sanfilippo syndrome): A survey of managing clinicians. *Clin. Genet.* **2002**, *62*, 418–421. [CrossRef] [PubMed]
9. Galimberti, C.; Madeo, A.; Di Rocco, M.; Fiumara, A. Mucopolysaccharidoses: Early diagnostic signs in infants and children. *Ital. J. Pediatr.* **2018**, *44*, 133. [CrossRef] [PubMed]
10. Krawiec, P.; Pac-Kożuchowska, E.; Mełges, B.; Mroczkowska-Juchkiewicz, A.; Skomra, S.; Pawłowska-Kamieniak, A.; Kominek, K. From Hypertransaminasemia to Mucopolysaccharidosis IIIA. *Ital. J. Pediatr.* **2014**, *40*, 97. [CrossRef]
11. Valstar, M.J.; Neijs, S.; Bruggenwirth, H.T.; Olmer, R.; Ruijter, G.J.; Wevers, R.A.; van Diggelen, O.P.; Poorthuis, B.J.; Halley, D.J.; Wijburg, F.A. Mucopolysaccharidosis type IIIA: Clinical spectrum and genotype-phenotype correlations. *Ann. Neurol.* **2010**, *68*, 876–887. [CrossRef] [PubMed]
12. Wijburg, F.A.; Węgrzyn, G.; Burton, B.K.; Tylki-Szymańska, A. Mucopolysaccharidosis type III (*Sanfilippo syndrome*) and misdiagnosis of idiopathic developmental delay, attention deficit/hyperactivity disorder or autism spectrum disorder. *Acta Paediatr.* **2013**, *102*, 462–470. [CrossRef] [PubMed]
13. Kubaski, F.; Poswar, F.D.O.; Michelin-Tirelli, K.; Burin, M.G.; Rojas-Málaga, D.; Brusius-Facchin, A.C.; Leistner-Segal, S.; Giugliani, R. Diagnosis of Mucopolysaccharidoses. *Diagnostics* **2020**, *10*, 172. [CrossRef] [PubMed]
14. Shapiro, E.G.; Nestrasil, I.; Delaney, K.A.; Rudser, K.; Kovac, V.; Nair, N.; Richard, C.W., 3rd; Haslett, P.; Whitley, C.B. A prospective natural history study of Mucopolysaccharidosis type IIIA. *J. Pediatr.* **2016**, *170*, 278–287. [CrossRef]
15. Andrade, F.; Aldámiz-Echevarría, L.; Llarena, M.; Couce, M.L. Sanfilippo syndrome: Overall review. *Pediatr. Int.* **2015**, *57*, 331–338. [CrossRef] [PubMed]
16. White, K.K.; Karol, L.A.; White, D.R.; Hale, S. Musculoskeletal manifestations of Sanfilippo Syndrome (Mucopolysaccharidosis type III). *J. Pediatr. Orthop.* **2011**, *31*, 594–598. [CrossRef]
17. Lavery, C.; Hendriksz, C.J.; Jones, S.A. Mortality in patients with Sanfilippo syndrome. *Orphanet J. Rare Dis.* **2017**, *12*, 1–7. [CrossRef] [PubMed]
18. Valstar, M.J.; Bruggenwirth, H.T.; Olmer, R.; Wevers, R.A.; Verheijen, F.W.; Poorthuis, B.J.; Halley, D.J.; Wijburg, F.A. Mucopolysaccharidosis type IIIB may predominantly present with an attenuated clinical phenotype. *J. Inherit. Metab. Dis.* **2010**, *33*, 759–767. [CrossRef]
19. Delgadillo, V.; O'Callaghan, M.D.M.; Gort, L.; Coll, M.J.; Pineda, M. Natural history of Sanfilippo syndrome in Spain. *Orphanet J. Rare Dis.* **2013**, *8*, 189. [CrossRef]
20. Ruijter, G.J.; Valstar, M.J.; van de Kamp, J.M.; van der Helm, R.M.; Durand, S.; van Diggelen, O.P.; Wevers, R.A.; Poorthuis, B.J.; Pshezhetsky, A.V.; Wijburg, F.A. Clinical and genetic spectrum of Sanfilippo type C (MPS IIIC) disease in The Netherlands. *Mol. Genet. Metab.* **2008**, *93*, 104–111. [CrossRef]
21. Van de Kamp, J.J.; Niermeijer, M.F.; von Figura, K.; Giesberts, M.A. Genetic heterogeneity and clinical variability in the Sanfilippo syndrome (types A., B., and C). *Clin. Genet.* **1981**, *20*, 152–160. [CrossRef]
22. Porter, K.A.; O'Neill, C.; Drake, E.; Parker, S.; Escolar, M.L.; Montgomery, S.; Moon, W.; Worrall, C.; Peay, H.L. Parent experiences of Sanfilippo Syndrome impact and unmet treatment needs: A qualitative assessment. *Neurol. Ther.* **2021**, *10*, 197–212. [CrossRef]
23. Government UK. *F66 Guidance for Doctors Completing Medical Certificates of Cause of Death in England and Wales*; Publishing Service Government: London, UK, 2008.
24. Ouzzani, M.; Hammady, H.; Fedorowicz, Z.; Elmagarmid, A. Rayyan—A web and mobile app for systematic reviews. *Syst. Rev.* **2016**, *5*, 210. [CrossRef] [PubMed]
25. Sun, A.; Hopwood, J.J.; Thompson, J.; Cederbaum, S.D. Combined Hurler and Sanfilippo syndrome in a sibling pair. *Mol. Genet. Metab.* **2011**, *103*, 135–137. [CrossRef] [PubMed]
26. Cleary, M.A.; Wraith, J.E. Management of Mucopolysaccharidosis type III. *Arch. Dis. Child.* **1993**, *69*, 403–406. [CrossRef] [PubMed]
27. Kurihara, M.; Kumagai, K.; Yagishita, S. Sanfilippo syndrome type C: A clinicopathological autopsy study of a long-term survivor. *Pediatr. Neurol.* **1996**, *14*, 317–321. [CrossRef]
28. Danks, D.M.; Campbell, P.E.; Cartwright, E.; Mayne, V.; Taft, L.I.; Wilson, R.G. The Sanfilippo syndrome: Clinical, biochemical, radiological, haematological and pathological features of nine cases. *Aust. Paediatr. J.* **1972**, *8*, 174–186. [CrossRef]
29. Bartsocas, C.; Gröbe, H.; van de Kamp, J.J.; von Figura, K.; Kresse, H.; Klein, U.; Giesberts, M.A. Sanfilippo type C disease: Clinical findings in four patients with a new variant of Mucopolysaccharidosis III. *Eur. J. Pediatr.* **1979**, *130*, 251–258. [CrossRef]
30. Valk, H.M.J.V.S.-D.; Van De Kamp, J.J.P.; Reynolds, J.F. Follow-up on seven adult patients with mild Sanfilippo B-disease. *Am. J. Med. Genet.* **1987**, *28*, 125–129. [CrossRef]
31. Jones, M.Z.; Alroy, J.; Rutledge, J.C.; Taylor, J.W.; Alvord, E.C., Jr.; Toone, J.; Applegarth, D.; Hopwood, J.J.; Skutelsky, E.; Ianelli, C.; et al. Human Mucopolysaccharidosis IIID: Clinical, biochemical, morphological and immunohistochemical characteristics. *J. Neuropathol. Exp. Neurol.* **1997**, *56*, 1158–1167. [CrossRef]
32. Jansen, A.C.; Cao, H.; Kaplan, P.; Silver, K.; Leonard, G.; De Meirleir, L.; Lissens, W.; Liebaers, I.; Veilleux, M.; Andermann, F.; et al. Sanfilippo syndrome type D: Natural history and identification of 3 novel mutations in the GNS Gene. *Arch. Neurol.* **2007**, *64*, 1629–1634. [CrossRef]
33. Moog, U.; Van Mierlo, I.; van Schrojenstein Lantman-de Valk, H.; Spaapen, L.; Maaskant, M.A.; Curfs, L.M. Is Sanfilippo type B in your mind when you see adults with mental retardation and behavioral problems? *Am. J. Med. Genet. C Semin. Med. Genet.* **2007**, *145*, 293–301. [CrossRef]

34. Malcolm, C.; Hain, R.; Gibson, F.; Adams, S.; Anderson, G.; Forbat, L. Challenging symptoms in children with rare life-limiting conditions: Findings from a prospective diary and interview study with families. *Acta Paediatr.* **2012**, *101*, 985–992. [CrossRef]
35. Velasco, H.M.; Sanchez, Y.; Martin, A.M.; Umaña, L.A. Natural history of Sanfilippo syndrome type, C. in Boyacá, Colombia. *J. Child Neurol.* **2017**, *32*, 177–183. [CrossRef] [PubMed]
36. Shapiro, E.; Ahmed, A.; Whitley, C.; Delaney, K. Observing the advanced disease course in Mucopolysaccharidosis, type IIIA; a case series. *Mol. Genet. Metab.* **2018**, *123*, 123–126. [CrossRef]
37. Malm, G.; Månsson, J.E. Mucopolysaccharidosis type III (Sanfilippo disease) in Sweden: Clinical presentation of 22 children diagnosed during a 30-year period. *Acta Paediatr.* **2010**, *99*, 1253–1257. [CrossRef]
38. Lin, H.Y.; Chuang, C.K.; Lee, C.L.; Tu, R.Y.; Lo, Y.T.; Chiu, P.C.; Niu, D.M.; Fang, Y.Y.; Chen, T.L.; Tsai, F.J.; et al. Mucopolysaccharidosis III in Taiwan: Natural history, clinical and molecular characteristics of 28 patients diagnosed during a 21-year period. *Am. J. Med. Genet. A* **2018**, *176*, 1799–1809. [CrossRef] [PubMed]
39. Do, L.; Pasalic, L. Lymphocytes in Sanfilippo syndrome display characteristic Alder-Reilly anomaly. *Blood* **2019**, *134*, 1194. [CrossRef]
40. Gatti, R.; Borrone, C.; Durand, P.; De Virgilis, S.; Sanna, G.; Cao, A.; von Figura, K.; Kresse, H.; Paschke, E. Sanfilippo type D disease: Clinical findings in two patients with a new variant of mucopolysaccharidosis III. *Eur. J. Pediatr.* **1982**, *138*, 168–171. [CrossRef] [PubMed]
41. Sibilio, M.; Miele, E.; Ungaro, C.; Astarita, L.; Turco, R.; Di Natale, P.; Pontarelli, G.; Vecchione, R.; Andria, G.; Staiano, A.; et al. Chronic diarrhea in Mucopolysaccharidosis IIIB. *J. Pediatr. Gastroenterol. Nutr.* **2009**, *49*, 477–480. [CrossRef]
42. Sivakumur, P.; Wraith, J.E. Bone marrow transplantation in mucopolysaccharidosis type IIIA: A comparison of an early treated patient with his untreated sibling. *J. Inherit. Metab. Dis.* **1999**, *22*, 849–850. [CrossRef]
43. Kong, W.; Meng, Y.; Zou, L.; Yang, G.; Wang, J.; Shi, X. Mucopolysaccharidosis III in Mainland China: Natural history, clinical and molecular characteristics of 34 patients. *J. Pediatr. Endocrinol. Metab.* **2020**, *33*, 793–802. [CrossRef]
44. Gordon, N.; Thursby-Pelham, D. The Sanfilippo syndrome: An unusual disorder of mucopolysaccharide metabolism. *Dev. Med. Child Neurol.* **1969**, *11*, 485–492. [CrossRef]
45. Lindor, N.M.; Hoffman, A.; O'Brien, J.F.; Hanson, N.P.; Thompson, J.N. Sanfilippo syndrome type A in two adult sibs. *Am. J. Med. Genet.* **1994**, *53*, 241–244. [CrossRef]
46. Hoffmann, B.; Keshav, S. Gastrointestinal symptoms in Fabry disease: Everything is possible, including treatment. *Acta Paediatr.* **2007**, *96*, 84–86. [CrossRef] [PubMed]
47. Pensabene, L.; Sestito, S.; Nicoletti, A.; Graziano, F.; Strisciuglio, P.; Concolino, D. Gastrointestinal symptoms of patients with Fabry disease. *Gastroenterol. Res. Pract.* **2016**, *2016*, 9712831. [CrossRef] [PubMed]
48. Amiri, M.; Kuech, E.-M.; Shammas, H.; Wetzel, G.; Naim, H.Y. The Pathobiochemistry of gastrointestinal symptoms in a patient with Niemann-Pick type C disease. *JIMD Rep.* **2015**, *25*, 25–29. [CrossRef] [PubMed]
49. Cavounidis, A.; Uhlig, H.H. Crohn's disease in Niemann–Pick disease type C1: Caught in the cross-fire of host-microbial interactions. *Dig. Dis. Sci.* **2018**, *63*, 811–813. [CrossRef] [PubMed]
50. Dike, C.R.; Bernat, J.; Bishop, W.; DeGeeter, C. Niemann-Pick disease type C presenting as very early onset inflammatory bowel disease. *BMJ Case Rep.* **2019**, *12*, e229780. [CrossRef]
51. Roberts, A.L.; Howarth, G.S.; Liaw, W.C.; Moretta, S.; Kritas, S.; Lymn, K.A.; Yazbeck, R.; Tran, C.; Fletcher, J.M.; Butler, R.N.; et al. Gastrointestinal pathology in a mouse model of mucopolysaccharidosis type IIIA. *J. Cell. Physiol.* **2009**, *219*, 259–264. [CrossRef]
52. Fu, H.; Bartz, J.D.; Stephens, R.L., Jr.; McCarty, D.M. Peripheral nervous system neuropathology and progressive sensory impairments in a mouse model of Mucopolysaccharidosis IIIB. *PLoS ONE* **2012**, *7*, e45992. [CrossRef]
53. Wraith, J.E.; Scarpa, M.; Beck, M.; Bodamer, O.A.; De Meirleir, L.; Guffon, N.; Meldgaard Lund, A.; Malm, G.; Van der Ploeg, A.T.; Zeman, J. Mucopolysaccharidosis type II (Hunter syndrome): A clinical review and recommendations for treatment in the era of enzyme replacement therapy. *Eur. J. Pediatr.* **2008**, *167*, 267–277. [CrossRef]
54. Mori, H.; Kobara, H.; Fujihara, S.; Nishiyama, N.; Kobayashi, M.; Masaki, T.; Izuishi, K.; Suzuki, Y. Rectal perforations and fistulae secondary to a glycerin enema: Closure by over-the-scope-clip. *World J. Gastroenterol.* **2012**, *18*, 3177–3180. [CrossRef]
55. Araghizadeh, F. Fecal impaction. *Clin. Colon Rectal Surg.* **2005**, *18*, 116–119. [CrossRef]
56. Datta, V.; Engledow, A.; Chan, S.; Forbes, A.; Cohen, C.R.; Windsor, A. The management of enterocutaneous fistula in a regional unit in the United kingdom: A prospective study. *Dis. Colon Rectum* **2010**, *53*, 192–199. [CrossRef] [PubMed]
57. Medicines.org.uk. *Loperamide 2 mg Capsules—Summary of Product Characteristics (SPC) (eMC)*; Aurobindo Pharma—Milpharm Ltd.: Middlesex, UK, 2019.
58. Tchan, M.C.; Sillence, D. Extrapyramidal symptoms and medication use in Mucopolysaccharidosis type III. *J. Intellect. Dev. Disabil.* **2009**, *34*, 275–279. [CrossRef] [PubMed]
59. Moudgal, R.; Schultz, A.W.; Shah, E.D. Systemic disease associations with disorders of gut-brain interaction and gastrointestinal transit: A review. *Clin. Exp. Gastroenterol.* **2021**, *14*, 249–257. [CrossRef] [PubMed]
60. Mahon, L.V.; Lomax, M.; Grant, S.; Cross, E.; Hare, D.J.; Wraith, J.E.; Jones, S.; Bigger, B.; Langford-Smith, K.; Canal, M. Assessment of sleep in children with Mucopolysaccharidosis type III. *PLoS ONE* **2014**, *9*, e84128. [CrossRef]

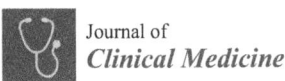

Article

Assessment of Dysphonia in Children with Pompe Disease Using Auditory-Perceptual and Acoustic/Physiologic Methods

Kelly D. Crisp [1], Amy T. Neel [2], Sathya Amarasekara [3], Jill Marcus [4], Gretchen Nichting [5], Aditi Korlimarla [5], Priya S. Kishnani [5] and Harrison N. Jones [1],*

[1] Department of Head and Neck Surgery & Communication Sciences, Duke University School of Medicine, Durham, NC 27710, USA; kelly.crisp@duke.edu
[2] Department of Speech and Hearing Sciences, University of New Mexico, Albuquerque, NM 87131, USA; atneel@unm.edu
[3] Duke Clinical Research Institute, Duke Health, Durham, NC 27710, USA; sathya.amarasekara@duke.edu
[4] Division of Speech Pathology and Audiology, Duke Health, Durham, NC 27710, USA; jill.marcus@duke.edu
[5] Department of Pediatrics, Division of Medical Genetics, Duke University School of Medicine, Durham, NC 27710, USA; gretchen.nichting@duke.edu (G.N.); aditi.korlimarla@duke.edu (A.K.); priya.kishnani@duke.edu (P.S.K.)
* Correspondence: harrison.jones@duke.edu; Tel.: +1-919-681-1852

Abstract: Bulbar and respiratory weakness occur commonly in children with Pompe disease and frequently lead to dysarthria. However, changes in vocal quality associated with this motor speech disorder are poorly described. The goal of this study was to characterize the vocal function of children with Pompe disease using auditory-perceptual and physiologic/acoustic methods. High-quality voice recordings were collected from 21 children with Pompe disease. The Grade, Roughness, Breathiness, Asthenia, and Strain (GRBAS) scale was used to assess voice quality and ratings were compared to physiologic/acoustic measurements collected during sustained phonation tasks, reading of a standard passage, and repetition of a short phrase at maximal volume. Based on ratings of grade, dysphonia was present in 90% of participants and was most commonly rated as mild or moderate in severity. Duration of sustained phonation tasks was reduced and shimmer was increased in comparison to published reference values for children without dysphonia. Specific measures of loudness were found to have statistically significant relationships with perceptual ratings of grade, breathiness, asthenia, and strain. Our data suggest that dysphonia is common in children with Pompe disease and primarily reflects impairments in respiratory and laryngeal function; however, the primary cause of dysphonia remains unclear. Future studies should seek to quantify the relative contribution of deficits in individual speech subsystems on voice quality and motor speech performance more broadly.

Keywords: pompe disease; speech; voice; dysphonia; acoustic; auditory-perceptual; GRBAS; respiratory

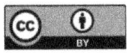

1. Introduction

Pompe disease, caused by a deficiency of the enzyme acid-alpha glucosidase (GAA), is characterized by an abnormal accumulation of glycogen in the lysosomes of multiple tissues, including skeletal, cardiac, and smooth muscles. Pompe disease is broadly classified into two groups: Infantile and late-onset Pompe disease. Infantile-onset Pompe disease (IOPD) represents the most severe end of the clinical spectrum. Children with IOPD present with hypertrophic cardiomyopathy and profound muscle weakness at or soon after birth. Symptom onset for patients with late-onset Pompe disease (LOPD) ranges from the first year of life to later adulthood. Individuals with LOPD generally exhibit a slower rate of disease progression and suffer less severe clinical outcomes than those with IOPD. Even within these categories, the disease exists along a continuum with variable clinical presentation related age of symptom onset, amount of residual GAA, and cross-reactive immune material (CRIM) status [1,2].

Since the introduction of enzyme replacement therapy (ERT) in 2006, children with IOPD are surviving longer [1]. The wide-spread adoption of newborn screening (NBS) programs has resulted in the identification of more children with Pompe disease, both with and without clinical symptoms. Accordingly, new phenotypes are emerging in the survivors of IOPD and children with LOPD. There is evidence of motor-based impairments that persist due to residual myopathy, including progressive skeletal muscle weakness, gait abnormalities, contractures, ptosis, and respiratory decline [3].

Dysarthria is a neuromuscular speech disorder in which damage to the central and/or peripheral nervous system or muscles affects speech production. Flaccid dysarthria results from weakness caused by damage to the motor unit and may arise from a variety of neurologic diseases and conditions including myopathy [4]. Characteristics of dysarthria associated with bulbar weakness include hypernasality, nasal emission, short phrases, reduced articulatory precision, and reduced speech intelligibility, all of which negatively impact affected individuals' communication abilities [4]. Dysarthria arising from bulbar weakness often includes changes in voice such as breathiness, reduced loudness, and hoarseness, which further reduce communicative effectiveness [4]. Previous reports describe articulation disorders, hypernasality, and impaired speech intelligibility consistent with flaccid dysarthria in children with Pompe disease [5–8]. However, speech disorders have received less attention in the literature than other motor-based impairments.

Though our clinical experiences suggest that dysphonia (abnormal vocal quality) is a common feature of dysarthria in children with Pompe disease, relatively little detailed information about the voice characteristics of this population is available. We previously identified the presence of dysphonia in 35% of auditory-perceptual assessments in 10 children with IOPD via retrospective analysis [5]. Szklanny and colleagues investigated laryngeal function and structure in ten adults and nine children with LOPD [9]. Based on electroglottography and acoustic analysis, vocal fold insufficiency attributed to laryngeal weakness was present in both groups, though these changes were greater in children than adults with LOPD.

Recent investigations have identified disease impact in both the central and peripheral nervous systems of individuals with IOPD and LOPD [10–15]. Understanding clinical signs resulting from neurological and motor impairments, both individually and in combination with each other, are critical to refining our understanding of disease phenotype. Speech disorders associated with neurological involvement result in activity limitations and participation restrictions that negatively impact quality of life for many children with Pompe disease and therefore merit investigation. Bulbar and respiratory weakness occur commonly in children with Pompe disease and frequently lead to dysarthria; however, associated changes in vocal quality are poorly described. In this study, our goal was to characterize the vocal function of children with Pompe disease using auditory-perceptual and physiologic/acoustic methods that permit objective quantification of various aspects of the acoustic signal. We expected that both auditory-perceptual and physiologic/acoustic assessments would reveal abnormalities in vocal function occur commonly in children with Pompe disease.

2. Materials and Methods

2.1. Participants

English-speaking participants between the ages of 5 and 18 years with a confirmed diagnosis of IOPD or LOPD were recruited from the Duke University Pompe Disease Clinic and Research Program as part of a larger study investigating cognitive and neurological pathologies in children with Pompe disease (Pro00072329). Exclusion criteria were inability to travel to Duke for study assessments or refusal of informed consent. Written consent for participation was given by the participants' parents or legal guardians. Verbal assent was obtained from children 6 to 11 years of age, and additional written assent was obtained from children 12 years of age and older. The study was approved by the Duke University Institutional Review Board and conducted in accordance with the Declaration of Helsinki.

2.2. Procedures

2.2.1. Auditory-Perceptual Assessment

The GRBAS (Grade, Roughness, Breathiness, Asthenia, and Strain) scale is a widely used and highly reliable perceptual scale to assess voice quality in individuals with voice disorders [16,17]. Each of five voice characteristics is rated on a Likert scale of 0–3 in which 0 = normal/no disorder, 1 = mild disorder, 2 = moderate disorder, and 3 = severe disorder. Two speech-language pathologists (SLPs) with ten years or more of clinical experience listened to recordings of a vowel prolongation task and used the GRBAS scale to make judgments regarding voice characteristics. High-quality acoustic recordings of a series of speech tasks were obtained from each participant using a Sony PCM M-10 recorder and an omnidirectional Countryman head-mounted microphone. The microphone headframe and the mic boom were adjusted to achieve a consistent mouth-to-microphone position approximately 0.25″ to 0.5″ from the corner of the participant's mouth when smiling. Analog signals were manually recorded at a sampling frequency of 44.1 kHz and 16 bit depth while the recording level and microphone sensitivity were held constant. The acoustic recordings were digitally encoded via linear PCM and saved on a microSD card, then transferred to a secure server on a lab computer where they were stored in WAV format. Lab personnel not otherwise involved in the research extracted recordings of the vowel prolongation task from the audio files of each study participant. Sample presentation was randomized using an online randomization sequence generator and the audio clips were compiled into a master audio file for auditory-perceptual assessment. In this master audio file, the vowel prolongation sample from each participant was presented five times in a row with a five-second break between each presentation, allowing raters to consider grade, roughness, breathiness, asthenia, and strain individually. A 10-s break followed the fifth presentation of each participant's sample.

Prior to collecting GRBAS scale ratings for analysis, the two raters completed a listener calibration session. After both raters reviewed the terms and definitions used in the GRBAS scale, approximately 20 samples of vowel prolongation were randomly selected from the data set. Each rater independently scored each sample using the GRBAS scale and then compared results, discussing the voice characteristics and their severity. The purposes of this training activity were to establish agreement regarding the definitions of the voice characteristics being evaluated and establish a joint reference for ratings of severity [18].

GRBAS scale ratings were collected for all participants in a single listening session. The master audio file was played in sound field for both raters simultaneously at a comfortable listening level over high-quality speakers in a quiet, carpeted room with <50 dB A of ambient noise. The raters scored the samples independently. After the listening session was completed, one of the two raters (HJ) compared the ratings for all samples and identified each GRBAS scale component that lacked exact agreement. One-month later, the two raters met again and re-listened to the samples in question. After discussing their impressions, a final consensus rating was recorded.

2.2.2. Physiologic/Acoustic Assessment

Instrumental assessment of voice was completed using the WEVOSYS lingWAVES measurement system and the lingWAVES Voice Protocol (version 3.2, WEVOSYS, Forchheim, Germany). Digital-acoustic voice data was collected using standardized hardware provided by the system manufacturer, which included a certified A meter/microphone set to C frequency and slow time weighting and the lingWAVES Connector USB containing its own high-quality sound card. The A meter/microphone was placed directly in front of the participant with the mic head 30 cm from the participant's mouth. Data were collected in a quiet, carpeted room with ambient noise < 50 dB A. The lingWAVES Voice Protocol includes standard instructions for assessment tasks which included sustained phonation tasks, reading of a standard passage (the Rainbow Passage), and repetition of a short phrase at maximal volume. Participants completed all assessment tasks while seated. Participants who were unable to read aloud fluently were excluded from completing the oral reading task. A variety of measurements were derived, including /s/duration; /z/duration; s/z ratio; maximum phonation time (MPT); jitter; shimmer; mean fundamental frequency; mean loudness; glottal-to-noise excitation (GNE); and dysphonia severity index (DSI) for sustained phonation; mean, minimum, and maximum loudness for spoken text; and maximum loudness. Calculations for these parameters were automatically performed by the lingWAVES algorithm. There were no additional manipulations of the signal prior to calculation.

2.3. Statistical Analysis

Descriptive statistics were calculated to describe the sample characteristics. Weighted kappa statistics were utilized to examine the interrater agreement of ordinal auditory perceptual ratings between the two raters. The results were assessed as <0 indicating less than chance agreement, 0.01–0.20 as slight agreement, 0.21–0.40 as fair agreement, 0.41–0.60 as moderate agreement, 0.61–0.80 as substantial agreement, and 0.81–0.99 as almost perfect agreement [19]. Multiple regression analysis models were used to assess the relationships among each voice protocol variable as the outcome and each auditory-perceptual feature as the predictor controlling for sex and age at assessment. The analyses were conducted using SAS/STAT software (version 9.4, SAS System for Windows, SAS Institute Inc., Cary, NC, USA, 2012). All analyses were two-tailed with a $p < 0.05$ deemed as statistically significant.

3. Results

Auditory-perceptual and physiologic/acoustic voice data were collected from 21 children with Pompe disease with a mean age of 9.9 years (median = 9.4, SD = 3.7, range 5.0–17.0) at the time of assessment. Seventeen of 21 participants were diagnosed with IOPD; 14 were CRIM positive and three were CRIM negative. Four of 21 participants were diagnosed with LOPD. All participants were on ERT at the time of assessment; 4/21 received standard of care (20 mg/kg biweekly) and 16/21 received doses ranging from 30–40 mg/kg weekly/biweekly. Complete demographic data for participants with IOPD and LOPD are provided in Table 1. Additional cohort characteristics are contained within the Supplementary Materials (Table S1).

Table 1. Baseline characteristics. Categorical variables presented as n, (%). Continuous variables presented as Mean (SD), median (Min-Max).

	IOPD (n = 17)	LOPD (n = 4)
Sex		
Male	8/17 (47%)	3/4 (75%)
Female	9/17 (53%)	1/4 (25%)
Race		
Caucasian	11/17 (65%)	2/4 (50%)
Black or African American	4/17 (24%)	1/4 (25%)
Asian	1/17 (6%)	1/4 (25%)
Other or more than one race	1/17 (6%)	-
Ethnicity		
Not Hispanic or Latino	15/17 (88%)	4/4 (100%)
Hispanic or Latino	2/17 (12%)	-
Age at diagnosis (years)	0.3 (0.3), 0.2 (0.0–1.1)	5.0 (4.5), 3.9 (1.1–11.1)
Age at assessment (years)	8.9 (3.8), 7.0 (5.0–17.0)	11.8 (2.2), 12.0 (9.0–14.0)
CRIM status		
Positive	14/17 (82%)	-
Negative	3/17 (18%)	-

Table 1. Cont.

	IOPD (n = 17)	LOPD (n = 4)
ERT history		
ERT Start Age (years)	0.3 (0.3), 0.3 (0.0–1.1)	5.3 (4.7), 4.0 (1.4, 11.7)
Time on ERT at assessment (years)	9.0 (3.8), 7.6 (5.0–16.9)	7.1 (5.1), 7.9 (0.1–12.3)
ERT dose at assessment		
20 mg/kg biweekly	2/17 (12%)	2/4 (50%)
30 mg/kg weekly	1/17 (6%)	-
40 mg/kg biweekly	4/17 (24%)	-
40 mg/kg weekly	9/17 (53%)	2/4 (50%)
Infused biweekly; dose not recorded	1/17 (6%)	-

IOPD = infantile-onset Pompe disease; LOPD = late-onset Pompe disease; CRIM = cross-reactive immunological status; ERT = enzyme replacement therapy.

3.1. Inter-Rater Agreement

The weighted kappa for each coefficient is provided in Table 2. In the first listening session, moderate agreement was achieved between the two raters for grade (0.51, $p < 0.01$), breathiness (0.45, $p = 0.02$), asthenia (0.58, $p < 0.01$) and strain (0.57, $p < 0.001$). Fair agreement was achieved for roughness (0.36, $p = 0.04$) [20]. Overall, samples from 17 of 21 participants (81%) required the two raters to re-listen to the sample to achieve consensus for one or more GRBAS component scores. Across the 210 individual GRBAS component scores provided by the two raters in the first listening session, 172 (82%) were in exact agreement after the first listen whereas 38 (18%) required re-listening. Original, independent ratings differed by 1 scale value in 36 (95%) of disagreements and by 2 scale values in 2 (5%) of disagreements.

Table 2. Interrater agreement for GRBAS scale. Kappa interrater agreement between two listeners in the first listening session across 21 participants.

	Weighted Kappa	95% CI	p-Value	Disagreements by 1 Scale Value	Disagreements by 2 Scale Values
Grade	0.51	(0.23, 0.79)	0.00 *	7	1
Roughness	0.36	(0.07, 0.64)	0.04 *	8	0
Breathiness	0.45	(0.13, 0.77)	0.02 *	8	0
Asthenia	0.58	(0.32, 0.85)	0.00 **	8	0
Strain	0.57	(0.26, 0.87)	0.00 ***	5	1

* $p < 0.05$, ** $p < 0.01$, *** $p < 0.001$.

3.2. Auditory-Perceptual Ratings

Auditory-perceptual ratings of grade (a proxy for overall dysphonia severity), roughness, breathiness, asthenia, and strain for 21 participants are presented in Table 3. Based on ratings of grade, dysphonia was present during vowel prolongation in 19/21 participants with IOPD and LOPD (90%). Across all five components of the GRBAS, deviations from normal were most commonly rated as mild or moderate in severity. Deviations from normal were infrequently rated as severe in the IOPD group, and none of the five GRBAS components were rated as severe in the LOPD group.

Table 3. Auditory-perceptual ratings of vocal quality.

	Normal	Mild	Moderate	Severe	Mean (SD)
IOPD (n = 17)					
Grade	1/17 (6%)	7/17 (41%)	7/17 (41%)	2/17 (12%)	1.59 (0.80)
Roughness	2/17 (12%)	9/17 (53%)	5/17 (29%)	1/17 (6%)	1.29 (0.77)
Breathiness	1/17 (6%)	11/17 (65%)	4/17 (24%)	1/17 (6%)	1.29 (0.69)
Asthenia	7/17 (41%)	6/17 (35%)	3/17 (18%)	1/17 (6%)	0.88 (0.93)
Strain	3/17 (18%)	13/17 (76%)	1/17 (6%)	-	0.88 (0.49)

Table 3. Cont.

	Normal	Mild	Moderate	Severe	Mean (SD)
LOPD (n = 4)					
Grade	1/4 (25%)	3/4 (75%)	-	-	0.75 (0.50)
Roughness	-	4/4 (100%)	-	-	1.00 (0.00)
Breathiness	-	3/4 (75%)	1/4 (25%)	-	1.25 (0.50)
Asthenia	-	4/4 (100%)	-	-	1.00 (0.00)
Strain	3/4 (75%)	1/4 (25%)	-	-	0.25 (0.50)
Overall (n = 21)					
Grade	2/21 (10%)	10/21 (48%)	7/21 (33%)	2/21 (10%)	1.43 (0.81)
Roughness	2/21 (10%)	13/21 (62%)	5/21 (24%)	1/21 (5%)	1.24 (0.70)
Breathiness	1/21 (5%)	14/21 (67%)	5/21 (24%)	1/21 (5%)	1.29 (0.64)
Asthenia	7/21 (33%)	10/21 (48%)	3/21 (14%)	1/21 (5%)	0.90 (0.83)
Strain	6/21 (29%)	14/21 (67%)	1/21 (5%)	-	0.76 (0.54)

Data presented as n, (%). Mean (SD) calculated where 0 = normal, 1 = mild, 2 = moderate, 3 = severe. IOPD = infantile-onset Pompe disease; LOPD = late-onset Pompe disease.

3.3. Physiologic/Acoustic Data

Summary statistics for physiologic/acoustic voice data are presented in Table 4. Individual physiologic/acoustic data for each participant is provided in the Supplementary Material (Tables S2–S4). Some participants were unable to complete all assessment tasks due to difficulty following task instructions or limitations in literacy. Equipment malfunction interfered with collection of physiologic/acoustic data in one participant.

Our data revealed mean sustained phonation time for the phonemes /s/, /z/, and /a/ was reduced in study participants when compared to published reference values [21–30]. Duration of sustained /s/ was shorter than the 8–12 s thresholds for typically developing children in 20/21 participants and sustained /a/ duration was shorter than 8 s in 18/21 participants. Only one participant, however, had an s/z ratio greater than 1.45, the threshold value for typical children. The majority of participants (18/20) had elevated mean shimmer values compared to pediatric normative threshold of 5%, but only 7 of 20 had jitter values that exceeded 0.5% [20,28,29]. The mean GNE value was 0.5 compared to the value of 0.90 found in children without dysphonia [31]. In our sample, GNE values were below this threshold in 18/20 subjects. The mean DSI value was −0.6 and these values ranged from 3.6 to −5.0. Pebbili and colleagues report mean DSI values in typically developing children without voice complaints to be 2.9 in males and 3.8 in females [32]. Based on these thresholds, DSI values were abnormal in 14/15 participants. Mean loudness values for the passage read aloud fell within the range of typical speakers reported by Corthals (69.39 dBA (4.08)) [22]. Seven of the 14 participants who completed the task had mean loudness values below 65 dB; two of those produced mean loudness values below 60 dB. Maximum loudness levels produced when participants repeated a short phrase as loudly as possible appeared consistent with pediatric norms reported by Weinrich et al. [23]. Three of the 21 participants produced maximum loudness values of less than 83 dB, below the range of typical children.

Table 4. Summary statistics for physiologic/acoustic data.

		All Participants	Group-Wise Analysis	
	Task	(n = 14 [†], 15 [x], 20 [‡], or 21)	IOPD (n = 10 [*], 12 [**], 16 [§], or 17)	LOPD (n = 3 [††], 4)
Sustained phonation tasks [21–33]	/s/duration (s)	2.9 (2.9); 0.5–9.4	2.6 (2.8); 0.5–9.4	4.0 (3.1); 1.4–8.3
	/z/duration (s)	3.7 (3.1); 0.7–11.3	3.5 (3.1); 0.7–11.3	4.5 (3.7); 1.0–9.5
	s/z ratio	0.8 (0.4); 0.3–2.0	0.7 (0.3); 0.3–1.1	1.1 (0.7); 0.5–2.0
	MPT (s)	5.9 (4.4); 0.7–14.6 [‡]	5.5 (4.5); 0.7–14.6	8.0 (3.6); 5.8–12.1 [††]
	Jitter (%)	0.7 (0.8); 0.1–2.8 [‡]	0.8 (0.9); 0.1–2.8 [§]	0.2 (0.1); 0.1–0.3
	Shimmer (%)	11.2 (8.9); 4.9–40.6 [‡]	11.9 (9.8); 5.0–40.6 [§]	8.3 (2.5); 4.9–10.4
	Mean F0 (Hz)	244.6 (67.7); 114.5–351.2 [‡]	246.5 (72.8); 114.5–351.2 [§]	237.1 (49.2); 202.9–309.6
	Mean loudness (dBA)	76.8 (7.8); 63.0–93.1 [‡]	77.7 (6.9); 66.5–93.1 [§]	73.3 (11.3); 63.0–89.1
	GNE	0.5 (0.4); 0.2–2.2 [‡]	0.5 (0.5); 0.2–2.2 [§]	0.5 (0.3); −0.1–0.8
	DSI	−0.6 (2.2); −5.0–3.6 [x]	−0.9 (2.4); −5.0–3.6 [**]	0.3 (0.5); −0.1–0.8 [††]
Spoken text (Rainbow Passage) [22]	Mean loudness (dBA)	65.3 (4.7); 56.7–73.5 [†]	65.9 (4.9); 56.7–73.5 [*]	63.9 (4.4); 59.2–68.8
	Max loudness (dBA)	71.9 (5.1); 65.0–81.2 [†]	72.8 (4.9); 65.3–81.2 [*]	69.7 (5.6); 65.0–77.0
	Min loudness (dBA)	55.7 (5.2); 46.0–61.8 [†]	55.8 (5.3); 46.0–61.8 [*]	55.4 (5.6); 47.5–59.6
Max loudness task [23]	Max loudness (dBA)	91.3 (10.8); 58.9–104.3	89.9 (11.1); 58.9–103.9	96.9 (7.8); 89.6–104.3

Data are presented as mean (SD); range. MPT = maximum phonation time, s = seconds, Hz = Hertz, min = minimum, max = maximum, dBA = decibels A-weighted (reference value = 20 µPa), F0 = fundamental frequency; GNE = glottal-to-noise excitation; DSI = dysphonia severity index. Note mean values that differ from published normative data for typically developing children are highlighted in gray.
[†] n = 14, [x] n = 15, [‡] n = 20; [*] n = 10, [**] n = 12, [§] n = 16; [††] n = 3.

3.4. Relationship between Auditory-Perceptual and Acoustic Data

We examined the relationship among auditory-perceptual and physiologic/acoustic outcomes using multiple regression models while controlling for sex and age at time of assessment (Tables 5 and 6). Data for participants with IOPD and LOPD were collapsed for statistical analysis as there were minimal differences in the physiologic/acoustic characteristics of the two groups. Statistically significant relationships were identified between loudness measures and auditory perceptual ratings of breathiness and asthenia, including: Mean loudness during spoken text and breathiness ($p < 0.01$) and asthenia ($p < 0.05$); minimum loudness during spoken text and breathiness ($p < 0.01$) and asthenia ($p = 0.03$); and maximum loudness during spoken text and breathiness ($p = 0.03$) and asthenia ($p = 0.04$). As loudness increased, breathiness and asthenia ratings decreased. Loudness during an isolated maximum performance task was significantly related to grade ($p < 0.01$), breathiness ($p = 0.02$) and asthenia ($p = 0.01$). In addition, the relationship between s/z ratio and strain was statistically significant ($p = 0.02$). As s/z ratio increased, strain ratings decreased. Relationships between consensus ratings and other instrumental data did not reach statistical significance.

Table 5. Relationship between physiologic/acoustic voice data from sustained phonation tasks and consensus ratings from GRBAS scale, controlled for age at assessment and sex.

Versus GRBAS		Sustained Phonation Tasks									
		/s/ Duration (s)	/z/ Duration (s)	s/z Ratio	MPT (s)	Jitter (%)	Shimmer (%)	Mean F0 (Hz)	Mean Loudness (dBA)	GNE	DSI
G	Mean Est	0.76	0.63	0.01	−0.30	0.44	3.93	−0.94	−3.26	0.09	−0.18
	p-value	0.30	0.45	0.89	0.83	0.07	0.13	0.96	0.21	0.56	0.70
R	Mean Est	0.68	0.90	−0.07	1.12	0.20	0.15	−11.16	−1.90	−0.01	−0.34
	p-value	0.37	0.29	0.46	0.43	0.46	0.96	0.55	0.50	0.97	0.48
B	Mean Est	−0.47	−0.88	0.03	−2.20	0.21	−2.08	27.82	−5.84	0.26	−0.82
	p-value	0.63	0.42	0.83	0.21	0.56	0.59	0.27	0.12	0.25	0.16
A	Mean Est	0.05	−0.30	0.09	−0.89	0.00	−3.35	10.39	−4.19	0.21	−0.15
	p-value	0.95	0.70	0.30	0.49	0.99	0.20	0.57	0.11	0.18	0.73
S	Mean Est	0.20	1.02	−3.0	3.19	0.57	−0.42	−26.28	0.27	−0.07	−0.24
	p-value	0.85	0.39	0.02 *	0.11	0.09	0.91	0.28	0.94	0.75	0.73

G = grade, R = roughness, B = breathiness, A = asthenia, S = strain; Mean Est = mean estimate; s = seconds; MPT = maximum phonation time; SV = sustained vowel; F0 = fundamental frequency; Hz = Hertz, dB A = decibels sound pressure level A-weighted (reference value = 20 µPa); GNE = glottal-to-noise excitation; DSI = dysphonia severity index. * $p < 0.05$. Note mean values that differ from published normative data for typically developing children are highlighted in gray.

Table 6. Relationship between acoustic voice data from spoken text and maximal loudness tasks and consensus ratings from GRBAS scale, controlled for age at assessment and sex.

	Versus GRBAS	Spoken Text (Rainbow Passage)			Maximum Loudness Task
		Mean Loudness (dBA)	Min Loudness (dBA)	Max Loudness (dBA)	Max Loudness (dBA)
G	Mean Est	−1.65	−2.65	−0.82	−9.39
	p-value	0.41	0.25	0.72	0.00 **
R	Mean Est	−0.67	0.27	−0.67	1.31
	p-value	0.73	0.91	0.76	0.71
B	Mean Est	−6.55	−7.68	−6.26	−9.57
	p-value	0.00 **	0.00 **	0.026 *	0.02 *
A	Mean Est	−4.59	−4.68	−4.44	−7.23
	p-value	0.01 *	0.03 *	0.04 *	0.01 *
S	Mean Est	4.69	5.01	4.63	6.5
	p-value	0.13	0.17	0.20	0.17

G = grade, R = roughness, B = breathiness, A = asthenia, S = strain; Mean Est = mean estimate; dB A = decibels sound pressure level A-weighted (reference value = 20 µPa); Min = minimum; Max = maximum. * $p < 0.05$, ** $p < 0.01$. Note mean values that differ from published normative data for typically developing children are highlighted in gray.

4. Discussion

These data provide a detailed description of vocal function in children with IOPD and LOPD using both a validated auditory-perceptual rating scale (GRBAS) and physiologic/acoustic measures. With 21 unique participants, our report also describes the voice features of the largest cohort of children with IOPD and LOPD in the literature to date.

Two experienced SLP raters achieved moderate-fair agreement in rating voice quality using the GRBAS scale, which is comparable to that reported in other studies [34]. Dysphonia was a common finding in children with IOPD and LOPD when using this scale to evaluate vocal quality during vowel prolongation. Across all 21 participants, dysphonia was present in 90% of the sample. Based on ratings of grade, one participant with IOPD and one participant with LOPD were not judged as dysphonic during vowel prolongation. Dysphonia was judged as mild or moderate in severity in more than 80% of participants with IOPD and mild in 75% of participants with LOPD. No voice quality feature was rated as severe in the LOPD group. Breathiness and roughness were the most prevalent voice quality features identified by the raters in participants with IOPD and LOPD. Asthenia was present in 4/4 participants with LOPD; however, strain was noted less frequently in comparison to participants with IOPD.

Overall, our physiologic/acoustic data suggest that MPT, /s/duration, and /z/duration are reduced and shimmer is increased in children with both IOPD and LOPD when compared to published reference values for children without dysphonia. The most obvious differences between our sample of children with Pompe disease and reference values for typically developing children were noted in sustained phonation tasks. Mean MPT was 5.9 s (4.4), lower than the range of reference values reported in typically developing children [23,24,27,30,35]. According to Finnegan, MPT < 8 s in females and <9 s in males should be considered abnormal [27]. Mean duration for sustained phonation of /s/ and /z/ phonemes (mean values of 2.9 s (2.9) and 3.7 s (3.1), respectively) was also reduced in comparison to published normative data [24–26]. Sustained phonation tasks, widely included in voice evaluations in both clinical and research settings, are intended to assess the integrity of the laryngeal and respiratory systems and the ability to coordinate respiration with phonation [24,36]. Airflow measures such as vital capacity have been linked to MPT [28,37] and recent publications have recommended the inclusion of pulmonary function tests in voice assessment [38]. Respiratory muscle weakness with early involvement of the diaphragm is a known complication of both IOPD and LOPD [1,39,40] and therefore our finding of reduced MPT in this sample of children with Pompe disease is not surprising.

The integrity of laryngeal valving, neuromuscular control of the larynx, and its ability to rapidly adjust to various configurations of the vocal tract are also related to performance on sustained phonation tasks [28,36,37]. The s/z ratio task compares the duration of sustained production of /s/, a consonant that does not require vocal fold vibration, to the duration of sustained production of /z/, a consonant that does require vocal fold vibration. Typical speakers are expected to produce ratios below 1.4, sustaining both consonants for roughly the same amount of time, while speakers with vocal fold pathology may have ratios above 1.4 due to increased ability to sustain the voiceless/s/ compared to the voiced/z/. In this study, while the duration of /s/ and /z/ were reduced in our sample, the s/z ratio, an indicator of glottal efficiency, was below the 1.4 threshold for all but one participant. This may indicate that respiratory function had a larger impact than laryngeal function on total duration of sustained phonation in these participants. Interestingly, eight of the participants produced s/z ratios of less than 0.6; that is, they sustained the voiced/z/ for much longer than the voiceless/s/. This pattern may reflect a complex interaction between laryngeal function, voluntary control of the articulators influencing the shape and size of the vocal tract, and respiratory support for voicing [36].

Vocal intensity, or loudness, is also known to be impacted by pulmonary function, airflow measures, and neuromuscular control of the larynx [37,38,41]. Reference values for loudness are limited by variability in the way in which intensity is measured. The literature generally reports the intensity of conversational speech to vary between 50 and 70 dBA [42]. Corthals measured mean sound pressure over time (Leq) while 92 children between 7 and 18 years of age read the Rainbow Passage [22]. The participants in our study read the Rainbow Passage aloud with a mean loudness of 65.3 dBA (4.7), reflecting function at the lower end of the range reported by Corthals (65.31 to 73.47 dBA). However, performance varied substantially across individual participants, with loudness values during spoken text ranging from 56.7 to 73.5 dBA. It is the authors' clinical impression that both overall loudness and loudness range are frequently reduced in children with Pompe disease.

Jitter and shimmer are objective acoustic measures of voice quality, indicating irregularities in vocal fundamental frequency and intensity. While jitter values for the participants in this study were within normal limits, mean values for shimmer, reflecting cycle-to-cycle variability in amplitude, were increased in our sample compared to published norms [29,30]. While increased shimmer may reflect vocal pathology, recent studies have shown that both shimmer and jitter are influenced by vocal loudness [43]. Less intense voices, like those of children with Pompe disease, are associated with higher shimmer and jitter values than louder ones.

Auditory-perceptual ratings of breathiness, asthenia, and grade were negatively correlated with loudness during spoken text and maximum loudness during an isolated maximal performance task. In other words, as loudness and glottal closure increased, perception of breathiness and asthenia decreased and grade, a proxy for overall dysphonia severity, improved. This suggests that participants with louder voices and more complete glottal closure were perceived to have less severe dysphonia; breathy and/or asthenic voices are unlikely to be loud. As noted above, mean loudness in our sample was comparable to available reference values for loudness in typically developing children [22,23]. Several types of acoustic measures were obtained, including measures of irregularity of vocal fold vibration (jitter, shimmer), inharmonic noise (GNE) and composite measures (DSI), but none were significantly related to auditory-perceptual ratings for these participants.

Prior descriptions of the speech and swallowing function of children with IOPD confirm that dysarthria and dysphagia are common and appear related to widespread involvement of the bulbar muscles [5–8,44–47]. Involvement of the central and/or peripheral nervous systems can influence bulbar muscle pathology and impact speech production [4,11–16]. The resulting signs and symptoms manifested in respiration, phonation, articulation, resonance, and prosody result in dysarthria that frequently persists despite speech treatment [8]. Hearing loss is also documented and may further impact speech [48] but does not fully explain the degree of speech impairment observed in affected patients [46]. Early diagnosis with early initiation of ERT [49], high-dose regimens of ERT [3,50], and adjunctive treatments like physical therapy and beta-2 adrenergic agonists [51] often result in improvements or stabilization of motor and pulmonary function. However, dysarthria frequently appears to remain. This study focused on vocal function in children with Pompe disease and our findings suggest that dysphonia primarily reflect impairments in respiratory support and laryngeal function. However, its clinical presentation is complex and the primary cause of dysphonia remains unclear.

Reduced duration of sustained phonation tasks suggests respiratory support compromised task performance, both in our study as well as in a detailed report of the speech and oromotor features of a cohort of 14 children with Pompe disease by Su and colleagues [7]. However, mean MPT of the children in our sample (5.9 s (4.4)) was shorter in duration than the mean MPT reported by Su (8.29 s (3.7)). The 12 children with IOPD in Su's cohort were all identified by NBS with ERT initiation within one month of birth; CRIM status of these children was not reported. In the 17 children with IOPD from our sample, 11 were diagnosed >1 month of age, the median age at start of ERT was three months (range 0–13 months), and three of the participants were CRIM negative. As noted above, early initiation of ERT has been reported to have a positive impact on pulmonary function [3,49,52], which would be expected to improve respiratory support for phonation. Furthermore, the children with IOPD in our sample (mean 8.9 years (3.8), range 5.0–17.0) were older than the children with IOPD in Su's cohort (mean 5.9 years (1.8), range 3.5–8.8). Since both respiratory muscle strength and sustained phonation duration are known to increase with age [53–55], this may indicate the children in our cohort had greater respiratory muscle weakness than those studied by Su.

The relationship between acoustic and auditory-perceptual analyses of voice quality for children with IOPD has not previously been explored; however, data describing the voice characteristics of children with LOPD are available for comparison and also provide evidence of laryngeal involvement. Szklanny and colleagues collected perceptual ratings using the GRBAS scale along with video-laryngoscopic examination, electroglottography, and acoustic recordings from 9 individuals with LOPD ranging from 7.5 to 25.6 years old [9,56]. Evidence of tense voice type, altered pitch, and dysphonia related to glottal insufficiency with incomplete focal fold closure during phonation was identified through video-laryngoscopic examination. However, overall grade was judged as normal in 75% (6/8) of ratings; mild or moderate breathiness, asthenia or strain were identified in 63% (5/8). In contrast, GRBAS scores from our cohort indicate both a higher rate of occurrence and greater severity of dysphonia. Overall grade was rated as normal in only 2/21 (9.5%) of our participants, while breathiness was present in >95%, roughness in >90%, strain in >70%, and asthenia in >65%. Diagnosis could account for this discrepancy, as 17/21 children in our sample were diagnosed with IOPD and could therefore be expected to present with greater disease severity than children with LOPD.

While clinicians might expect disease phenotype to have some relationship to the presence and severity of dysphonia, the small sample size of our study overall ($n = 21$) as well as the unequal distribution of participants with IOPD ($n = 17$) and LOPD ($n = 4$) precluded statistical analysis of such a relationship. Some of our acoustic and auditory-perceptual data suggest the presence of a relationship between disease phenotype and dysphonia severity and merit further study. For example, duration of sustained phonation tasks, DSI, and severity of overall grade ratings suggest the presence of more significant dysphonia in our participants with IOPD than those with LOPD. Longitudinal assessment of speech and voice characteristics within and across a larger sample of patients over time is needed to better understand the developing phenotypes of IOPD and LOPD.

Our findings suggest that the GRBAS scale can be used clinically to identify dysphonia in children with Pompe disease. We elected to use the GRBAS scale for auditory-perpetual assessment due its reliability and validity, widespread use in both clinical and research settings, and ease of administration. However, other scales such as the CAPE-V should be considered in future research. Compared to the GRBAS, the CAPE-V may be a better tool for the auditory-perceptual assessment of voice quality due to slightly improved intra- and inter-rater reliability, ability for its use in parametric statistical analysis, and the incorporation of additional parameters (e.g., pitch, loudness) which may enhance understanding of voice patterns [17].

The findings also emphasize the importance of collecting both auditory perceptual and physiologic/acoustic data when assessing voice as these measures provide complementary information about the presence and severity of dysphonia that will guide development of a treatment plan. The relationship between loudness during spoken text and maximum loudness during an isolated maximal performance task was statistically significant for dysphonia severity (overall grade) as well as ratings of breathiness and asthenia. It is possible that efforts to improve respiratory support, such as respiratory muscle training, combined with behavioral techniques to increase breath support and loudness during speech production may reduce the perceived severity of dysphonia in some children with Pompe disease. Loudness is an acoustic variable that is quick and easy to measure in most clinical settings and may be a useful objective data point to track alongside changes in perceptual ratings.

Alternative explanations for our findings and limitations of the present study must be considered. One limitation of this study was the relatively limited range of dysphonia severity present in our subjects, as 12 of 21 were judged to have normal voice quality or mild dysphonia. However, the range of dysphonia severity in this sample was greater than in previous research in this area [9,56]. Though our data reflect moderate-fair inter-rater agreement on GRBAS ratings, we did not assess intra-rater reliability.

It is possible that we failed to capture accurate physiologic/acoustic data and identify relationships between auditory-perceptual and acoustic parameters due to measurement error, reduced participant effort, or the use of relatively novel equipment lacking robust age- and gender-specific norms. We attempted to interpret our acoustic/physiologic data using reference values reported by other investigators; however, thresholds for acoustic parameters differ among studies based on the analysis methods and algorithms employed by the equipment used for data collection [57]. This may limit the validity of our comparisons between the acoustic parameters collected from our participants and threshold values reported by other authors for typically developing children. Furthermore, sex, age, and puberty stage as well as differences in recording environment, assessment tasks, and task instructions are known to impact acoustic findings and therefore limit comparison of findings among studies [23,36,57–60]. For example, both shimmer and jitter have been shown to be influenced by vocal loudness; analysis of quieter voices may artificially inflate jitter and shimmer values [43].

Barties and De Bodt point out that a major limitation of many studies is the lack of correspondence between acoustic data collected from sustained phonation tasks and acoustic data collected during running speech [57]. Recent recommendations for preferred practice patterns for instrumental assessment from the American Speech-Language-Hearing Association endorse the use of connected speech tasks for analysis of habitual loudness, fundamental frequency range, and noise in the acoustic signal [61]. Cepstral-based measures, such as cepstral peak prominence (CPP), long-term averaged spectral measurements such as low-versus high-spectral ratio (LHR), and the cepstral and spectral index of dysphonia (CSID) may be better correlated with auditory-perceptual judgments of dysphonia than time-based spectral measures such as jitter and shimmer [62–64]. These analyses will be used in subsequent studies. Inclusion of laryngeal videostroboscopy and aerodynamic measures are also recommended for comprehensive instrumental assessment of dysphonia [61,65,66]; however, these measures were not collected in this preliminary study. We did not assess puberty stage in our male participants, which is known to affect fundamental frequency [67]. Though all audio recordings were obtained using consistent techniques in the same environment, recording in a sound booth or with a head-mounted microphone would have strengthened the quality of our data by optimizing the signal-to-noise ratio [57]. While correlations between physiologic/acoustic data and perceptual voice features have been identified by some authors [31,68,69], vocal quality is a multidimensional perceived construct and evidence of these correlations in both adults and children is inconsistent [57,70]. These and other data support the idea that neither auditory-perceptual nor physiologic/acoustic measures can stand alone, and a battery approach to clinical assessment of voice is necessary to fully describe the features of dysphonia, the extent of its functional impact, and evidence of benefit from intervention [70–72].

While these findings extend our knowledge of the voice characteristics of children with Pompe disease, we were unable to associate the presence and severity of dysphonia with impairment in a particular speech subsystem. Lack of respiratory and nasalance data limited our ability to attempt such an analysis. Future research should seek to quantify the relative contributions of deficits in resonance, respiration, and phonation to overall dysphonia severity. For example, useful insights may be obtained by comparing relationships among measures of pulmonary function and the acoustic and instrumental parameters that reflect the contribution of the respiratory system, such as MPT and loudness. Similarly, videostroboscopy or electroglottography should be utilized to provide additional information about the pattern of vocal fold vibration and glottal closure that could be associated with acoustic findings. Additional acoustic parameters such as the normalized amplitude quotient (NAQ), peak slope (PS), cepstral peak prominence (CPP), and harmonic richness factor (HRF) have shown value in prior research investigating the effects of Pompe disease on voice function and should be included in future research to better differentiate and describe dysphonic voices [9,56]. Hypernasality is widely reported to be the most commonly occurring deviant speech feature in children with Pompe disease [5,7,8,73] and the relationship between disorders of resonance and reduced speech intelligibility in other populations is well documented [30,74]. Quantifying the relative impact of deficits in individual speech subsystems in children with Pompe disease who exhibit dysarthria and dysphonia might allow clinicians to focus their interventions to maximize benefit from therapy and achieve optimal clinical outcomes. This is an important goal, as the presence of a communication disorder negatively impacts quality of life for many children with Pompe disease. Use of a patient-reported outcome tool such as the VHI-10 may provide additional insight into the functional impact of dysphonia on communication and should be included in future studies.

5. Conclusions

In summary, this study reveals that dysphonia is common in children with Pompe disease, and symptoms appear primarily related to dysfunction in the respiratory and laryngeal systems. However, with the exception of specific measures of loudness, the predictive relationship between our physiologic/acoustic data and auditory perceptual ratings was poor. The impact of dysfunction spread across the motor speech system is nearly certain and likely confounded our efforts to determine associations between auditory perceptual and acoustic voice data. The complex interrelationship between the various subsystems supporting voice production should be evaluated by adding electroglottographic, nasalance, and respiratory assessments. Comparison of these findings to measures of articulation and speech intelligibility will paint a more complete picture of speech disturbances in children with Pompe disease.

Supplementary Materials: The following are available online at https://www.mdpi.com/2077-0383/10/16/3617/s1, Table S1: Additional cohort characteristics; Table S2: Physiologic data from sustained phonation tasks for individual study participants; Table S3: Acoustic data from sustained phonation tasks for individual study participants; Table S4: Acoustic data from spoken text and maximal loudness tasks for individual study participants.

Author Contributions: Conceptualization, P.S.K., H.N.J., K.D.C., A.K.; methodology, P.S.K., H.N.J., K.D.C.; formal analysis, S.A., H.N.J., A.T.N., K.D.C.; investigation, J.M., K.D.C., G.N.; data curation, K.D.C., J.M., S.A.; writing—original draft preparation, K.D.C., H.N.J.; writing—review & editing, K.D.C., J.M., S.A., A.K., P.S.K., H.N.J., A.T.N., G.N.; visualization, K.D.C., A.T.N., H.N.J.; supervision, H.N.J., P.S.K.; project administration, G.N., K.D.C., J.M.; funding acquisition, P.S.K., H.N.J. All authors have read and agreed to the published version of the manuscript.

Funding: This study was funded in part by Sanofi Genzyme, MA, under a collaborative study agreement with the Duke Center of Excellence Research. The authors also acknowledge the generous support of The Lucas Garrett Pompe Foundation, Inc., which provided philanthropic funding for this research. The APC was funded by Sanofi Genzyme, MA.

Institutional Review Board Statement: The study was conducted according to the guidelines of the Declaration of Helsinki, and approved by the Institutional Review Board of Duke University (Pro00072329).

Informed Consent Statement: Informed consent for participation was given by the participants' parents or legal guardians. Verbal assent was obtained from children 6 to 11 years of age, and additional written assent was obtained from children 12 years of age and older.

Data Availability Statement: The data presented in this study are available in the Supplementary Materials.

Conflicts of Interest: P.S.K. has received research/grant support from Sanofi Genzyme, Valerion Therapeutics, and Amicus Therapeutics and consulting fees and honoraria from Sanofi Genzyme, Amicus Therapeutics, Maze Therapeutics, J.C.R. Pharmaceutical and Asklepios Biopharmaceutical, Inc. (AskBio, Research Triangle, NC, USA). P.S.K. is member of the Pompe and Gaucher Disease Registry Advisory Board for Sanofi Genzyme, Amicus Therapeutics, and Baebies. P.S.K. has equity in Asklepios Biopharmaceutical, Inc. (AskBio), which is developing gene therapy for Pompe disease and Maze Therapeutics, which is developing small molecule in Pompe disease. H.N.J. has received research grant support from Sanofi Genzyme. K.C., A.N., J.M., G.N., S.A. and A.K. have no conflicts to disclose. The funders had no role in the design of the study; in the collection, analyses, or interpretation of data; in the writing of the manuscript, or in the decision to publish the results.

References

1. Kishnani, P.S.; Hwu, W.L.; Mandel, H.; Nicolino, M.; Yong, F.; Corzo, D.; Infantile-Onset Pompe Disease Natural History Study Group. A retrospective, multinational, multicenter study on the natural history of infantile-onset Pompe disease. *J. Pediatr.* **2006**, *148*, 671–676. [CrossRef]
2. Li, C.; Desai, A.K.; Gupta, P.; Dempsey, K.; Bhambhani, V.; Hopkin, R.J.; Ficicioglu, C.; Tanpaiboon, P.; Craigen, W.J.; Rosenberg, A.S.; et al. Transforming the clinical outcome in CRIM-negative infantile Pompe disease identified via newborn screening: The benefits of early treatment with enzyme replacement therapy and immune tolerance induction. *Genet. Med.* **2021**, *23*, 845–855. [CrossRef] [PubMed]
3. Khan, A.A.; Case, L.E.; Herbert, M.; DeArmey, S.; Jones, H.; Crisp, K.; Zimmerman, K.; ElMallah, M.K.; Young, S.P.; Kishnani, P.S. Higher dosing of alglucosidase alfa improves outcomes in children with Pompe disease: A clinical study and review of the literature. *Genet. Med.* **2020**, *22*, 898–907. [CrossRef] [PubMed]
4. Duffy, J.R. *Motor Speech Disorders: Substrates, Differential Diagnosis, and Management*; Elsevier: St. Louis, MO, USA, 2019.
5. Muller, C.W.; Jones, H.N.; O'Grady, G.; Suarez, A.H.; Heller, J.H.; Kishnani, P.S. Language and speech function in children with infantile Pompe disease. *J. Pediatr. Neurol.* **2009**, *7*, 147–156.
6. Van Gelder, C.M.; van Capelle, C.I.; Ebbink, B.J.; Moor-van Nugteren, I.; van den Hout, J.M.P.; Hakkesteegt, M.M.; van Doorn, P.A.; de Coo, I.F.M.; Reuser, A.J.J.; de Gier, H.H.W.; et al. Facial-muscle weakness, speech disorders and dysphagia are common in patients with classic infantile Pompe disease treated with enzyme therapy. *J. Inherit. Metab. Dis.* **2012**, *35*, 505–511. [CrossRef] [PubMed]
7. Su, H.; Wang, L.; Yang, C.; Lee, L.; Brajot, F. Language, speech, and oromotor function in children with Pompe disease. *Neuromuscul. Disord.* **2020**, *30*, 400–412. [CrossRef]
8. Zeng, Y.; Hwu, W.; Torng, P.; Lee, N.; Shieh, J.; Lu, L.; Chien, Y. Longitudinal follow-up to evaluate speech disorders in early-treated patients with infantile-onset Pompe disease. *Eur. J. Paediatr. Neurol.* **2017**, *21*, 485–493. [CrossRef]
9. Szklanny, K.; Gubrynowicz, R.; Iwanicka-Pronicka, K.; Tylki-Szymańska, A. Analysis of voice quality in patients with late-onset Pompe disease. *Orphanet J. Rare Dis.* **2016**, *11*, 99. [CrossRef]
10. Hobson-Webb, L.D.; Austin, S.L.; Jain, S.; Case, L.E.; Greene, K.; Kishnani, P.S. Small-fiber neuropathy in Pompe disease: First reported cases and prospective screening of a clinic cohort. *Am. J. Case Rep.* **2015**, *16*, 196–201. [CrossRef]
11. McIntosh, P.T.; Hobson-Webb, L.D.; Kazi, Z.B.; Prater, S.N.; Banugaria, S.G.; Austin, S.; Wang, R.; Enterline, D.S.; Frush, D.P.; Kishnani, P.S. Neuroimaging findings in infantile Pompe patients treated with enzyme replacement therapy. *Mol. Genet. Metab.* **2018**, *123*, 85–91. [CrossRef]
12. Hahn, A.; Schänzer, A. Long-term outcome and unmet needs in infantile-onset Pompe disease. *Ann. Transl. Med.* **2019**, *7*, 283. [CrossRef]
13. Spiridigliozzi, G.A.; Keeling, L.A.; Stefanescu, M.; Li, C.; Austin, S.; Kishnani, P.S. Cognitive and academic outcomes in long-term survivors of infantile-onset Pompe disease: A longitudinal follow-up. *Mol. Genet. Metab.* **2017**, *121*, 127–137. [CrossRef]
14. Korlimarla, A.; Spiridigliozzi, G.A.; Crisp, K.; Herbert, M.; Chen, S.; Malinzak, M.; Stefanescu, M.; Austin, S.L.; Cope, H.; Zimmerman, K.; et al. Novel approaches to quantify CNS involvement in children with Pompe disease. *Neurology* **2020**, *95*, e718–e732. [CrossRef]

15. Korlimarla, A.; Lim, J.; Kishnani, P.S.; Sun, B. An emerging phenotype of central nervous system involvement in Pompe disease: From bench to bedside and beyond. *Ann. Transl. Med.* **2019**, *7*, 289. [CrossRef] [PubMed]
16. Hirano, M. "GRBAS" scale for evaluating the hoarse voice & frequency range of phonation. *Clin. Exam. Voice* **1981**, *5*, 83–89.
17. Zraick, R.I.; Kempster, G.B.; Connor, N.P.; Thibeault, S.; Klaben, B.K.; Bursac, Z.; Thrush, C.R.; Glaze, L.E. Establishing validity of the Consensus Auditory-Perceptual Evaluation of Voice (CAPE-V). *Am. J. Speech Lang. Pathol.* **2011**, *20*, 14–22. [CrossRef]
18. Iwarsson, J.; Petersen, N.R. Effects of Consensus Training on the Reliability of Auditory Perceptual Ratings of Voice Quality. *J. Voice* **2012**, *26*, 304–312. [CrossRef] [PubMed]
19. Landis, J.R.; Koch, G.G. The measurement of observer agreement for categorical data. *Biometrics* **1977**, *33*, 159–174. [CrossRef]
20. Cohen, J. A Coefficient of Agreement for Nominal Scales. *Educ. Psychol. Meas.* **1960**, *20*, 37–46. [CrossRef]
21. Voice Protocol Norms. Available online: https://mmsp.com.au/mmsp/wp-content/uploads/2019/08/lingWAVES_Voice_Protocol_Norms_2017_09_25.pdf (accessed on 29 April 2021).
22. Corthals, P. Sound pressure level of running speech: Percentile level statistics and equivalent continuous sound level. *Folia Phoniatr. Logop.* **2004**, *56*, 170–181. [CrossRef]
23. Weinrich, B.; Brehm, S.B.; Knudsen, C.; McBride, S.; Hughes, M. Pediatric normative data for the KayPENTAX phonatory aerodynamic system model 6600. *J. Voice* **2013**, *27*, 46–56. [CrossRef]
24. Tavares, E.L.M.; Brasolotto, A.G.; Rodrigues, S.A.; Pessin, A.B.B.; Martins, R.H.G. Maximum phonation time and s/z ratio in a large child cohort. *J. Voice* **2012**, *26*, 675.e1–675.e4. [CrossRef]
25. Eckel, F.C.; Boone, D.R. The S/Z ratio as an indicator of laryngeal pathology. *J. Speech Hear. Disord.* **1981**, *46*, 147–149. [CrossRef]
26. Tait, N.A.; Michel, J.F.; Carpenter, M.A. Maximum duration of sustained /s/ and /z/ in children. *J. Speech Hear. Disord.* **1980**, *45*, 239–246. [CrossRef]
27. Finnegan, D.E. Maximum phonation time for children with normal voices. *J. Commun. Disord.* **1984**, *17*, 309–317. [CrossRef]
28. Kent, R.D.; Kent, J.F.; Rosenbek, J.C. Maximum performance tests of speech production. *J. Speech Hear. Disord.* **1987**, *52*, 367–387. [CrossRef] [PubMed]
29. Teixeira, J.P.; Oliveira, C.; Lopes, C. Vocal acoustic analysis—Jitter, shimmer and HNR parameters. *Procedia Technol.* **2013**, *9*, 1112–1122. [CrossRef]
30. Kent, R.D.; Eichhorn, J.T.; Vorperian, H.K. Acoustic parameters of voice in typically developing children ages 4–19 years. *Int. J. Pediatri. Otorhinolaryngol.* **2021**, *142*, 110614. [CrossRef] [PubMed]
31. Lopes, L.W.; Lima, I.L.B.; Almeida, L.N.A.; Cavalcante, D.P.; de Almeida, A.A.F. Severity of voice disorders in children: Correlations between perceptual and acoustic data. *J. Voice* **2012**, *26*, 819.e7–819.e12. [CrossRef] [PubMed]
32. Pebbili, G.K.; Kidwai, J.; Shabnam, S. Dysphonia Severity Index in Typically Developing Indian Children. *J. Voice* **2017**, *31*, 125.e1–125.e6. [CrossRef] [PubMed]
33. Wuyts, F.L.; De Bodt, M.S.; Molenberghs, G.; Remacle, M.; Heylen, L.; Millet, B.; Van Lierde, K.; Raes, J.; Van de Heyning, P.H. The dysphonia severity index: An objective measure of vocal quality based on a multiparameter approach. *J. Speech Lang. Hear. Res.* **2000**, *43*, 796–809. [CrossRef]
34. De Bodt, M.S.; Wutys, F.L.; Van de Heyning, P.H.; Croux, C. Test-retest study of the GRBAS scale: Influence of experience and professional background on perceptual ratings of voice quality. *J. Voice* **1997**, *11*, 74–80. [CrossRef]
35. Knuijt, S.; Kalf, J.; Van Engelen, B.; Geurts, A.; de Swart, B. Reference values of maximum performance tests of speech production. *Int. J. Speech Lang. Pathol.* **2019**, *21*, 56–64. [CrossRef]
36. Gilman, M. Revisiting Sustained Phonation Time of /s/, /z/, and /a/. *J. Voice* **2020**. [CrossRef] [PubMed]
37. Solomon, N.P.; Garlitz, S.J.; Milbrath, R.L. Respiratory and laryngeal contributions to maximum phonation duration. *J. Voice* **2000**, *14*, 331–340. [CrossRef]
38. Tong, J.Y.; Sataloff, R.T. Respiratory Function and Voice: The Role for Airflow Measures. *J. Voice* **2020**. [CrossRef]
39. ElMallah, M.K.; Desai, A.K.; Nading, E.B.; DeArmey, S.; Kravitz, R.M.; Kishnani, P.S. Pulmonary outcome measures in long-term survivors of infantile Pompe disease on enzyme replacement therapy: A case series. *Pediatr. Pulmonol.* **2020**, *55*, 674–681. [CrossRef]
40. Jones, H.N.; Crisp, K.D.; Moss, T.; Strollo, K.; Robey, R.; Sank, J.; Canfield, M.; Case, L.E.; Mahler, L.; Kravitz, R.M.; et al. Effects of respiratory muscle training (RMT) in children with infantile-onset Pompe disease and respiratory muscle weakness. *J. Pediatr. Rehabil. Med.* **2014**, *7*, 255–265. [CrossRef]
41. Baker, K.K.; Ramig, L.O.; Sapir, S.; Luschei, E.S.; Smith, M.E. Control of Vocal Loudness in Young and Old Adults. *J. Speech Lang. Hear. Res.* **2001**, *44*, 297. [CrossRef]
42. Zraick, R.I.; Marshall, W.; Smith-Olinde, L.; Montague, J.C. The effect of task on determination of habitual loudness. *J. Voice* **2004**, *18*, 176–182. [CrossRef]
43. Brockmann-Bauser, M.; Beyer, D.; Bohlender, J.E. Clinical relevance of speaking voice intensity effects on acoustic jitter and shimmer in children between 5;0 and 9;11 years. *Int. J. Pediatr. Otorhinolaryngol.* **2014**, *78*, 2121–2126. [CrossRef]
44. Swift, G.; Cleary, M.; Grunewald, S.; Lozano, S.; Ryan, M.; Davison, J. Swallow Prognosis and Follow-Up Protocol in Infantile Onset Pompe Disease. *JIMD Rep.* **2017**, *33*, 11–17. [CrossRef]
45. Prater, S.N.; Banugaria, S.G.; DeArmey, S.M.; Botha, E.G.; Stege, E.M.; Case, L.E.; Jones, H.N.; Phornphutkul, C.; Wang, R.Y.; Young, S.P.; et al. The emerging phenotype of long-term survivors with infantile Pompe disease. *Genet. Med.* **2012**, *14*, 800–810. [CrossRef]

46. Rohrbach, M.; Klein, A.; Köhli-Wiesner, A.; Veraguth, D.; Scheer, I.; Balmer, C.; Lauener, R.; Baumgartner, M.R. CRIM-negative infantile Pompe disease: 42-month treatment outcome. *J. Inherit. Metab. Dis.* **2010**, *33*, 751–757. [CrossRef]
47. Jones, H.N.; Muller, C.W.; Lin, M.; Banugaria, S.G.; Case, L.E.; Li, J.S.; O'Grady, G.; Heller, J.H.; Kishnani, P.S. Oropharyngeal dysphagia in infants and children with infantile Pompe disease. *Dysphagia* **2010**, *25*, 277–283. [CrossRef]
48. Van Capelle, C.I.; Goedegebure, A.; Homans, N.C.; Hoeve, H.L.J.; Reuser, A.J.; van der Ploeg, A.T. Hearing loss in Pompe disease revisited: Results from a study of 24 children. *J. Inherit. Metab. Dis.* **2010**, *33*, 597–602. [CrossRef] [PubMed]
49. Chien, Y.; van der Ploeg, A.; Jones, S.; Byrne, B.; Vellodi, A.; Leslie, N.; Mengel, E.; Shankar, S.P.; Tanpaiboon, P.; Stockton, D.W.; et al. Survival and Developmental Milestones among Pompe Registry Patients with Classic Infantile-Onset Pompe Disease with Different Timing of Initiation of Treatment with Enzyme Replacement Therapy. *J. Neuromuscul. Dis.* **2015**, *2*, S61–S62. [CrossRef] [PubMed]
50. Spada, M.; Pagliardini, V.; Ricci, F.; Biamino, E.; Mongini, T.; Porta, F. Early higher dosage of alglucosidase alpha in classic Pompe disease. *J. Pediatr. Endocrinol. Metab.* **2018**, *31*, 1343–1347. [CrossRef] [PubMed]
51. Chien, Y.; Hwu, W.; Lee, N.; Tsai, F.; Koeberl, D.D.; Tsai, W.; Chiu, P.; Chang, C. Albuterol as an adjunctive treatment to enzyme replacement therapy in infantile-onset Pompe disease. *Mol. Genet. Metab. Rep.* **2017**, *11*, 31–35. [CrossRef]
52. Kronn, D.F.; Day-Salvatore, D.; Hwu, W.; Jones, S.A.; Nakamura, K.; Okuyama, T.; Swoboda, K.J.; Kishnani, P.S. Management of Confirmed Newborn-Screened Patients with Pompe Disease across the Disease Spectrum. *Pediatrics* **2017**, *140*, S24–S45. [CrossRef] [PubMed]
53. Heinzmann-Filho, J.P.; Vidal, P.C.V.; Jones, M.H.; Donadio, M.V.F. Normal values for respiratory muscle strength in healthy preschoolers and school children. *Respir. Med.* **2012**, *106*, 1639–1646. [CrossRef]
54. Hulzebos, E.; Takken, T.; Reijneveld, E.A.; Mulder, M.M.G.; Bongers, B.C. Reference Values for Respiratory Muscle Strength in Children and Adolescents. *Respiration* **2018**, *95*, 235–243. [CrossRef] [PubMed]
55. Patil, P.; Deodhar, A.; Jadhav, S. Respiratory Muscle Strength in Children in Age Group 7-12 Years: A Cross-Sectional Observational Pilot Study. *Int. J. Health Sci. Res.* **2020**, *10*, 145–156.
56. Szklanny, K.; Tylki-Szymańska, A. Follow-up analysis of voice quality in patients with late-onset Pompe disease. *Orphanet J. Rare Dis.* **2018**, *13*, 189. [CrossRef] [PubMed]
57. Barsties, B.; De Bodt, M. Assessment of voice quality: Current state-of-the-art. *Auris Nasus Larynx* **2015**, *42*, 183–188. [CrossRef]
58. Karnell, M.P.; Hall, K.D.; Landahl, K.L. Comparison of fundamental frequency and perturbation measurements among three analysis systems. *J. Voice* **1995**, *9*, 383–393. [CrossRef]
59. Gelfer, M.P.; Pazera, J.F. Maximum duration of sustained /s/ and /z/ and the s/z ratio with controlled intensity. *J. Voice* **2006**, *20*, 369–379. [CrossRef]
60. McAllister, A.; Sundberg, J. Data on subglottal pressure and SPL at varied vocal loudness and pitch in 8- to 11-year-old children. *J. Voice* **1998**, *12*, 166–174. [CrossRef]
61. Patel, R.R.; Awan, S.N.; Barkmeier-Kraemer, J.; Courey, M.; Deliyski, D.; Eadie, T.; Paul, D.; Svec, J.G.; Hillman, R. Recommended protocols for instrumental assessment of voice: American Speech-Language-Hearing Association expert panel to develop a protocol for instrumental assessment of vocal function. *Am. J. Speech Lang. Pathol.* **2018**, *27*, 887–905. [CrossRef]
62. Shim, H.; Jung, H.; Koul, R.; Ko, D. Spectral and Cepstral Based Acoustic Features of Voices with Muscle Tension Dysphonia. *Clin. Arch. Commun. Disord.* **2016**, *1*, 42–47. [CrossRef]
63. Watts, C.R.; Awan, S.N. Use of spectral/cepstral analyses for differentiating normal from hypofunctional voices in sustained vowel and continuous speech contexts. *J. Speech Lang. Hear. Res.* **2011**, *54*, 1525–1537. [CrossRef]
64. Garrett, R.K.M. *Cepstral- and Spectral-Based Acoustic Measures of Normal Voices*; ProQuest Dissertations Publishing: Ann Arbor, MI, USA, 2013; Available online: https://dc.uwm.edu/etd/217/ (accessed on 9 August 2021).
65. Friedrich, G.; Dejonckere, P.H. The voice evaluation protocol of the European Laryngological Society (ELS)—First results of a multicenter study. *Laryngorhinootologie* **2005**, *84*, 744–752. [CrossRef]
66. Cohen, W.; Wynne, D.M.; Kubba, H.; McCartney, E. Development of a minimum protocol for assessment in the paediatric voice clinic. Part 1: Evaluating vocal function. *Logop. Phoniatr. Vocol.* **2012**, *37*, 33–38. [CrossRef]
67. Harries, M.L.; Walker, J.M.; Williams, D.M.; Hawkins, S.; Hughes, I.A. Changes in the male voice at puberty. *Arch. Dis. Child.* **1997**, *77*, 445–447. [CrossRef]
68. Bhuta, T.; Patrick, L.; Garnett, J.D. Perceptual evaluation of voice quality and its correlation with acoustic measurements. *J. Voice* **2004**, *18*, 299–304. [CrossRef]
69. Dejonckere, P.H.; Remacle, M.; Fresnel-Elbaz, E.; Woisard, V.; Crevier-Buchman, L.; Millet, B. Differentiated perceptual evaluation of pathological voice quality: Reliability and correlations with acoustic measurements. *Rev. Laryngol. Otol. Rhinol.* **1996**, *117*, 219–224.
70. Kreiman, J.; Gerratt, B.R. Perceptual assessment of voice quality: Past, present, and future. *Perspect. Voice Voice Disord.* **2010**, *20*, 62–67. [CrossRef]
71. Fujiki, R.B.; Thibeault, S.L. The Relationship between Auditory-Perceptual Rating Scales and Objective Voice Measures in Children with Voice Disorders. *Am. J. Speech Lang. Pathol.* **2021**, *30*, 228–238. [CrossRef]
72. Roy, N.; Barkmeier-Kraemer, J.; Eadie, T.; Sivasankar, M.P.; Mehta, D.; Paul, D.; Hillman, R. Evidence-based clinical voice assessment: A systematic review. *Am. J. Speech Lang. Pathol.* **2013**, *22*, 212–226. [CrossRef]

73. Jones, H.N.; Fernandes, S.; Hannah, W.B.; Kansagra, S.; Raynor, E.M.; Kishnani, P.S. Adenotonsillectomy should be avoided whenever possible in infantile-onset Pompe disease. *Mol. Genet. Metab. Rep.* **2020**, *23*, 100574. [CrossRef] [PubMed]
74. Kummer, A.W. Speech therapy for errors secondary to cleft palate and velopharyngeal dysfunction. *Semin. Speech Lang.* **2011**, *32*, 191–198. [CrossRef] [PubMed]

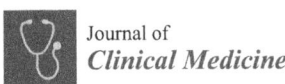

Article

Secondary Hyperparathyroidism in Children with Mucolipidosis Type II (I-Cell Disease): Irish Experience

Ritma Boruah [1,*], Ahmad Ardeshir Monavari [1,2], Tracey Conlon [2,3], Nuala Murphy [2,3], Andreea Stroiescu [4], Stephanie Ryan [4], Joanne Hughes [1], Ina Knerr [1,2], Ciara McDonnell [3] and Ellen Crushell [1,2]

1 National Centre for Inherited Metabolic Diseases (NCIMD), Children's Health Ireland at Temple Street, D01 XD99 Dublin, Ireland; ahmad.monavari@cuh.ie (A.A.M.); joanne.hughes@cuh.ie (J.H.); ina.knerr@cuh.ie (I.K.); ellen.crushell@cuh.ie (E.C.)
2 School of Medicine, University College Dublin, D04 V1W8 Dublin, Ireland; tracey.conlon@cuh.ie (T.C.); nuala.murphy@cuh.ie (N.M.)
3 Department of Endocrinology, Children's Health Ireland at Temple Street, D01 XD99 Dublin, Ireland; ciara.mcdonnell@cuh.ie
4 Department of Radiology, Children's Health Ireland at Temple Street, D01 XD99 Dublin, Ireland; andreeastroiescu@gmail.com (A.S.); stephanie.ryan99@gmail.com (S.R.)
* Correspondence: ritma.boruah@cuh.ie

Citation: Boruah, R.; Monavari, A.A.; Conlon, T.; Murphy, N.; Stroiescu, A.; Ryan, S.; Hughes, J.; Knerr, I.; McDonnell, C.; Crushell, E. Secondary Hyperparathyroidism in Children with Mucolipidosis Type II (I-Cell Disease): Irish Experience. J. Clin. Med. 2022, 11, 1366. https://doi.org/10.3390/jcm11051366

Academic Editors: Karolina M. Stepien and Sylvia Lee-Huang

Received: 6 January 2022
Accepted: 25 February 2022
Published: 2 March 2022

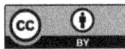

Copyright: © 2022 by the authors. Licensee MDPI, Basel, Switzerland. This article is an open access article distributed under the terms and conditions of the Creative Commons Attribution (CC BY) license (https://creativecommons.org/licenses/by/4.0/).

Abstract: Mucolipidosis type II (ML II) is an autosomal recessive lysosomal targeting disorder that may present with features of hyperparathyroidism. The aim of this study was to describe in detail the clinical cases of ML II presenting to a tertiary referral centre with biochemical and/or radiological features of hyperparathyroidism. There were twenty-three children diagnosed with ML II in the Republic of Ireland from July 1998 to July 2021 inclusive (a 23-year period). The approximate incidence of ML II in the Republic of Ireland is, therefore, 1 per 64,000 live births. Medical records were available and were reviewed for 21 of the 23 children. Five of these had been identified as having biochemical and/or radiological features of hyperparathyroidism. Of these five, three children were born to Irish Traveller parents and two to non-Traveller Irish parents. All five children had radiological features of hyperparathyroidism (on skeletal survey), with evidence of antenatal fractures in three cases and an acute fracture in one. Four children had biochemical features of secondary hyperparathyroidism. Three children received treatment with high dose Vitamin D supplements and two who had antenatal/acute fractures were managed with minimal handling. We observed resolution of secondary hyperparathyroidism in all cases irrespective of treatment. Four of five children with ML II and hyperparathyroidism died as a result of cardiorespiratory failure at ages ranging from 10 months to 7 years. Biochemical and/or radiological evidence of hyperparathyroidism is commonly identified at presentation of ML II. Further studies are needed to establish the pathophysiology and optimal management of hyperparathyroidism in this cohort. Recognition of this association may improve diagnostic accuracy and management, facilitate family counseling and is also important for natural history data.

Keywords: mucolipidosis type II; ML II; I-cell disease; hyperparathyroidism

1. Introduction

Mucolipidosis type II (ML II) (OMIM #252500) or inclusion cell disease (I-cell disease) is a rare autosomal recessive lysosomal enzymetargeting disease due to deficiency of uridine diphosphate-N-acetylglucosamine: lysosomal enzyme N-acetylglucosamine-1-phosphotransferase (GlcNac-1-phosphotransferase). This enzyme is involved in the first step of the mannose 6-phosphate signal, which allows specific targeting of lysosomal acid hydrolase from the trans-Golgi network to lysosomes. The enzyme deficiency precludes the generation of the common phosphomannosyl recognition marker of lysosomal enzymes [1]. Subsequently, newly synthesized lysosomal enzymes are secreted into the extracellular space rather than targeted to the lysosomes. Thus, affected lysosomes are secondarily deficient in most acid hydrolases; undigested junk materials accumulate within the lysosomes [1,2]. ML II was first described as inclusion-cell (I-cell) disease by Leroy and Demars in 1967 [3], because the fibroblasts derived from patients contain abundant 'inclusions' (now recognized as swollen lysosomes) within the cytoplasm. These inclusions are observed not only in cultured skin fibroblasts, but also in a variety of other cell types in vivo, including peripheral blood lymphocytes [2].

The term "mucolipidosis" was introduced in 1970 by Spranger and Wiedemann to describe several conditions with features both of mucopolysaccharidoses (MPS) and sphingolipidoses [4]. ML II is a progressive multi-organ disease, usually with prenatal clinical onset and fatal outcome within the first decade of life due to cardiopulmonary complications [5]. It is characterized by coarse facial features, short stature, hyperplastic gums, organomegaly, retarded psychomotor development and skeletal deformities, which may include shortened limbs, flexion contractures and talipes [6,7]. Secondary hyperparathyroidism is a recognized feature of ML II [1,7–11]. Reported biochemical features of secondary hyperparathyroidism include elevated parathyroid hormone (PTH), serum calcium (Ca), alkaline phosphatase (ALP) levels and low levels of phosphate (P) [8,11–14], Radiographic findings in neonates resemble changes of rickets and/or hyperparathyroidism. These changes include osteopenia, subperiosteal resorption, poor cortical delineation, periosteal new bone formation with 'cloaking' (linear periosteal new bone parallel to the shaft of the bone but widely separated from the bone), metaphyseal irregularity and submetaphyseal lucent bands and later develop into Hurler-type dysostosis multiplex. Congenital long bone and rib fractures are rare and likely the result of severe osteopenia and disorganized bone formation [9,12,15–17]. Bone changes can precede elevations in biochemical markers [12]; therefore, regular monitoring in infancy is required and skeletal radiographs should be performed regardless of initial biochemical findings.

Clinical suspicion is the first step in establishing a diagnosis of ML II, with typical clinical features often apparent at birth or otherwise manifesting in the first year of life [12]. An indirect diagnosis is usually established by measurement of lysosomal hydrolases, both in white blood cells, where their levels should be low, and their surrounding extracellular environment (e.g., plasma), where their levels should be high [18]. The diagnosis is confirmed by *GNPTAB* gene molecular analysis; this is particularly important in cases when biochemical testing is inconclusive or carrier detection is required [11,19]. There are at least 258 mutations reported in the *GNPTAB* gene, the most prevalent being c.3503_3504del. Despite increased prevalence of homozygous mutations, particularly in highly consanguineous populations, the autosomal recessive inheritance of MLII means a high number of compound heterozygous *GNPTAB* sequence alterations [5]. ML II is a multi-ethnic disease. It has been identified in many different ethnic groups [9,11,19–25], with reported prevalence as follows: Portugal—approximately 1:123, 500 live births [22], Japan—1:252, 500 live births [23] and 1:625, 500 live births in Netherlands [24].

ML II has a very high incidence of 1 per 909 live births in the Irish Traveller community [26]. Irish Travellers are an endogamous grouup who have cultural values and customs quite distinct from that of the "settled community", i.e., the non-Traveller Irish population. Cultural traditions within the community include a preference to marry within their own community (often resulting in consanguineous unions), young age at marriage and large families [26].

Hyperparathyroidism is not universal but has been observed in patients with MLII [1,7–12,14,27]. The biochemical and radiological features of hyperparathyroidism in infants with ML II vary in the literature [9,10,12,15,16,27,28], with resolution of these findings observed in many cases, even in the absence of active management [14,17,27]. It is known that, following this initial early period where features of hyperparathyroidism or rickets may be observed, children with ML II experience a progressive osteodystrophy [9]. Recognition and active management of hyperparathyroidism may prevent complications such as bone fractures and, thus, improve quality of life for the affected children. It is also important to recognize hyperparathyroidism in this cohort for natural history data. Here, we describe clinical, biochemical, radiological and molecular findings in five children with ML II and hyperparathyroidism from 5 unrelated families.

2. Materials and Methods

This study was performed in The National Centre for Inherited Metabolic Diseases, Children's Health Ireland (CHI) at Temple Street in the Republic of Ireland. A retrospective chart review of ML II patients born between July 1998 and July 2021 inclusive was performed, providing a twenty-three-year cohort. A database was compiled documenting clinical features, focusing on those consistent with hyperparathyroidism. For those diagnosed with hyperparathyroidism, biochemical, radiological and molecular data were recorded. This study was approved by the Research and Ethics Committee of CHI at Temple Street (protocol code 21. 013).

3. Results

We identified 23 patients with ML II from 14 families, born between 1 July 1998 and 1 July 2021. This gives an approximate national incidence of 1 per 64,000 live births in the Republic of Ireland. Medical records were available for 21 out of 23 children. Of the 23 identified, 19 were from the Irish Traveller community, confirming the very high incidence within the Traveller community, in line with previously reported figure of 1 in 909 [26]. In this cohort, five patients from five families had biochemical and/or radiological evidence of hyperparathyroidism, three of these children were born to Irish Traveller parents.

3.1. Diagnosis of ML II—Biochemical and Molecular Genetic Features

The diagnosis of ML II was based on clinical features and biochemical testing by detecting increased activity of alpha mannosidase and beta hexosaminidase in plasma. In all cases, the diagnosis was confirmed by molecular genetic testing; these patients were found to be homozygous for a common mutation c.3503_3504delTC (p.L1168Qfs*5) in *GNPTAB* gene.

3.2. Biochemical Features of Hyperparathyroidism

All five patients had been tested for hyperparathyroidism within the first few weeks of life and four had increased levels of parathyroid hormone (PTH). Calcium (Ca) and phosphate (P) levels were normal; however, alkaline phosphatase (ALP) levels were markedly raised in four of five cases (Patients 2, 3, 4, 5). Vitamin D levels were checked in four cases (Patients 2, 3, 4, 5) and were normal in three, with one (Patient 5) having a suboptimal level of 30 nmol/L (normal range is >50 nmol/L).

3.3. Radiological Abnormalities Identified

Skeletal radiographs in the first week of life were available for four patients and at 2 months of age for one patient (Patient 3). Follow up radiographs were available for four out five patients. Early radiographs already showed marked changes of hyperparathyroidism in all five infants including osteopenia, subperiosteal resorption, poor cortical delineation, periosteal new bone formation with 'cloaking' (linear periosteal new bone parallel to the shaft of the bone but widely separated from the bone), metaphyseal irregularity and submetaphyseal lucent bands (Figures 1 and 2).

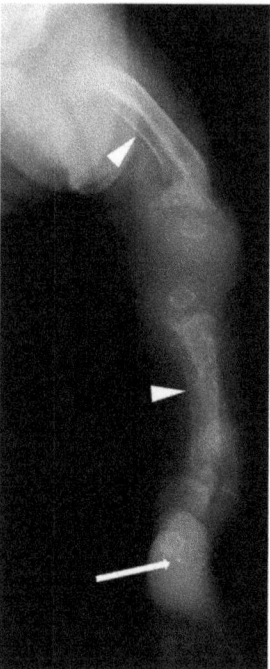

Figure 1. Acute findings of hyperparathyroidism and rickets. Patient 1, left leg radiograph day 1 demonstrates features of hyperparathyroidism including reduced bone density, subperiosteal resorption and poor cortical delineation (see medial tibia) as well as diaphyseal cloaking of the femur and tibia (arrowheads). Features of rickets are seen with cupped, splayed and frayed metaphyses especially in the distal femur. Diaphyseal angulation consistent with antenatal fractures is seen in the distal femur and tibia. Additionally, talocalcaneal stippling, a feature of I-cell disease is also present (white arrow).

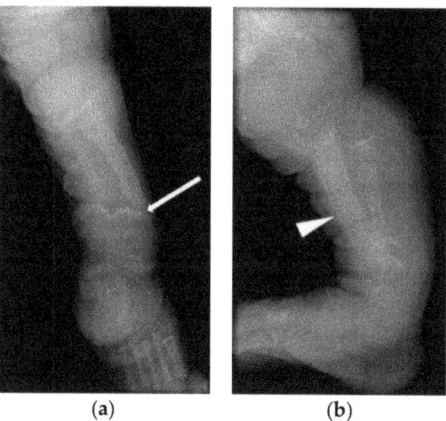

(a) (b)

Figure 2. Acute findings of hyperparathyroidism and of rickets. Patient 2, right leg radiograph day 4 (**a**) frontal and (**b**) lateral views show features of hyperparathyroidism (best seen on the lateral view) including reduced bone density, subperiosteal resorption and poor cortical delineation as well as diaphyseal cloaking of the tibia (arrowheads). Features of rickets are seen with cupped, splayed and frayed metaphyses in all the bones. A submetaphyseal lucent band is seen in the tibia (white arrow). Talocalcaneal stippling is also present.

All early radiographs also showed features of rickets, with metaphyseal cupping, fraying and splaying (Figures 1 and 2). There was evidence of antenatal long bone fractures in Patients 1, 2 and 4. Patient 4 also had an acute fracture of the proximal left humeral neck (Figure 3). Further radiographic findings of ML II including talocalcaneal stippling were identified in Patients 1, 2 and 5, and an abnormal appearance of the vertebral bodies with increased height; rounding and sclerosis were seen in Patients 1, 2 and 4.

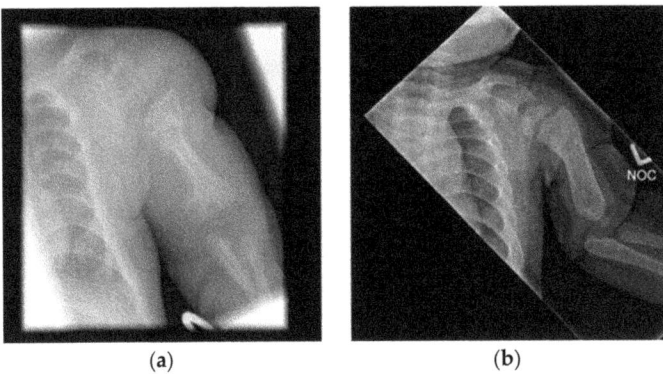

Figure 3. Acute fracture with healing at 4 months. Patient 4 (**a**) radiograph of left humerus on day 1 shows a transverse fracture of the left humerus. (**b**) Follow-up radiograph 4 months later showing interval healing of the fracture and resolution of the periosteal cloaking. There are already emerging features of dysostosis multi-plex with widening of the shaft and short length of the humerus and coarse trabecular markings as well as thickening of the ribs.

Follow-up radiographs in all but the most recent patient showed resolution of the features of hyperparathyroidism and rickets, with interval healing of the fractures. There was progression of skeletal features to those of dysostosis multiplex, the constellation of radiographic abnormalities classically seen in mucopolysaccharidoses (MPS), including coarse trabecular markings, broadening of the ribs (oar/paddle shaped ribs), flared iliac wings, constricted inferior iliac bodies and dysplastic femoral heads (Figures 3 and 4).

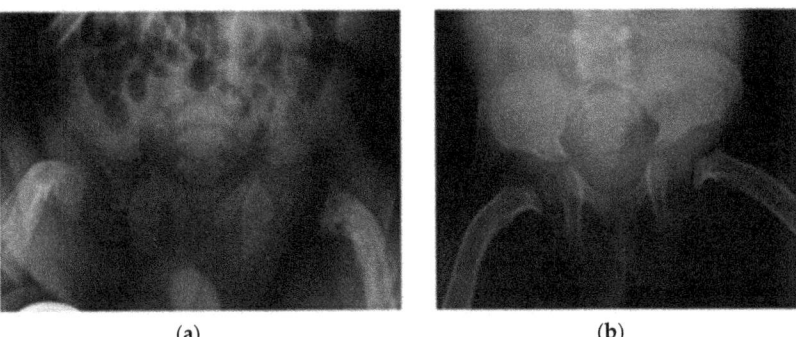

Figure 4. Progression to dysostosis multiplex. Patient 4 (**a**) Radiograph of pelvis on day 1 shows a reduced bone density and irregularity of the proximal femora with periosteal cloaking. (**b**) Follow-up radiograph at 2 years old shows normal bone density. The pelvis now has a typical shape of dysostosis multiplex with constriction of the lower part of the iliac bones. There has been interval healing of the rickets of the proximal femora and resolution of the periosteal cloaking.

Follow up radiographs in Patient 1 showed resolution of the acute changes, including the periosteal reaction and subperiosteal erosion, but development of a progressive erosive osteodystrophy with erosion of the humeral and femoral necks and also erosion of the necks of the ribs was observed (Figure 5).

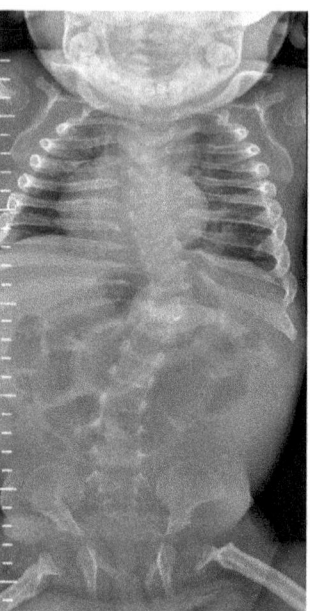

Figure 5. Progressive erosive osteodystrophy in Patient 1 at 6 years. Resolution of the acute changes seen in Figure 1. Development of a progressive erosive osteodystrophy with erosion of the heads and necks of the ribs, erosion of the lower part of the iliac bones, erosion of the ischial and pubic bones and of the femoral necks.

3.4. Management and Clinical Course

Two of the infants who had evidence of antenatal fractures (Patients 1, 4), including the one with an acute fracture (Patient 1), received treatment with increased Vitamin D supplementation of 600 IU per day and guidance around minimal handling, including a lie flat car seat, lying supported on the side and avoidance of walkers and bouncers. In the case of Patient 4, the previously abnormal biochemical parameters normalized within five months of treatment with vitamin D; the dose was then reduced to the standard supplementation dose of 200 IU/day, with handling liberalized successfully. A follow-up left humeral radiograph 4 months later showed interval healing of the humeral neck fracture (Figure 3). Patient 1 was followed up at a local hospital and vitamin D dose was reduced to 200 IU/day and handling liberalized at 1 year.

Patients 2 and 3 were monitored without specific treatment. In Patient 2, PTH level had spontaneously returned to normal at 10 months. In the case of Patient 3, the previously abnormal biochemical marker (ALP) had normalized at 10 months of age (during an admission to Pediatric Intensive Care unit with respiratory failure). No further fractures were observed. Patient 5 was started on high dose Vitamin D supplementation of 1000 IU/day with interval re-evaluation planned.

Four of the five affected infants died from progressive cardiopulmonary decline at ages ranging from 10 months to 7 years. Summary of clinical, biochemical, radiological features of secondary hyperparathyroidism, Vitamin D levels at diagnosis and treatment can be found in Table 1.

Table 1. Summary Summary of clinical, biochemical, radiological features of secondary hyperparathyroidism and Vitamin D levels at diagnosis and treatment.

	Clinical Features	PTH Reference Range: 11–25 ng/L	Ca Reference Range: 2.15–2.65 mmol/L	P Reference Range: 1.2–2.0 mmol/L	ALP Reference Range: 60–550 IU/L	Vitamin D Reference Range: >50 nmol/L	Radiological Features	Treatment
Patient 1	Antenatal fractures of long bones	25	2.46	1.65	434	Not available in medical notes	All patients had features of HPT (Figures 1 and 2), including: • Osteopenia • Subperiosteal resorption • Poor cortical delineation • Periosteal new bone formation with 'cloaking' (linear periosteal new bone parallel to the shaft of the bone but widely separated from the bone) • Metaphyseal irregularity • Submetaphyseal lucent bands	Vitamin D 600 IU, minimal handling until 1 year of age
Patient 2	Antenatal fractures of long bones	119 ↑	2.36	1.17	1540 ↑	66.7		None
Patient 3	No fractures	72 ↑	2.45	1.96	1063 ↑	48 (reference range > 15 mmol/L)		None
Patient 4	Acute fracture of the proximal left humeral neck (Figure 3a), antenatal fractures	252 ↑	2.32	1.62	1007 ↑	121		Vitamin D 600 IU, minimal handling for 5 month
Patient 5	No fractures	110 ↑	2.31	1.3	1256 ↑	30 ↓		Vitamin D 1000 IU, re-evaluation planned in due course

↑ raised level; ↓ reduced level.

4. Discussion

Patients with ML II have been reported to present in the neonatal period with features of "metabolic" bone disease [9,27]. While features of dysostosis multiplex (the constellation of radiographic abnormalities classically seen in mucopolysaccharidoses) are seen in older children with ML II, the skeleton in ML II in the young infant is characterized by an osteodystrophy which has clinical and radiographic features of hyperparathyroidism and rickets and these changes have been reported in ML II as early as 19 weeks of gestation [28].

Osteoporosis, fractures, periosteal new bone formation and cupped epiphyses have been described in neonates and infants [9]. Radiological and histological features of both rickets and hyperparathyroidism (subperiosteal bone resorption and loss of bone mass) have been documented in babies with I-cell disease [15,16]. Biochemical evidence of hyperparathyroidism is more variable but had been reported in some affected neonates [9].

In our study, none of the patients had abnormal serum calcium or phosphate levels. Similar findings were reported by David-Vizcarra et al. [9]. Four out of five of our patients had increased levels of ALP and PTH. All children had early skeletal x-rays with radiographic evidence of hyperparathyroidism, including osteopenia, subperiosteal bone resorption, poor cortical delineation, periosteal new bone formation, metaphyseal irregularity and submetaphyseal lucent bands. Three had evidence of antenatal fractures. All early radiographs also had features of rickets, with metaphyseal cupping, fraying and splaying.

Sathasivam et al. [10] previously described similar findings in a female neonate with neonatal hyperparathyroidism and rickets-like radiographic changes. Alfadhel et al. [11] reported two children with raised PTH and ALP, normal calcium levels who also had radiographic changes consistent with rickets/hyperparathyroidism. Some authors speculate that the presence of severe skeletal changes related to secondary hyperparathyroidism indicate that the abnormal elevation of PTH starts in utero [8].

The exact etiology of secondary hyperparathyroidism in ML II remains unclear. It has been suggested that the active transplacental transport of calcium is interrupted by ML II. The syncytiotrophoblastic layer where active transplacental calcium transport is regulated demonstrates generalized cytoplasmic vacuolization in patients with ML II. This suggests that the enzymatic abnormalities related to ML II interfere in some way with transplacental calcium transport. PTH secretion is thought to increase to maintain extracellular calcium at the expense of the skeleton [27]. This, however, does not explain skeletal changes in those with normal PTH levels.

David-Vizcarra et al. [9] observed that, following birth, biochemical hyperparathyroidism in ML II resolves, but a progressive erosive osteodystrophy develops after 4 months of age. We saw this progressive erosive osteodystrophy in one patient whose early PTH levels were not increased. They proposed that tissue hypersensitivity to circulating PTH ("pseudohyperparathyroidism") may be a factor. They confirmed that circulating levels of parathyroid related protein (PTHrP) were normal and postulated that, postnatally, the radiographic features could be consistent with an increased sensitivity of skeletal tissue to normal circulating levels of PTH. A more recent study by Kollmann et al. [29], however, refuted tissue hypersensitivity to PTH as a pathogenetic mechanism for the osteopenia, since the secretion of Rankl (pro-osteoclastogenic cytokine) in osteoblasts from ML II mice was not affected in response to PTH stimulation.

The above demonstrates the need for further studies regarding the pathophysiology of bone disease in patients with ML II.

Optimal management of the secondary hyperparathyroidism in this patient cohort is also controversial, as changes may be self-limiting and might represent the natural history of ML II [14,17,27].

Unger et al. [27] described three patients with bone disease, increased serum PTH and ALP, but normal calcium levels. Two were treated with Vitamin D and calcium supplements, while one received no treatment and secondary hyperparathyroidism resolved in all cases. Another report by Leyva et al. [8] described a patient with secondary hyperparathyroidism (with biochemical and radiographic changes), in whom a spontaneous normalization of previously elevated PTH was observed in the absence of treatment, however the ALP level remained high and radiographic follow up was not reported.

In contrast, a patient reported by Khan et al. [12] had low serum phosphate, normal vitamin D and PTH levels at birth and radiographic findings of rickets/hyperparathyroidism. Initially, after parents declined vitamin D supplementation, ALP and PTH levels rose significantly. At 4 months of age, parents agreed to vitamin D supplementation and, within a month, serum phosphate, PTH and ALP levels normalized. This indicates that bone disease can precede the elevations in biochemical markers and highlights the importance of regular biochemical monitoring, even if initial PTH levels are normal. We recommend checking for biochemical and radiographic features of secondary hyperparathyroidism at diagnosis of ML II by checking levels of PTH, Ca, P, ALP, Vitamin D and by performing skeletal survey. We suggest monitoring of biochemical markers at least 6–12 monthly during infancy; however, such monitoring intervals are arbitrary and would depend on the initial levels. Similarly, the frequency of radiological monitoring would depend on initial clinical and radiographic findings, e.g., sooner re-imaging for those with bone fractures. Rapid normalization of biochemical markers post commencement of vitamin D supplementation may indicate that this supplement has a role in the treatment of secondary hyperparathyroidism in some patients with ML II. Currently, in our centre, we recommend high dose Vitamin D supplements in those with biochemical features of secondary hyperparathyroidism and/or bone fractures and low/suboptimal Vitamin D levels. Minimal handling, including a lie flat car seat, lying supported on the side and avoidance of walkers and bouncers would be recommended for children with bone fractures.

Antiresorptive therapy has also been suggested as a therapeutic option, but this is usually reserved for individuals with a high fracture risk and this treatment is controversial in ML II, given the multisystem involvement and overall poor prognosis [29].

Unger et al. [27] summarized that most children with a neonatal presentation of ML II and perinatal bone disease have a shortened life expectancy, i.e., most die before the age of 2 years. In our cohort with secondary hyperparathyroidism, all patients had perinatal bone disease confirmed by skeletal survey and two died before the age of 2 years.

Given the rarity of ML II, extensive sequential assessment of five patients with secondary hyperparathyroidism from a clinical, radiological and biochemical perspective provides important information regarding natural history of the condition. Our paper also provides recommendations on diagnostics and management of secondary hyperparathyroidism in this cohort; we believe that these would help to improve diagnostic accuracy and to optimize management of these patients. In addition, our paper contains interesting figures depicting clinical and radiological course of the disease and provides an up-to-date incidence of ML II in Republic of Ireland.

While we identified five members of the cohort as having secondary HPT, not all infants were systematically investigated for the same; therefore, it is likely that there is under-ascertainment.

5. Conclusions

Children with ML II may have varying degrees of radiological and biochemical features of hyperparathyroidism at presentation. It is important to recognize this association, as this may improve diagnostic accuracy and management. It is also important for appropriate family counseling and natural history data. In this cohort, resolution of abnormal biochemical findings was observed in all cases, irrespective of management. Further studies are needed to establish the etiology and pathophysiology of the bony changes observed in ML II and the potential benefit of Vitamin D supplementation in this cohort.

Author Contributions: Conceptualization, E.C. and R.B.; methodology, R.B.; data curation, R.B.; clinical data—I.K., J.H. and C.M.; writing—original draft preparation, R.B.; radiology images and legends—S.R. and A.S.; writing—review and editing, E.C., N.M., T.C., A.A.M., S.R. and A.S.; supervision, E.C. All authors have read and agreed to the published version of the manuscript.

Funding: This research received no external funding.

Institutional Review Board Statement: The study was conducted in accordance with the Declaration of Helsinki and approved by the Research and Ethics Committee of Children's Health Ireland at Temple Street, Dublin (protocol code 21. 013).

Informed Consent Statement: This study was approved as a retrospective chart review under the Health Research Regulations, 2018 and patient consent is not required.

Data Availability Statement: The data presented in this study are available on request from the corresponding author. The data are not publicly available due to privacy restrictions.

Acknowledgments: We acknowledge the care given by colleagues on multidisciplinary teams at NCIMD and across the country who look after these special children. We thank staff at Willink laboratory in Manchester for diagnostic assistance, and last, but not least we thank our patients and their parents as without them this manuscript would not be possible.

Conflicts of Interest: The authors declare no conflict of interest.

References

1. Heo, J.S.; Choi, K.Y.; Sohn, S.H.; Kim, C.; Kim, Y.J.; Shin, S.H.; Lee, J.M.; Lee, J.; Sohn, J.A.; Lim, B.C.; et al. A case of mucolipidosis II presenting with prenatal skeletal dysplasia and severe secondary hyperparathyroidism at birth. *Korean J. Pediatr.* **2012**, *55*, 438–444. [CrossRef]
2. Yokoi, A.; Niida, Y.; Kuroda, M.; Imi-Hashida, Y.; Toma, T.; Yachie, A. B-cell-specific accumulation of inclusion bodies loaded with HLA class II molecules in patients with mucolipidosis II (I-cell disease). *Pediatr. Res.* **2018**, *86*, 85–91. [CrossRef] [PubMed]
3. Leroy, J.G.; DeMars, R.I. Mutant Enzymatic and Cytological Phenotypes in Cultured Human Fibroblasts. *Science* **1967**, *157*, 804–806. [CrossRef] [PubMed]
4. Spranger, J.W.; Wiedemann, H.-R. The genetic mucolipidoses. *Qual. Life Res.* **1970**, *9*, 113–139. [CrossRef]
5. Velho, R.V.; Harms, F.L.; Danyukova, T.; Ludwig, N.F.; Friez, M.J.; Cathey, S.S.; Filocamo, M.; Tappino, B.; Gunes, N.; Tuysuz, B.; et al. The lysosomal storage disorders mucolipidosis type II, type III alpha/beta, and type III gamma: Update on GNPTAB and GNPTG mutations. *Hum. Mutat.* **2019**, *40*, 842–864. [PubMed]
6. Sly, W.; Sundaram, V. The I-Cell model: The molecular basis for abnormal lysosomal enzyme transport in mucolipidosis II and mucolipidosis III. In *Genetic and Metabolic Disease in Pediatrics*; Lloyd, K.K.; Scriver, C.R., Eds.; Butterworths: London, UK, 1985; pp. 91–110.
7. Ammer, L.S.; Oussoren, E.; Muschol, N.M.; Pohl, S.; Rubio-Gozalbo, M.E.; Santer, R.; Stuecker, R.; Vettorazzi, E.; Breyer, S.R. Hip Morphology in Mucolipidosis Type II. *J. Clin. Med.* **2020**, *9*, 728. [CrossRef]
8. Leyva, C.; Buch, M.; Wierenga, K.J.; Berkovitz, G.; Seeherunvong, T. A neonate with mucolipidosis II and transient secondary hyperparathyroidism. *J. Pediatr. Endocrinol. Metab.* **2019**, *32*, 1399–1402. [CrossRef]
9. David-Vizcarra, G.; Briody, J.; Ault, J.; Fietz, M.; Fletcher, J.; Savarirayan, R.; Wilson, M.; McGill, J.; Edwards, M.; Munns, C.; et al. The natural history and osteodystrophy of mucolipidosis types II and III. *J. Paediatr. Child Health* **2010**, *46*, 316–322. [CrossRef]
10. Sathasivam, A.; Garibaldi, L.; Murphy, R.; Ibrahim, J. Transient Neonatal Hyperparathyroidism: A Presenting Feature of Mucolipidosis Type II. *J. Pediatr. Endocrinol. Metab.* **2006**, *19*, 859–862. [CrossRef]
11. Alfadhel, M.; Alshehhi, W.; Alshaalan, H.; Al Balwi, M.; Eyaid, W. Mucolipidosis II: First report from Saudi Arabia. *Ann. Saudi Med.* **2013**, *33*, 382–386, Erratum in *Ann. Saudi Med.* **2014**, *34*, 91. [CrossRef]
12. Khan, A.; Ho, J.; Pender, A.; Wei, X.; Potter, M. I-Cell Disease (Mucolipidosis II) Presenting as Neonatal Fractures: A Case for Continued Monitoring of Serum Parathyroid Hormone Levels. *Clin. Pediatr. Endocrinol.* **2008**, *17*, 81–85. [CrossRef] [PubMed]
13. Lin, M.H.-C.; Pitukcheewanont, P. Mucolipidosis type II (I-cell disease) masquerading as rickets: Two case reports and review of literature. *J. Pediatr. Endocrinol. Metab.* **2012**, *25*, 191–195. [CrossRef] [PubMed]
14. Alegra, T.; Cury, G.; Todeschini, L.A.; Schwartz, I.V. Should neonatal hyperparathyroidism associated with mucolipidosis II/III be treated pharmacologically? *J. Pediatr. Endocrinol. Metab.* **2013**, *26*, 1011–1013. [CrossRef]
15. Pazzaglia, U.E.; Beluffi, G.; Campbell, J.B.; Bianchi, E.; Colavita, N.; Diard, F.; Gugliantini, P.; Hirche, U.; Kozlowski, K.; Marchi, A.; et al. Mucolipidosis II: Correlation between radiological features and histopathology of the bones. *Pediatr. Radiol.* **1989**, *19*, 406–413. [CrossRef] [PubMed]
16. Pazzaglia, U.E.; Beluffi, G.; Castello, A.; Coci, A.; Zatti, G. Bone changes of mucolipidosis II at different ages. Postmortem study of three cases. *Clin. Orthop. Relat. Res.* **1992**, *276*, 283–290. [CrossRef]
17. Pazzaglia, U.E.; Beluffi, G.; Danesino, C.; Frediani, P.V.; Pagani, G.; Zatti, G. Neonatal mucolipidosis 2. The spontaneous evolution of early bone lesions and the effect of vitamin D treatment. *Pediatr. Radiol.* **1989**, *20*, 80–84. [CrossRef]
18. Kornfeld, S.; Sly, W. I-cell disease and pseudo-Hurler polydystrophy: Disorders of lysosomal enzyme phosphorylation and localization. In *The Metabolic and Molecular Bases of Inherited Disease*; Scriver, C.H., Beaudet, A., Sly, W., Valle, D., Eds.; McGraw-Hill, Inc.: New York, NY, USA, 2001; pp. 3469–3482.

19. Alegra, T.; Koppe, T.; Acosta, A.; Sarno, M.; Burin, M.; Kessler, R.G.; Sperb-Ludwig, F.; Cury, G.; Baldo, G.; Matte, U.; et al. Pitfalls in the prenatal diagnosis of mucolipidosis II alpha/beta: A case report. *Meta Gene* **2014**, *2*, 403–406. [CrossRef]
20. Ma, G.-C.; Ke, Y.-Y.; Chang, S.-P.; Lee, D.-J.; Chen, M. A compound heterozygous GNPTAB mutation causes mucolipidosis II with marked hair color change in a Han Chinese baby. *Am. J. Med. Genet. Part A* **2011**, *155*, 931–934. [CrossRef]
21. Coutinho, M.F.; Santos, L.D.S.; Girisha, K.M.; Satyamoorthy, K.; Lacerda, L.; Prata, M.J.; Alves, S. Mucolipidosis type II α/β with a homozygous missense mutation in the GNPTAB gene. *Am. J. Med. Genet. Part A* **2012**, *158A*, 1225–1228. [CrossRef]
22. Pinto, R.R.; Caseiro, C.; Lemos, M.; Lopes, L.; Fontes, A.; Ribeiro, H.; Pinto, E.; Silva, E.; Rocha, S.; Marcão, A.; et al. Prevalence of lysosomal storage diseases in Portugal. *Eur. J. Hum. Genet.* **2003**, *12*, 87–92. [CrossRef]
23. Okada, S.; Owada, M.; Sakiyama, T.; Yutaka, T.; Ogawa, M. I-cell disease: Clinical studies of 21 Japanese cases. *Clin. Genet.* **2008**, *28*, 207–215. [CrossRef]
24. Poorthuis, B.; Wevers, R.; Kleijer, W.; Groener, J.; De Jong, J.; Van Weely, S.; Niezen-Koning, K.; Van Diggelen, O. The frequency of lysosomal storage diseases in The Netherlands. *Qual. Life Res.* **1999**, *105*, 151–156. [CrossRef]
25. Kovacevic, A.; Schranz, D.; Meissner, T.; Pillekamp, F.; Schmidt, K.G. Mucolipidosis II complicated by severe pulmonary hypertension. *Mol. Genet. Metab.* **2011**, *104*, 192–193. [CrossRef] [PubMed]
26. McElligott, F.; Beatty, E.; O'Sullivan, S.; Hughes, J.; Lambert, D.; Cooper, A.; Crushell, E. Incidence of I-cell disease (muco-lipidosis type II) in the irish population. *J. Inherit. Metab. Dis.* **2011**, *34*, S206.
27. Unger, S.; Paul, D.A.; Nino, M.C.; McKay, C.P.; Miller, S.; Sochett, E.; Braverman, N.; Clarke, J.T.R.; Cole, D.E.C.; Superti-Furga, A. Mucolipidosis II presenting as severe neonatal hyperparathyroidism. *Eur. J. Pediatr.* **2004**, *164*, 236–243. [CrossRef] [PubMed]
28. Babcock, D.S.; Bove, K.E.; Hug, G.; Dignan, P.S.J.; Soukup, S.; Warren, N.S. Fetal mucolipidosis II (I-cell disease): Radiologic and pathologic correlation. *Pediatr. Radiol.* **1986**, *16*, 32–39. [CrossRef]
29. Kollmann, K.; Pestka, J.M.; Kühn, S.C.; Schöne, E.; Schweizer, M.; Karkmann, K.; Otomo, T.; Catala-Lehnen, P.; Failla, A.V.; Marshall, R.P.; et al. Decreased bone formation and increased osteoclastogenesis cause bone loss in mucolipidosis II. *EMBO Mol. Med.* **2013**, *5*, 1871–1886. [CrossRef]

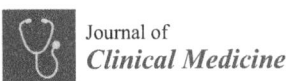

Article

Attention Deficits and ADHD Symptoms in Adults with Fabry Disease—A Pilot Investigation

Nadia Ali [1,*], Amanda Caceres [2], Eric W. Hall [3] and Dawn Laney [1]

1. Department of Human Genetics, Emory University School of Medicine, Atlanta, GA 30322, USA; Dawn.Laney@emory.edu
2. AdventHealth Cancer Institute, Orlando, FL 32804, USA; Aehodgkins24@gmail.com
3. Department of Epidemiology, Rollins School of Public Health, Emory University, Atlanta, GA 30322, USA; Eric.W.Hall@emory.edu
* Correspondence: Nadia.Ali@emory.edu

Abstract: The present pilot study examines subjective reported symptoms of attention-deficit/ hyperactivity (AD/H) in adults with Fabry disease (FD) in comparison with existing normative control data. Existing data from 69 adults with FD via the Achenbach System of Empirically Based Assessment Adult Self-Report questionnaire were analyzed. The results demonstrated a higher prevalence of AD/H symptoms in adults with FD than in the general United States population, with a roughly equal endorsement of Inattention/Attention Deficit symptoms (AD), Hyperactivity-Impulsivity (H-I) symptoms, and Combined Inattention/hyperactivity-impulsivity (C) symptoms. No gender differences were observed. While all subjects endorsing H-I symptoms fell into the symptomatic range on the AD/H scale, only two-thirds of subjects endorsing AD did so. This suggests that attention difficulties with FD are not solely explained by ADHD. Adults with FD who endorsed the AD, H-I, and C symptoms were also more likely to report mean adaptive functioning difficulties. These findings support the growing literature regarding attention difficulties in adults with FD, as well as suggesting a previously unrecognized risk of AD/H symptoms. Future research involving the objective assessment of ADHD in adults with FD is recommended. When serving adults with FD clinically, healthcare professionals should address multiple areas of care, including physical, psychological, and cognitive arenas.

Keywords: Fabry disease; attention; Attention Deficit/Hyperactivity; cognition

Citation: Ali, N.; Caceres, A.; Hall, E.W.; Laney, D. Attention Deficits and ADHD Symptoms in Adults with Fabry Disease—A Pilot Investigation. *J. Clin. Med.* **2021**, *10*, 3367. https://doi.org/10.3390/jcm10153367

Academic Editors: Karolina M. Stepien, Christian J. Hendriksz and Gregory M Pastores

Received: 26 June 2021
Accepted: 24 July 2021
Published: 29 July 2021

Publisher's Note: MDPI stays neutral with regard to jurisdictional claims in published maps and institutional affiliations.

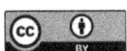

Copyright: © 2021 by the authors. Licensee MDPI, Basel, Switzerland. This article is an open access article distributed under the terms and conditions of the Creative Commons Attribution (CC BY) license (https:// creativecommons.org/licenses/by/ 4.0/).

1. Introduction

Fabry disease (FD) is an X-linked lysosomal storage disorder (LSD) caused by mutations in the *GLA* gene, leading to a deficiency of α-galactosidase A (α-gal A; EC 3.2.1.22) and resulting in the storage of globotriaosylceramide (GL3) and related lipids in the lysosome. Its incidence has historically been estimated at 1:40,000 male live births; however recent data suggests as high as 1:3000 [1], with a range of 1250–117,000 worldwide [2]. The symptoms and complications include acroparesthesia, fatigue, anhidrosis, angiokeratomas, gastrointestinal symptoms, kidney failure, cardiovascular problems, and stroke [3–7]. The standard of care treatment is enzyme replacement therapy (ERT) or chaperone therapy (in individuals with amenable *GLA* mutations).

Historically, research has focused on somatic manifestations of FD, with less attention paid to neuropsychological manifestations. However, recent research suggests difficulties with cognitive functioning, particularly in the realm of attention and concentration, with implications for central nervous system (CNS) functioning in patients with FD.

The initial neuropsychological screening studies of patients with FD reported contradictory results due to varying testing methods and small sample sizes. One initial study found patients with FD performed marginally better on tasks of attention than normal controls and slightly worse on tasks measuring language skills, with unimpaired performances in other cognitive domains [8], while another found patients with FD performed mildly worse on tasks of attention than normal controls [9]. Although the patients initially appeared to perform worse on executive functioning tasks, this difference disappeared once corrected for the effects of depression and remained absent in a subset of patients eight years later [10]. The subsequent early research found that patients with FD performed worse on some tests of attention (especially those involving information processing speed) [11–13], as well as some measures of executive functioning [11,13].

The first study to examine neurocognitive functioning in FD using comprehensive and well-validated neuropsychological measures rather than screening tools found that males with FD demonstrated a slower information processing speed and reduced performance on measures of executive functioning compared to both females with FD and 15 age-matched normal controls [14]. However, several confounds were present. None of the females with FD had experienced a stroke or transient ischemic attacks compared to 33% of the males. Males with FD were also more likely to report symptoms of anxiety and depression, which is known to have delirious effects on cognition, including attention, memory, and executive functioning [15]. Taken together with a low sample size and correlational analyses suggesting a link between the cognition and clinical measures of disease severity, these confounds compromised the generalizability.

A more recent study found 29.3% of Danish patients with FD to have cognitive difficulties, with attention, psychomotor speed, and executive functioning once again being the most frequently impaired [16]. Neither depression, disease severity, nor gender predicted objective cognitive impairment; however, depression was associated with the subjective perception of cognition. The subjective perception of cognition was lower than the actual cognitive performance among subjects.

In comparison, subjective perceptions of cognitive impairment among Dutch subjects with FD were found to be much greater (64%) than the objective evidence of impairment (16%) [17]. Objective impairment was found primarily in males, especially those with classical FD. Follow-up testing one year later, however, demonstrated a worsening objective cognitive impairment in only 5.3% of subjects and was found more often among women (three women and one man) [18]. Subjective impairment was prevalent in both genders and correlated with depression [16,17].

Given the increasing evidence of the role of FD in aspects of attention, anecdotal patient reports regarding the use of medication for Attention Deficit Hyperactivity Disorder (ADHD) should perhaps not come as a surprise. Previously referred to as Attention Deficit Disorder (ADD) in the Diagnostic and Statistical Manual of Mental Disorders 3rd Edition (DSM III) [19], one of the core symptoms is a deficiency in attention. The updated label of ADHD in DSM IV and DSM-5 is an umbrella term for a wide range of symptoms and consists of three main types: Inattentive/Attention Deficit (AD), Hyperactive-Impulsive (H-I), and Combination (C) types [20,21]. While attention-deficit/hyperactivity (AD/H) symptoms in patients with FD have been shown to be associated with poorer adaptive functioning (AF) [22], no further exploration of AD/H symptoms in FD has been done. A pilot study specifically documenting and exploring patient reports of attention deficits will be beneficial as a prequel to more in-depth studies of attention deficits in patients with FD.

The present pilot study examines the self-reported symptoms of attention deficits/hyperactivity in adults with FD in comparison with the existing normative control data, as well as potential differences in the frequency between symptoms of attention deficits and symptoms of hyperactivity. In addition, we explored the possible association between attention-deficit/hyperactivity symptoms and poorer adaptive functioning in patients with FD.

2. Materials and Methods

Data was derived from a subset of data in existence at the Emory Lysosomal Storage Disease Center. Specifically, data concerning Attention Deficit/Hyperactivity, Attention,

Inattention, Hyperactivity-impulsivity, Somatic Symptoms, Depression, Anxiety, and Mean Adaptive Functioning were utilized from the Achenbach System of Empirically Based Assessment (ASEBA) Adult Self-Report (ASR) questionnaires completed by patients with FD between January 2005 and July 2013. Approval from the Institutional Review Board was granted through Emory University (IRB00068700).

The ASEBA ASR is a reliable, validated measure of social-adaptive and psychological functioning in adults aged 18–59 and the OASR for ages 60–90+ [23]. Norms represent the mix of ethnicities, socioeconomic status, urban–rural–suburban residency, and geography within the US. Raw scores are converted to T-scores to permit comparisons with the general population. Scale scores are normed by gender and age and categorized as normal (<93rd percentile), borderline-clinical (93rd–97th percentiles), or clinical (>97th percentile). The ASEBA is used with a wide variety of medical conditions, including cystic fibrosis, Fabry, Morquio, Turner, Williams, Angelman, and Prader-Willi syndromes [22–25].

Data Analysis

ASEBA ASR raw data was entered into assessment data manager (ADM, version 9.0) ASEBA scoring software (https://adm-assessment-data-manager.software.informer.com/9.0/, accessed on 1 June 2021), which produces detailed profiles on multiple aspects of psychological functioning. For this study, data from the DSM-Oriented Scale for AD/H, as well as the Attention Problem Syndrome scale, Depression scale, Somatic Complaints scale, and Mean Adaptive Functioning scale, were utilized. Subjects with T-scores in the borderline-clinical and clinical ranges were considered to have symptoms for the purposes of this study.

All data analysis was done using SAS 9.4 (SAS Institute, Cary, NC, USA). Demographic participant characteristics were summarized using frequencies and proportions. Chi-square and Fisher's exact tests were used to assess the associations between mean adaptive functioning and demographic variables of interest. Similarly, chi-square tests were used to assess the association between depressive symptoms and gender, AD/H symptoms, H-I symptoms, and AD symptoms. The prevalence of AD/H in our study sample was compared to the most recent estimated prevalence of AD/H among the US adult population [26] using Fisher's exact test. All statistical tests were assessed using an alpha = 0.05.

3. Results

Existing data from 69 adults with FD who completed the ASEBA ASR questionnaire was examined. The demographic information is presented in Table 1. The ages ranged from 18 to 61 years.

Table 1. Demographic characteristics of the subjects.

	n	%
Gender		
Female	38	55.1
Male	31	44.9
Race		
African American	4	5.8
Caucasian	61	88.4
Other	4	5.8
Education		
Some High School	5	7.3
High School or GED degree	13	18.8
Some college	24	34.8
College degree or higher	27	39.1
Employment		
Yes	32	46.4
No	23	33.3
Disability	4	5.8
Student	10	14.5

Of the 69 subjects who completed the ASEBA ASR, twenty (29%) endorsed symptoms within the borderline-clinical-to-clinical range on the AD/H problems scale (Figure 1). This represents a significantly higher prevalence of AD/H symptoms in our population of adults with FD than in the general population ($p < 0.001$), using the most recently estimated prevalence (4.4%) of adult ADHD in the United States [26].

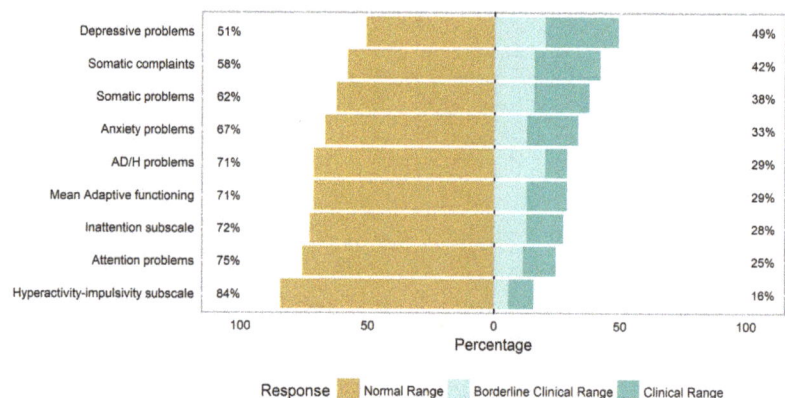

Figure 1. Prevalence of ASEBA symptoms in adults with Fabry disease.

Among the twenty subjects endorsing symptoms within the borderline-clinical-to-clinical range on the AD/H scale, the source of those scores was almost equally balanced between the symptomatic endorsement of AD items, H-I items, and combined AD/H items, with a final three subjects whose endorsement of items was evenly split such that they fell within the normal ranges on the individual subscales while still falling within the symptomatic range on the overall combined AD/H scale (Table 2). All subjects endorsing the H-I symptoms within borderline-clinical-to-clinical range also scored in the borderline-clinical-to-clinical range on the AD/H scale; however, only 12/19 (63.2%) subjects endorsing AD symptoms also scored in the borderline-clinical-to-clinical range on the AD/H scale.

Table 2. Subscale breakdown among adults with FD endorsing AD/H symptoms ($n = 20$).

Subscale within Symptomatic Range	n	Column%
Combined Attention Deficit/Hyperactivity	6	30.0
Attention Deficit/Inattention only	6	30.0
Hyperactivity-impulsivity only	5	25.0
None (items evenly split)	3	15.0

Almost half of the adults with FD (49%) were also noted to self-report depressive symptoms in the borderline-clinical-to-clinical range on the ASEBA ASR, with no significant differences between the male and female subjects ($p = 0.537$). A third of the adults with FD (33%) self-reported symptoms of anxiety, with no significant differences between the male and female subjects ($p = 0.0870$). Almost a third of adults with FD (29%) self-reported difficulties in adaptive functioning, with no significant differences between the male and female subjects ($p = 0.060$). Over a third of adults with FD (38%) self-reported somatic symptoms in the borderline-clinical-to-clinical range, with no significant differences between the male and female subjects ($p = 0.2468$).

Adults who scored in the borderline-clinical-to-clinical range on the AD/H scale, AD subscale, and H-I subscale were significantly more likely to self-report both depressive symptoms and somatic problems (Table 3). Adults scoring in the borderline-clinical-to-clinical range on the AD/H scale and H-I scale were significantly more likely to self-report anxiety symptoms as well (Table 3). There were no differences between males and females in any of these categories.

Table 3. Association between the comorbid symptoms and symptoms of AD/H, AD, and H-I in adults with FD when using the ASEBA Adult Self-Report.

		AD/H					Inattention					Hyperactivity-Impulsivity				
		Clinical/Borderline		Normal			Clinical/Borderline		Normal			Clinical/Borderline		Normal		
	N	n	col %	n	col %	p-Value	n	col %	n	col %	p-Value	n	col %	n	col %	p-Value
Depressive Problems	34	17	85.0	17	34.70	<0.001	15	79	19	38.0	0.002	10	90.9	24	41.4	0.003
No depressive problems	35	3	15.0	32	65.30		4	21.1	31	62.0		1	9.1	34	58.6	
Anxiety problems	23	13	65.0	10	20.4	<0.001	9	47.4	14	28.0	0.127	7	63.6	16	27.6	0.034
No anxiety problems	46	7	35.0	39	79.6		10	52.6	36	72.0		4	36.4	42	72.4	
Somatic problems	26	12	60.0	14	28.6	0.015	11	57.9	15	30.0	0.033	8	72.7	18	31.0	0.015
No somatic problems	43	8	40.0	35	71.4		8	42.1	35	70.0		3	27.3	40	69.0	
Female	38	13	65.0	25	51	0.290	8	42.1	30	60.0	0.182	7	63.6	31	53.5	0.743
Male	31	7	35.0	24	49		11	57.9	20	40.0		4	36.4	27	46.6	

There were no significant demographic differences between those with and without AF deficits; however, the adults with FD who self-reported AD problems, AD/H symptoms, depressive symptoms, and anxiety were also significantly more likely to report AF difficulties (Table 4).

Table 4. Association between psychological symptoms and adaptive functioning in adults with FD when using the ASEBA Adult Self-Report.

		Mean Adaptive Functioning				
		Normal Range		Borderline/Clinical Range		
Demographic Characteristics	N	n	Row %	n	Row %	p-Value
Sex						0.06
Female	38	23	60.5	15	39.5	
Male	31	26	83.9	5	16.1	
Race						0.137
African American	4	3	75	1	25	
Caucasian	61	45	73.8	16	26.2	
Other	4	1	25	3	75	
Education						0.269
Some High School	5	3	60	2	40	
High School or GED degree	13	7	53.9	6	46.2	
Some college	24	17	70.8	7	29.2	
College degree or higher	27	22	81.5	5	18.5	
Employment						0.702
Yes	32	23	71.9	9	28.1	
No	23	15	65.2	8	34.8	
Disability	4	4	100	0	0	
Student	10	7	70	3	30	
ASR Conditions						
Attention problems	17	5	29.4	12	70.6	<0.001
Normal range	52	44	84.6	8	15.4	
AD/H problems	20	7	35	13	65	<0.001
Normal range	49	42	85.7	7	14.3	
Somatic problems	26	15	57.7	11	42.3	0.099
Normal range	43	34	79.1	9	20.9	
Depressive problems	34	15	44.1	19	55.9	<0.001
Normal range	35	34	97.1	1	2.9	
Anxiety problems	23	11	47.8	12	52.2	0.005
Normal range	46	38	82.6	8	17.4	
Somatic complaints	29	17	58.6	12	41.4	0.065
Normal range	40	32	80	8	20	
H-I subscale	11	3	27.3	8	72.7	0.001
Normal range	58	46	79.3	12	20.7	
AD subscale	19	11	22	9	47.4	0.072
Normal range	50	39	78	10	52.6	

p-values calculated using chi-sq or Fisher's exact test.

4. Discussion

The present study is a pilot exploration of self-reported attention deficit symptoms in adults with Fabry disease. The results demonstrate a higher prevalence of AD/H symptoms in adults with FD than in the general United States population, with a roughly equal numbers of adults with FD endorsing AD symptoms, H-I symptoms, and Combined symptoms. While ADHD is more common in men than women in the general population [26], and some studies have found greater evidence of cognitive impairment in men with FD than women [14,17], our study found no gender differences in the rate of AD/H, H-I, or AD symptoms amongst adults with FD.

While all subjects endorsing H-I symptoms fell within the symptomatic range on the AD/H scale, only two-thirds of subjects endorsing AD symptoms did so. The remaining third endorsing AD without AD/H symptoms suggests that attention difficulties within FD are not solely linked to AD/H and lends credence to prior research outlining cognitive difficulties in attention in FD [9,11,13,16]. However, the reverse is also true; the endorsement of an equally high rate of H-I symptoms among our FD population suggests a previously unrecognized prevalence of such symptoms among adults with FD separate from attention deficits.

Of note, almost half of adults with FD in the present study endorsed symptoms of depression (49%), with no significant differences between men and women. This replicates the previously reported high rates of depression among adults with FD, with prevalence estimates ranging from 15% to 62% [9,13,25,27–29]. The present study likewise supported research demonstrating that depression in FD does not follow gender norms, with males reporting equal or greater rates than females [14,27]. While the most common factor associated with depression in FD is chronic pain [13,27,30], economic status, relationship status, specific coping styles, and somatic symptoms such as anhidrosis and acroparaesthesia have also been associated with depression and a lower QOL [27,30,31].

While depression can have deleterious effects on attention [15], its interaction with hyperactivity-impulsivity goes in the opposite direction; it is more likely to be a consequence of ADHD than a cause. Thus, while adults with FD who reported symptoms of AD/H, AD and H-I were more likely to also report symptoms of depression, this is consistent with previous research demonstrating that people with ADHD are at risk for depression and anxiety as a result of living with ADHD [26,32–34].

Finally, the present study found adults with FD-endorsing AD symptoms, AD/H symptoms, depressive symptoms, and anxiety were also significantly more likely to endorse adaptive functioning (AF) difficulties. An indication of the effectiveness with which individuals cope with the demands of everyday tasks and responsibilities as parents, students, employees, etc., AF is measured via evaluations such as the ASEBA focused on individuals' relationships, jobs, education, substance use, psychological issues, and coping skills. These findings corroborate earlier research in which FD patients had a higher rate of mean AF deficits compared to population norms, with poorer AF associated with greater rates of AD/H, depression, and anxiety [22].

All of the above findings make clear the need to pay attention to the psychological symptoms associated with FD, including the possibility of symptoms of AD/H, and expand our standard of care to include mental health treatments, if necessary. Of note, of the 20 people who self-reported AD/H symptoms in our sample, four had been prescribed medication typically used for ADHD at some point in their life, though only one had undergone a clinical diagnosis for their symptoms. As symptoms of ADHD are more heterogeneous and subtle in adults than children [35,36], with only 25% of adults with ADHD receiving treatment [26], it is possible that ADHD symptoms in adults with FD are being overlooked amidst the urgency of the other symptoms of FD.

The limitations of this study include the use of self-reported symptoms at a single point in time; however, adults with ADHD have been found to be quite reliable in identifying their own symptoms via self-reported measures [35], and an earlier study found that adults with FD were, if anything, more likely to underreport than overreport neurocognitive complaints [16]. Another limitation is the comparison between self-reported symptoms (FD population) and diagnosis (US population). To our knowledge, there is no nationally representative database of self-reported symptoms of AD/H, as compared to the frequency of diagnosis. Previous research has likewise used self-reported ADHD symptoms rather than diagnoses and presented evidence for the use of such as an effective tool [37]. Finally, this study included data primarily from Caucasian adults with FD and may not be generalizable to adults with FD of other ethnicities.

The implications of this study include the need for greater attention to cognitive and psychological health in people with FD, particularly in the areas of attention, AD/H-like symptoms, depression, anxiety, and adaptive functioning. Genetic counselors and other healthcare providers should address such issues in their annual clinic appointments and make referrals as needed to maximize overall treatment for patients with FD.

The recommendations for future research include a more objective assessment of AD/H symptoms in patients with FD, as well as further in-depth neurocognitive studying of attention/concentration in FD. Such research should utilize objective neuropsychological tests with the existing normative data with the general population.

5. Conclusions

In conclusion, the present study suggests that adults with FD are at a higher risk than the general population for attention deficits, as well as symptoms of ADHD, with equal rates among men and women. When serving adults with FD clinically, genetic counselors and other healthcare professionals should address multiple areas of care, including the physical, psychological, and cognitive issues that may accompany the disease.

Author Contributions: Conceptualization, N.A; methodology, N.A., A.C. and D.L.; software, E.W.H.; formal analysis, E.W.H.; writing—original draft preparation, N.A.; writing review and editing, N.A., A.C., E.W.H. and D.L.; and funding acquisition, N.A. All authors have read and agreed to the published version of the manuscript.

Funding: This research was funded by Pfizer Inc., grant number WI194299.

Institutional Review Board Statement: This study was conducted according to the guidelines of the Declaration of Helsinki and approved by the Institutional Review Board of Emory University (IRB00068700).

Informed Consent Statement: Informed consent was obtained from all subjects involved in the study.

Data availability Statement: The data for this study are available by contacting the corresponding author.

Acknowledgments: The authors wish to thank all patients with Fabry who participate so generously in this research regarding Fabry disease and their lived experiences.

Conflicts of Interest: Nadia Ali, Ph.D. received research support from Sanofi Genzyme, Shire Takeda, BioMarin, Amicus, and Pfizer, as well as lecturers' honoraria from Sanofi Genzyme, BioMarin, Amicus, and Vitaflo. These activities were monitored and in compliance with the conflicts of interest policies at Emory University. Amanda Caceres, M.MSc, CGC received research support from Genzyme and Pfizer. Eric W Hall, Ph.D. has no conflicts of interest to report. Dawn Laney, M.S., CGC consults for Genzyme, Amicus, and Shire and is a study coordinator in clinical trials sponsored by Genzyme, Amicus, and Protalix. She is a co-founder of ThinkGenetic, Inc. She also received research funding from Alexion, Amicus, Genzyme, Pfizer, Retrophin, Shire, and Synageva. These activities are monitored and are in compliance with the conflicts of interest policies at Emory University. The funders had no role in the design of the study; in the collection, analyses, or interpretation of the data; in the writing of the manuscript; or in the decision to publish the results.

References

1. Hopkins, P.V.; Campbell, C.; Klug, T.; Rogers, S.; Raburn-Miller, J.; Kiesling, J. Lysosomal Storage Disorder Screening Implementation: Findings from the First Six Months of Full Population Pilot Testing in Missouri. *J. Pediatr.* **2015**, *166*, 172–177. [CrossRef] [PubMed]
2. Laney, D.A.; Peck, D.S.; Atherton, A.M.; Manwaring, L.; Christensen, K.M.; Shankar, S.P.; Grange, D.K.; Wilcox, W.R.; Hopkin, R.J. Fabry disease in infancy and early childhood: A systematic literature review. *Genet. Med.* **2015**, *17*, 323–330. [CrossRef] [PubMed]
3. Desnick, R.J.; Brady, R.; Barranger, J.; Collins, A.J.; Germain, D.P.; Goldman, M.; Grabowski, G.; Packman, S.; Wilcox, W.R. Fabry Disease, an Under-Recognized Multisystemic Disorder: Expert Recommendations for Diagnosis, Management, and Enzyme Replacement Therapy. *Ann. Intern. Med.* **2003**, *138*, 338–346. [CrossRef]
4. MacDermot, K.D.; Holmes, A.; Miners, A.H. Anderson-Fabry disease: Clinical manifestations and impact of disease in a cohort of 60 obligate carrier females. *J. Med Genet.* **2001**, *38*, 769–775. [CrossRef]
5. D'Arco, F.; Hanagandi, P.; Ganau, M.; Krishnan, P.; Taranath, A. Neuroimaging Findings in Lysosomal Disorders. *Top. Magn. Reson. Imaging* **2018**, *27*, 259–274. [CrossRef] [PubMed]
6. Ortiz, A.; Germain, D.P.; Desnick, R.J.; Politei, J.; Mauer, M.; Burlina, A.; Eng, C.; Hopkin, R.J.; Laney, D.; Linhart, A.; et al. Fabry disease revisited: Management and treatment recommendations for adult patients. *Mol. Genet. Metab.* **2018**, *123*, 416–427. [CrossRef] [PubMed]
7. Mishra, V.; Banerjee, A.; Gandhi, A.B.; Kaleem, I.; Alexander, J.; Hisbulla, M.; Kannichamy, V.; Subas, S.V.; Hamid, P. Stroke and Fabry Disease: A Review of Literature. *Cureus* **2020**, *12*, 312083.
8. Low, M.; Nicholls, K.; Tubridy, N.; Hand, P.; Velakoulis, D.; Kiers, L.; Mitchell, P.; Becker, G. Neurology of Fabry disease. *Intern. Med. J.* **2007**, *37*, 436–447. [CrossRef]
9. Schermuly, I.; Müller, M.J.; Müller, K.-M.; Albrecht, J.; Keller, I.; Yakushev, I.; Beck, M.; Fellgiebel, A. Neuropsychiatric symptoms and brain structural alterations in Fabry disease. *Eur. J. Neurol.* **2011**, *18*, 347–353. [CrossRef]
10. Lelieveld, I.M.; Böttcher, A.; Hennermann, J.B.; Beck, M.; Fellgiebel, A. Eight-Year Follow-Up of Neuropsychiatric Symptoms and Brain Structural Changes in Fabry Disease. *PLoS ONE* **2015**, *10*, e0137603. [CrossRef]
11. Segal, P.; Kohn, Y.; Pollak, Y.; Altarescu, G.; Galili-Weisstub, E.; Raas-Rothschild, A. Psychiatric and cognitive profile in Anderson-Fabry patients: A preliminary study. *J. Inherit. Metab. Dis.* **2010**, *33*, 429–436. [CrossRef]
12. Elstein, D.; Doniger, G.M.; Altarescu, G. Cognitive testing in Fabry disease: Pilot using a brief computerized assessment tool. *Isr. Med Assoc. J. IMAJ* **2012**, *14*, 624–628. [PubMed]
13. Bolsover, F.E.; Murphy, E.; Cipolotti, L.; Werring, D.J.; Lachmann, R.H. Cognitive dysfunction and depression in Fabry disease: A systemic review. *J. Inherit. Metab. Dis.* **2014**, *37*, 177–187. [CrossRef]
14. Sigmundsdottir, L.; Tchan, M.C.; Knopman, A.A.; Menzies, G.C.; Batchelor, J.; Sillence, D.O. Cognitive and Psychological Functioning in Fabry Disease. *Arch. Clin. Neuropsychol.* **2014**, *29*, 642–650. [CrossRef] [PubMed]
15. Rock, P.L.; Roiser, J.P.; Riedel, W.J.; Blackwell, A.D. Cognitive impairment in depression: A systematic review and meta-anlysis. *Psychol. Med.* **2014**, *44*, 2029–2040. [CrossRef] [PubMed]
16. Loeb, J.; Feldt-Rasmussen, U.; Madsen, C.V.; Vogel, A. Cognitive Impairments and Subjective Cognitive Complaints in Fabry Disease: A Nationwide Study and Review of the Literature. *J. Inherit. Metab. Dis. Rep.* **2018**, *41*, 73–80.
17. Körver, S.; Geurtsen, G.J.; Hollak, C.E.; van Schaik, I.N.; Longo, M.G.; Lima, M.R.; Langeveld, M. Predictors of objective cognitive complaints in patients with Fabry disease. *Sci. Rep.* **2019**, *9*, 188. [CrossRef]
18. Körver, S.; Geurtsen, G.J.; Hollak, C.E.; van Schaik, I.N.; Longo, M.G.; Lima, M.R.; Langeveld, M. Cognitive functioning and depressive symptoms in Fabry disease: A follow-up study. *J. Inherit. Metab. Dis.* **2020**, *43*, 1070–1081. [CrossRef]
19. *Diagnostic and Statistical Manual of Mental Disorders*, 3rd ed.; American Psychiatric Association: Washington, DC, USA, 1980.
20. *Diagnostic and Statistical Manual of Mental Disorders*, 4th ed.; American Psychiatric Association: Washington, DC, USA, 1994.
21. *Diagnostic and Statistical Manual of Mental Disorders*, 5th ed.; American Psychiatric Association: Washington, DC, USA, 2013.
22. Laney, D.A.; Gruskin, D.J.; Fernhoff, P.M.; Cubells, J.F.; Ousley, O.Y.; Hipp, H.; Mehta, A.J. Social-adaptive and psychological functioning of patients affected by Fabry disease. *J. Inherit. Metab. Dis.* **2010**, *33* (Suppl. 3), S73–S81. [CrossRef]
23. Achenbach, T.M.; Rescorla, L.A. *Manual for the ASEBA Adult Forms and Profiles*; University of Vermont, Research Center for Children, Youth, and Families: Burlington, VT, USA, 2003.
24. Ali, N.; Cagle, S. Psychological health in adults with Morquio syndrome. *J. Inherit. Metab. Dis. Rep.* **2015**, *20*, 87–93. [CrossRef]
25. Ali, N.; Gillespie, S.; Laney, D.A. Treatment of depression in adults with Fabry disease. *J. Inherit. Metab. Dis. Rep.* **2017**, *38*, 13–21.
26. Kessler, R.C.; Adler, L.; Barkley, R.; Biederman, J.; Conners, C.K.; Demler, O.; Faraone, S.V.; Greenhill, L.L.; Howes, M.J.; Secnik, K.; et al. The prevalence and correlates of adult ADHD in the United States: Results from the National Comorbidity Survey Replication. *Am. J. Psychiatry* **2006**, *163*, 716–723. [CrossRef] [PubMed]
27. Cole, A.L.; Lee, P.J.; Hughes, D.; Deegan, P.; Waldek, S.; Lachmann, R. Depression in adults with Fabry disease: A common and under-diagnosed problem. *J. Inherit. Metab. Dis.* **2007**, *30*, 943–951. [CrossRef] [PubMed]
28. Laney, D.A.; Bennett, R.L.; Clarke, V.; Fox, A.; Hopkin, R.J.; Johnson, J.; O'Rourke, E.; Sims, K.; Walter, G. Fabry Disease Practice Guidelines: Recommendations of the National Society of Genetic Counselors. *J. Genet. Couns.* **2013**, *22*, 555–564. [CrossRef] [PubMed]
29. Löhle, M.; Hughes, D.; Milligan, A.; Richfield, L.; Reichmann, H.; Mehta, A.; Schapira, A. Clinical prodromes of neurodegeneration in Anderson-Fabry disease. *Neurology* **2015**, *84*, 1454–1464. [CrossRef]

30. Körver, S.; Geurtsen, G.J.; Hollak, C.E.M.; Van Schaik, I.N.; Longo, M.G.F.; Lima, M.R.; Vedolin, L.; Dijkgraaf, M.G.W.; Langeveld, M. Depressive symptoms in Fabry disease: The importance of coping, subjective health perception and pain. *Orphanet J. Rare Dis.* **2020**, *15*, 28. [CrossRef]
31. Gold, K.; Pastores, G.; Botteman, M.; Yeh, J.; Sweeney, S.; Aliski, W.; Pashos, C. Quality of life of patients with Fabry disease. *Qual. Life Res.* **2002**, *11*, 317–327. [CrossRef]
32. Chronis-Tuscano, A.; Molina, B.S.; Pelham, W.E.; Applegate, B.; Dahlke, A.; Overmyer, M.; Lahey, B.B. Very early predictors of adolescent depression and suicide attempts in children with attention-deficit/hyperactivity disorder. *Arch. Gen. Psychiatry* **2010**, *67*, 1044–1051. [CrossRef]
33. Furczyk, K.; Thome, J. Adult ADHD and suicide. *Atten. Def. Hyp. Disord.* **2014**, *6*, 153–158. [CrossRef]
34. Biederman, J.; Ball, S.W.; Monuteaux, M.C.; Mick, E.; Spencer, T.J.; McCREARY, M.; Cote, M.; Faraone, S. New Insights into the Comorbidity Between ADHD and Major Depression in Adolescent and Young Adult Females. *J. Am. Acad. Child Adolesc. Psychiatry* **2008**, *47*, 426–434. [CrossRef]
35. De Quiros, G.B.; Kinsbourne, M. Adult AHDH: Analysis of self-ratings on a behavior questionnaire. *Ann. N. Y. Acad. Sci.* **2001**, *931*, 140–147. [CrossRef] [PubMed]
36. Wender, P.H.; Wolf, L.E.; Wasserstein, J. Adults with ADHD. An overview. *Ann. N. Y. Acad. Sci.* **2001**, *931*, 1–16. [CrossRef] [PubMed]
37. Park, S.; Cho, M.J.; Chang, S.M.; Jeon, H.J.; Cho, S.-J.; Kim, B.-S.; Bae, J.N.; Wang, H.-R.; Ahn, J.H.; Hong, J.P. Prevalence, correlates, and comorbidities of adult ADHD symptoms in Korea: Results of the Korean epidemiologic catchment area study. *Psychiatry Res.* **2011**, *186*, 378–383. [CrossRef] [PubMed]

Article

Hyo-Mental Angle and Distance: An Important Adjunct in Airway Assessment of Adult Mucopolysaccharidosis

Chaitanya Gadepalli [1,*], Karolina M. Stepien [2] and Govind Tol [3]

1. Ear Nose and Throat Department, Salford Royal NHS Foundation Trust, Manchester M6 8HD, UK
2. Adult Inherited Metabolic Department, Salford Royal NHS Foundation Trust, Manchester M6 8HD, UK; karolina.stepien@srft.nhs.uk
3. Anaesthetics Department, Salford Royal NHS Foundation Trust, Manchester M6 8HD, UK; govind.tol@srft.nhs.uk
* Correspondence: cgadepalli@gmail.com

Abstract: Background: Mucopolysaccharidosis (MPS) is a rare congenital lysosomal storage disorder with complex airways. High anterior larynx is assessed by thyromental distance (TMD) nasendoscopy. A simpler method to assess this hyoid bone is described. The distance between the central-hyoid and symphysis of the mandible (hyo-mental distance; HMD) and inclination of this line to the horizontal axis (hyo-mental angle; HMA) in neutrally positioned patients is investigated. Methods: HMA, HMD in MPS, and non-MPS were compared, and their correlation with height and weight were assessed. Results: 50 adult MPS patients (M = 32, F = 18, age range = 19–66 years; mean BMI = 26.8 kg/m^2) of MPS I, II, III, IV, and VI were compared with 50 non-MPS (M = 25, F = 25; age range = 22–84 years; mean BMI = 26.5 kg/m^2). Mean HMA in MPS was 25.72° (−10 to +50) versus 2.42° (−35 to +28) in non-MPS. Mean HMD was 46.5 (25.7–66) millimeters in MPS versus 41.8 (27–60.3) in non-MPS. HMA versus height and weight showed a moderate correlation (r = −0.4, $p < 0.05$) in MPS and no significant correlation (r < 0.4, $p > 0.05$) in non-MPS. HMD versus height and weight showed no correlation (r < 0.4, $p > 0.05$) in both groups. Conclusions: HMA seems more acute in MPS despite nearly the same HMD as non-MPS, signifying a high larynx, which may be missed by TMD.

Keywords: mucopolysaccharidosis; airway management; radiology; hyoid bone; chin; intubation; intratracheal

1. Introduction

Mucopolysaccharidosis are a group of inherited congenital multisystem diseases due to a deficiency in enzymes required for the breakdown of complex mucopolysaccharides. Mucopolysaccharidoses (MPSs) are rare, inherited, lysosomal storage diseases with a combined incidence of 1 in 22,000 [1]. The disease is characterized by the accumulation of glycosaminoglycans (GAGs) in almost all parts of the body. There are seven types of MPS depending on the type of enzyme deficiency (Table 1). The manifestations of this disease are multisystemic, resulting in shortened longevity [2]. Along with other systems, airways are commonly involved. Knowledge about the airway abnormalities is important as these patients can pose airway problems. With advances in treatment modalities, such as hematopoietic stem cell transplantation (HSCT) [3] and enzyme replacement therapy (ERT) [4], the longevity of these patients has increased posing newer problems. Most of these patients will need general anesthetic for surgery at some point in their lifetime due to multi-system involvement. In our experience, we noted that most adult MPS patients have a large and bulky tongue, large lower jaw, and short neck [5]. A high or anterior larynx poses difficulty in access to the airway. A difficult laryngoscopy is defined as an inability to visualize any part of the vocal cords on conventional laryngoscopy [6]. Various bedside measures have been described to assess a high or anterior larynx. The method commonly used to assess a high or anterior larynx are measurement of the thyromental distance TMD [7], nasendoscopy, or cross-sectional imaging. TMD is the distance between the chin, also called the mentum, and prominence of the thyroid cartilage with the neck extended. TMD [7] is about 6.5 cm measured with an intubation gauze or three finger breadths. Direct visualization of the oropharynx and larynx via a fiber optic scope, also called nasendoscopy, can also estimate a high larynx. Figure 1 shows a nasendoscopy picture of a patient with a normal larynx. Figure 2 shows a nasendoscopy picture in an MPS I patient and Figure 3 shows a nasendoscopy picture in an MPS II patient. Cross-sectional imaging either with a computer tomography scan (CT) or magnetic resonance imaging (MRI) provides a detailed evaluation of the head and neck in a neutral position. Many times, these scans have been performed in MPS patients for their co-morbidities. We propose a simpler and possibly more accurate method of assessing a high or anterior larynx using existing cross-section imaging of the neck. This information is very helpful in planning any airway intervention or general anesthetic. We use the body of the hyoid bone as a stable landmark: the distance from the center of the body of hyoid to the symphysis mentum of the mandible is the hyomental distance (HMD). The inclination or declination of HMD to the horizontal axis is the hyomental angle (HMA). The HMD quantifies the anterior larynx and HMA identifies the high larynx. Figure 4 shows a sagittal section diagram showing the landmarks and Figure 5 shows HMA and HMD on a CT scan in a non-MPS and MPS patient. Figure 6 is a three-dimensional reconstruction of the upper body skeleton, showing the level of the hyoid bone in a non-MPS and MPS patient in relation to the mandible. The primary aim of this study was to identify a different and possibly a more accurate method to assess a high or anterior larynx and discuss its usefulness in airway management in adult MPS. The secondary aim was to assess the relationship of the body habitus to a high and anterior larynx.

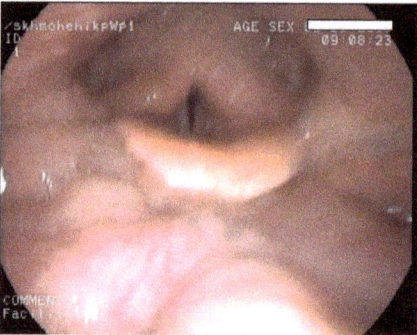

Figure 1. Nasendoscopy pictures showing a normal larynx: the vallecula, epiglottis, glottic inlet, and posterior larynx can be clearly seen.

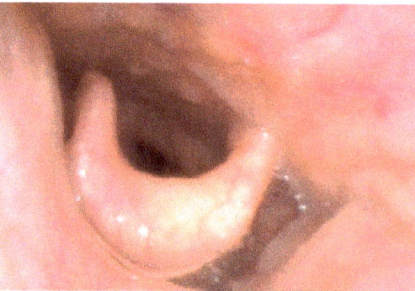

Figure 2. Nasendoscopy picture in MPS I showing a high larynx, large epiglottis touching the soft palate, vallecula cannot be seen, and only the posterior glottis is visible.

Table 1. Various types of MPS; reproduced with permission from Braunlin et al. [8], who compiled data from Neufeld et al. [9] and Valayannopoulos et al. [10]. AR: autosomal recessive; CS: chondroitin sulfate; DS: dermatan sulfate; GAG: glycosaminoglycan; H: Hurler syndrome; HS: heparan sulfate; H-S: Hurler–Scheie syndrome; KS: keratan sulfate; S: Scheie syndrome; XR: X-linked recessive. * only 1 patient reported in the literature (Natowicz et al. 1996); ** death can occur in utero with hydrops fetalis.

MPS Type (Eponym)	Incidence per 10^5 Live Births; Inheritance Pattern	Typical Age at Diagnosis	Typical Life Expectancy If Untreated	Enzyme Deficiency	GAG
MPS I Hurler (H) MPS I Hurler-Scheie (H-S) MPS I Scheie (S)	0.11–1.67; AR	H: <1 year H-S: 3–8 years S: 10–20 years	H: death in childhood H-S: death in teens or early adulthood S: normal to slightly reduced lifespan	α-L-iduronidase	DS, HS
MPS II (Hunter)	0.1–1.07; XR	1–2 years when rapidly progressing	rapidly progressing: death < 15 years slowly progressing: death in adulthood	iduronate-2-sulfatase	DS, HS
MPS III (Sanfilippo) A-B-C-D	0.39–1.89; AR	4–6 years	death in puberty or early adulthood	heparan sulfamidase (A) N-acetyl-α-D-glucosaminidase (B) acetyl-CoA-α-glucosaminidase N-acetyltransferase (C) N-acetylglucosamine-6-sulfatase (D)	HS
MPS IV (Morquio) A-B	0.15–0.47; AR	1–3 years	death in childhood-middle age	N-acetylgalactosamine-6-sulfatase (A) β-galactosidase (B)	CS, KS (A) KS (B)
MPS VI (Maroteaux-Lamy)	0–0.38; AR	rapidly progressing: 1–9 years slowly progressing: >5 years	rapidly progressing: death in 2nd–3rd decade slowly progressing: death in 4–5th decade	N-acetylgalactosamine-4-sulfatase	DS
MPS VII (Sly)	0–0.29; AR	neonatal to adulthood	death in infancy-4th decade **	β-D-glucuronidase	CS, DS, HS
MPS IX (Natowicz) *	unknown	adolescence	unknown	hyaluronidase	CS

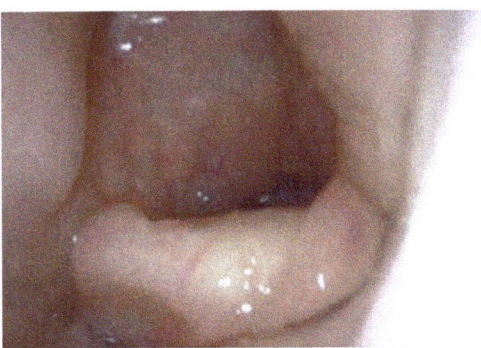

Figure 3. Nasendoscopy picture of MPS II showing a high and anterior larynx, epiglottis is touching the soft palate, vallecula is not seen, and only posterior pharyngeal wall is seen.

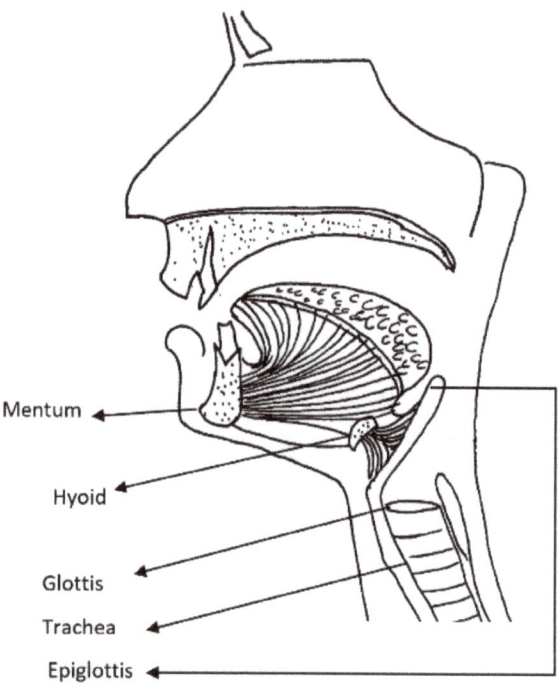

Figure 4. Line diagram sagittal section of the head and neck showing the upper airway and landmarks.

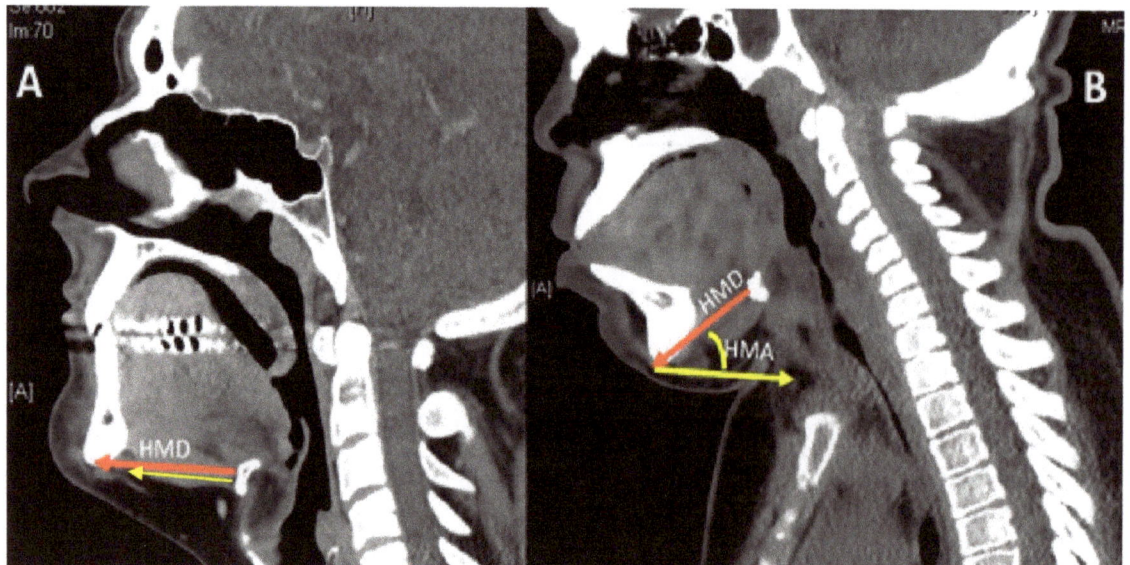

Figure 5. Shows the hyomental distance (HMD) and hyomental angle (HMA) in adult non-MPS marked (**A**) on the left and adult MPS patient marked (**B**) on the right, taken from a computer tomography (CT) scan of the neck in the neutral position. Red arrow represents the HMD and yellow arrow represents the horizontal.

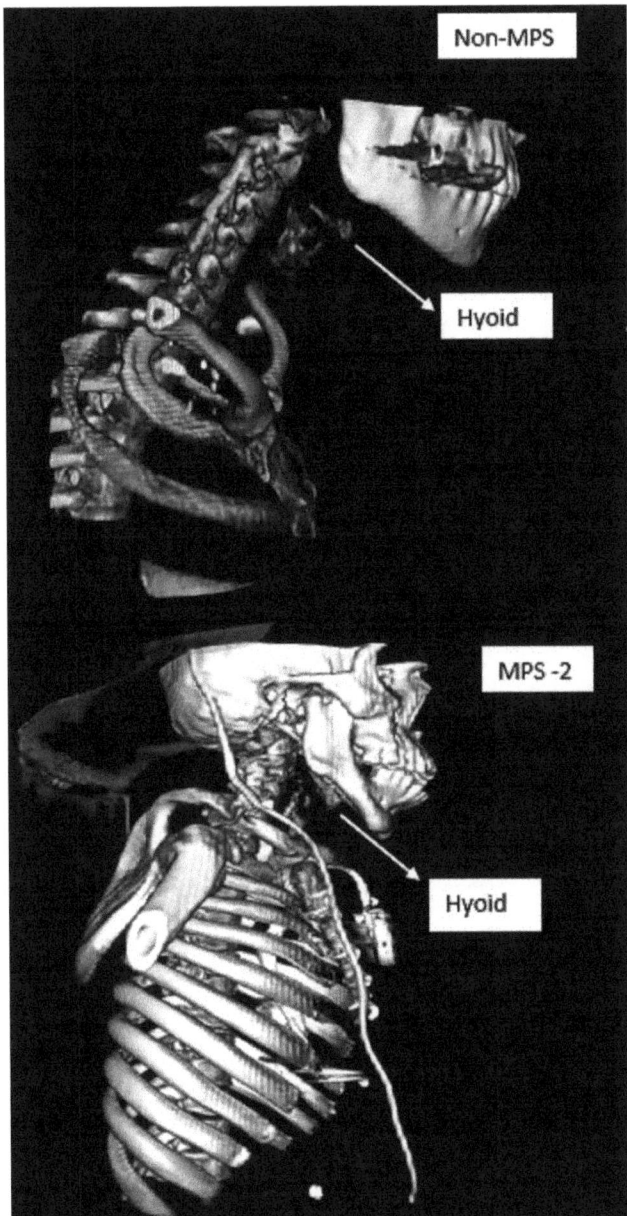

Figure 6. Three-dimensional reconstruction of the upper body skeleton, showing the level of hyoid bone in a non-MPS (top panel) and MPS-2 patient (lower panel) in relation to the mandible. A ventriculoperitoneal shunt and pacemaker are seen in the MPS patient. MPS- Mucopolysaccharidosis.

2. Materials and Methods

Retrospective analysis of case notes and radiological investigations was performed as part of routine care of 50 adult MPS patients and comparison with 50 healthy adults of similar age, gender, and body mass index (BMI). Ethical approval was obtained from the local research and innovation department, Salford Royal NHS Foundation Trust, Northern Care Alliance, United Kingdom, reference: S20HIP40. HMD and HMA were calculated for each group calculated in the picture archiving communications system (PACS) using the ruler tool. A smaller HMD was considered to be an anterior larynx and acute inclination of the HMA to the horizontal axis was considered to represent a high larynx. Both HMD and HMA reflect the difficulty in accessing an airway. The impact of body habitus on a high or anterior larynx was investigated by calculating the Pearsons correlation between HMD, HMD, and weight and height.

3. Results

Radiological cross-sectional images of 50 MPS and 50 non-MPS patients were included in the study. The MPS group included patients with types I, II, III, IV, and VI. Table 2 depicts the demographics in both groups. It may be noted that even though age does not match between both groups, BMI is comparable. The non-MPS group of patients included a range of patients of various ENT (ear, nose, and throat) pathologies who had imaging studies. All the patients in the non-MPS group had no pathology in the oral cavity, neck, oropharynx, supraglottis, and hypopharynx. The non-MPS group had a normal supra-glottic airway. This enabled us to investigate the abnormal hyomental region in MPS patients. Table 3 depicts the pathology subtypes in both groups. The HMA and HMD were calculated and compared between the two groups.

Table 2. Demographics of the study in both the MPS and non-MPS groups.

	MPS	Non-MPS
Number of patients	50	50
Males	32	25
Females	18	25
Age range in years	19–66	22–84
Mean age in years	31.7	59.9
Mean Body Mass index	26.8	26.5

MPS—Mucopolysaccharidosis.

Table 3. Clinical diagnosis of different patients in the MPS and non-MPS groups. MPS—Mucopolysaccharidosis.

Pathology	Number	Males	Females
MPS group			
MPSI	16	8	8
MPSII	13	13	0
MPSIII	1	1	0
MPSIV	14	6	8
MPSVI	6	4	2
Total	50	32	18
Non-MPS group			
Subglottic stenosis	10	1	9
Tracheal stenosis	8	5	3
Vasculitis	7	4	3
Malignancy not involving supraglottis, oropharynx	16	12	4
Bilateral vocal fold immobility	5	0	5
Vocal cord leukoplakia	4	3	1
Total	50	25	25

MPS—Mucopolysaccharidosis.

Table 4 depicts HMA and HMD in both MPS and non-MPS groups. It may be noted that the HMD is slightly less in the MPS depicting slightly anterior larynx in the MPS group. The HMA is more acute in the MPS group compared to the non-MPS group, depicting that larynx is higher in the MPS groups. The MPS group have a shorter stature and lower body mass, this is a recognized feature of MPS due to multisystemic involvement of the disease.

Table 4. HMD and HMA in the MPS and non-MPS groups.

	Age in Years	HMD in Millimeters	HMA in Degrees	Height in Centimeters	Weight in Kilograms	Body Mass Index
MPS						
N = 50						
Mean	31.74	46.5	27.6	135.8	50.47	26.8
Median	29.50	48.5	25.0	136.8	48	25.7
Range	19–66	25.7–66.0	−10.0 to 50	91.0–182	17.4–125.2	16.5–43.6
Non-MPS						
N = 50						
Mean	59.9	41.9	2.420	166.1	72.6	26.5
Median	63	40.9	0.0	166.0	71.9	26.9
Range	22–99	27.0–60.3	−35.0 to 28	150.0–188	39.3–130	14.2–47.3

HMD—Hyomental distance, HMA—Hyomental angle. MPS—Mucopolysaccharidosis.

It can be assumed that a bulky upper airway may be attributable to BMI, thereby affecting HMA or HMD. To test this hypothesis, the Pearson correlation between the BMI versus HMA and HMD was calculated and Table 5 depicts the results. HMD shows no correlation with height, weight, and BMI in the non-MPS group but reveals a statistically significant correlation with height and weight in MPS ($p = 0.05$; $p = 0.009$). It must be noted that the rho value in the MPS group is only 0.3 at best. The Pearson correlation between HMA versus height and weight showed a moderate negative correlation in the MPS group and no correlation in the non-MPS group. Thus, HMA shows a better correlation with height and weight in the MPS group, compared to HMD. The significant results are highlighted in the table.

Table 5. Pearson correlation between HMA, HMD, height, weight, and BMI in both the MPS and non-MPS groups.

		HMD	HMA	HT	WT	BMI
Correlations MPS						
HMD	rho	1	−0.2	0.28 *	0.3 *	0.2
	p-value		0.15	0.05 *	0.009 *	0.13
HMA	rho	−0.2	1	−0.45 *	−0.41 *	−0.1
	p-value	0.146		0.0001 *	0.003 *	0.73
Correlations Non-MPS						
HMD	rho	1	0.15	0.1	0.35	0.27
	p-value		0.3	0.49	0.014	0.06
HMA	rho	0.15	1	−0.03	−0.03	0.02
	p-value	0.296		0.85	0.862	0.91

* Represents significant results. HMA—Hyomental angle, HMD—Hyomental distance, HT—height, WT—weight, BMI—Body Mass Index, rho—Pearsons correlation coefficient value.

4. Discussion

4.1. Difficult Airway

Airway complications are a common feature of MPS I, II, IV, and VI and considerably contribute to morbidity and premature mortality [11,12]. Airway assessment is ideally performed holistically, taking into account all the factors in the upper and lower airways with various methods, including medical history, clinical examination, radiological evaluation, and endoscopy [13]. A high and anterior larynx is one of the important aspects in the upper airway, which can lead to difficult intubation due to poor access, also called difficult laryngoscopy. Failure to recognize airway problems pre-operatively or during the planning of airway intervention can lead to unfavorable outcomes. MPS is a rare disease, and awareness amongst health professionals regarding adult MPS patients is poor. Once a patient is paralyzed and anaesthetized, the tongue falls backwards, and the oropharynx collapses inwards. In this situation, a high or an anterior larynx makes access to the larynx difficult if not impossible. In a patient who is paralyzed and anaesthetized, this can lead to situation of "cannot intubate- cannot ventilate". The Difficult Airway Society (DAS; UK) has produced guidelines on this difficult situation [14]. This difficult situation can be prevented by recognition of the problem of difficult access by existing cross-section images. Metanalysis of 35 studies representing 50,760 patients revealed the incidence of difficult intubation is about 5.8 % in normal patients, 3.1% in obstetric patients, and 14.8 in obese patients [15]. This may be higher in MPS due to deposition of GAGs in the soft tissues and musculoskeletal system, leading to bulky upper airways and bony abnormalities. A combination of abnormalities in the soft tissue, cervical spine, and skull leads to a high larynx and anterior larynx, resulting in difficulty accessing the airway. In our study, an attempt was made to match the MPS and non-MPS groups. It is not possible to obtain an exact match as age-related changes are faster in the MPS group with a shortened life span. Most of the MPS patients have short stature; however, it can be noted that both MPS and non-MPS groups have nearly similar BMI. We must also understand that MPS patients have a short stature and have truncal obesity [16], and non-MPS patients in our group are taller. Hence, BMI may be a misleading airway health measure in MPS patients. The PACS has in-built tools to measure the distances and angles in the cross-sectional images. As this measurement tool is computerized, we can assume that inter or intra-rater variability is reduced. Bias may be observed if the landmarks are not correctly identified by the clinician. In situations where the clinician does not have access to PACS, an angle measure and a ruler can be used to obtain HMD or HMA on existing cross-sectional imaging. In our study, we note that HMD was slightly less in the MPS group, indicating that the larynx is mildly anterior. The overall difference, however, in HMD in the MPS and non-MPS groups is minimal. On the other hand, HMA was more acute in the MPS group, indicating that the larynx is higher in the MPS group. It is interesting to note that HMA can vary in the MPS group despite nearly the same HMD as non-MPS.

Moreover, it was observed that some MPS patients did not have acute HMA and nearly the same HMD as non-MPS. The reasons for this could be multifactorial. Firstly, 16 results from MPS type I had milder upper airway abnormalities; secondly, the severity of MPS is dependent on mutations, the length, or their therapies, such as enzyme replacement therapy (ERT) or hematopoietic stem cell transplantation (HSCT). ERT in MPS I Hurler–Scheie (HS) and Scheie, II, IVA, and VI and HSCT in MPS I Hurler (H) have demonstrated organ-specific and systemic metabolic correction [17–20]; hence, the severity of the disease is variable. Advances in treatment strategies have improved life expectancy, and the average age of our cohort was 31.7 years. So, our study may be representative of varied MPS phenotypes and younger adult MPS patients.

4.2. Clinical Measures of Difficult Airway

TMD is a commonly used tool in airway assessment. The sensitivity of TMD is about 25% (95% confidence interval: 23–28) and specificity is 90.2% (95% confidence interval: 90–91) [21]. In MPS patients, the lower jaw may be disproportionately large, resulting in a normal thyromental distance despite a high and anterior larynx. TMD may also be of limited use in patients with facial and skeletal dysmorphism, and bulky soft tissues of the neck and sub mental region as commonly noted in adult MPS. The sternomental distance (SMD) [22] is calculated by measuring the distance between the mentum and the manubrium sternum with the mouth closed. It may indicate the degree of neck extension, which is important in access to the airway. The authors [22] conclude that a sternomental distance of 13.5 cm or less was 66.7% sensitive and 71.1% specific, and the positive and negative predictive values were 7.6% and 98.4%, for difficult laryngoscopy [22]. In their study, there was no association between sternomental distance and age, weight, height, or BMI. Sternomental distance may indirectly reflect a high larynx, and further research can be done to invesitgate this association. The TMD and SMD may be normal in MPS patients due to a large lower jaw, giving a false sense of security of a normal airway. The distance between the hyoid and thyroid prominence may not be as variable, so HMD and TMD may represent the same measure. HMD may be more accurate as it does not take into account the sub cutaneous soft tissue of the neck. In our study, we observed that the HMD is nearly the same in the MPS and non-MPS groups but the HMA was more acute. This may indicate that HMA is a more accurate measure of a high or anterior larynx than HMD or TMD. The results of this study showed that there is no correlation between the HMA and HMD in both the MPS and non-MPS groups, suggesting that HMA may be a completely independent entity, not related to the distance between the mentum to the laryngeal framework. The HMA correlates negatively with height and weight but has no correlation with BMI. This is because correlation is a linear measure and BMI is weight divided by height squared. Hence, observing the weight and height independently may be more useful than BMI in airway assessments. This may be more relevant to the MPS population as they are known to have short stature and central obesity [23,24]. The other commonly used bedside airway assessments methods are neck movements, neck circumference, Wilson's score [25], mallampati [26], and modified mallampati grade [27]. Mallampati and modified mallampati grade assess the size of the tongue in relation to the opened oral cavity. Dalewski [28] et al., in a study of 129 adults, suggested the combination of Mallampati grade, CT scan upper airway volume, and Berlin score to calculate snoring and breathlessness. The authors noted a positive correlation between high modified mallampati grade, BMI, and reduced oxygen saturations and upper airway volume. The pre-operative assessment aims to assess the difficult airway and plan a difficult situation. Based on laryngoscopy views, Cormack [29] graded the airway into three grades: grade 1 being full view of the glottis, grade 2—partial view of the glottis, grade 3—only epiglottis is visible, and grade 4—neither epiglottis nor glottis are visible. Modifications [25,30] of grade 2 resulted in 2a being part of the glottis visible and 2b being arytenoids or posterior cords only just visible. Cook [31] suggested the grading system as "E" as easy view—grade 1 and 2a "R" restricted view—grade 2b and 3a and "D" difficult view—grade 3b and 4, where the grade being epiglottis can be elevated with a gum elastic bougie and 3b being epiglottis cannot be elevated by a gum elastic bougie. Knowledge of a grade R or D prior to intubation in the pre-assessment clinics is very useful; HMD and HMA will provide this information. Radiology plays an important role in airway assessment for an anesthetist [32]. Although lateral radiographs, chest X-rays, and ultrasonography [33,34] are useful, in our experience, we found that the use of MRI scans is helpful in upper airways and CT scans in lower airways. The images from CT and MRI scans can be used to perform three-dimensional reconstruction of the airways in MPS [35] and perform virtual endoscopy. We also found nasendoscopy to be very useful in adult MPS [36]. Imaging of the airway is not routinely performed for unsuspected airway problems. Any additional investigations should be carefully considered, keeping patient comfort in mind. Although HMD has been reported [37] as a predictor of difficult airway in patients with cervical spondylosis, HMA, to the best of our knowledge, has not been reported so far. We feel that this easily available tool is an adjunct to airway assessment and can be adopted in adult MPS and any other difficult airway situation. In our personal experience of adult airway assessment, we feel HMA close to zero or less than zero indicates a larynx that is not high. HMA could be considered as another important adjunct in upper airway assessment; however, holistic airway assessment should include both upper and lower airways.

4.3. Limitations of the Study

4.3.1. Head and Neck Position

Most of our MPS patients had cervical spine issues so we chose to take radiological images at the neutral position of the head, keeping patient comfort as the priority. To keep the upper airway open, the natural instinct of any patient is to adopt a sniffing posture. In all our MPS patients, some form of airway and cervical spine abnormality was noted, which may have prompted patients to adopt a comfortable posture. These factors could have skewed some of our measurements. It may be argued that HMA, which is acute in the neutral comfortable position in MPS compared to non-MPS, may be more acute in a standard position of the head and neck. Future studies could include standardization of head positions to obtain radiological images to obtain accurate measures of the HMA and HMD to test this hypothesis. Extension of the neck will improve laryngoscopic views. Future studies could also incorporate measurement of HMA and HMD in maximum extension and comparison with HMA and HMD in the neutral position to assess the degree of improvement of laryngoscopy views by neck extension.

4.3.2. Thyro-Hyoid Distance

We made the assumption that the distance between the hyoid and thyroid is small enough to assume that HMD and TMD reflect the same measure of a high or anterior larynx. Future studies could also assess the thyrohyoid distance in flexion and extension of the neck to test this hypothesis.

4.3.3. Numbers

Our cohort examined only 50 adult MPS patients of various types and varying severity, which was compared with 50 adults with no upper airway issues. Considering the rarity of the disease, this may appear a significant number; however, a larger study group could have produced more significant results. Future studies may incorporate larger number of patients in both pediatric and adult MPS by a multi-center collaboration.

4.4. Wider Implications

HMD and HMA application can be extended to wider use of difficult airway assessment in any patient due to its simplicity in use. This may play a special role in those with cervical spine or any craniofacial anomalies.

5. Conclusions

HMA and HMD are useful measurements that can be obtained from existing cross-section imaging, providing important information about an anterior or high larynx. This is very helpful in pre-planning during airway assessment as part of the pre-operative work-up. HMA may be a better indicator than HMD in MPS patients. The use of HMA and HMD can be extrapolated to airway assessments in other patients with or without head and neck dysmorphism. This simple airway assessment tool is a useful adjunct in the management of complex airways, such as adult MPS. Further investigation into the sensitivity and specificity of HMA and HMA with a standardized head position and its correlation with difficult intubation will be useful.

Author Contributions: Authors C.G. (Otolaryngologist), K.M.S. (Adult inherited Metabolic Medicine), G.T. (Anesthetist) come from different specialties with common interest in adult Mucopolysaccharidosis (MPS). C.G., G.T. have special interest with airway diseases came up with the conceptualization of this unique idea airway assessment in MPS. The methodology of the study was devised by C.G. and K.M.S. Formal analysis of the data was performed by C.G., K.M.S. The resources, data curation was performed by C.G., K.M.S., G.T.; writing original draft preparation by C.G.; writing—review and editing was performed by C.G., K.M.S., G.T. Visualization of the project was planned by C.G., K.M.S. The project was supervised by C.G. All authors contributed towards project administration. All authors have read and agreed to the published version of the manuscript.

Funding: This research received no external funding, the article processing fee was supported by BioMarin Pharmaceutical Inc.

Institutional Review Board Statement: The study was conducted according to the guidelines of the Declaration of Helsinki, and Ethical approval from the local research and development department form Salford Royal NHS Foundation trust, Manchester, UK was obtained, reference: S20HIP40. The study did not involve any animals. This study was retrospective case notes review of adult patients.

Informed Consent Statement: Informed consent was obtained from all subjects involved in the study. However, no personal identifiable information has been used in this study.

Data Availability Statement: All the data required to understand and the data supporting reported results this project has been provided in the paper.

Acknowledgments: We would like to thank Amit Herwadkar, Consultant Radiologist, Salford Royal NHS foundation Trust, Manchester, UK, for his expertise in this project.

Conflicts of Interest: The authors declare no conflict of interest.

References

1. Mehta, A.B.; Winchester, B. *Lysosomal Storage Disorders: A Practical Guide*; Wiley-Blackwell Chichester: Hoboken, NJ, USA, 2012.
2. Mucopolysaccharidoses Fact Sheet. Available online: https://www.ninds.nih.gov/Disorders/Patient-Caregiver-Education/Fact-Sheets/Mucopolysaccharidoses-Fact-Sheet (accessed on 31 July 2020).
3. Taylor, M.; Khan, S.; Stapleton, M.; Wang, J.; Chen, J.; Wynn, R.; Yabe, H.; Chinen, Y.; Boelens, J.J.; Mason, R.W. Hematopoietic stem cell transplantation for mucopolysaccharidoses: Past, present, and future. *Biol. Blood Marrow Transplant.* **2019**, *25*, e226–e246. [CrossRef] [PubMed]
4. Concolino, D.; Deodato, F.; Parini, R. Enzyme replacement therapy: Efficacy and limitations. *Ital. J. Pediatrics* **2018**, *44*, 117–126. [CrossRef] [PubMed]
5. Gadepalli, C.; Stepien, K.M.; Sharma, R.; Jovanovic, A.; Tol, G.; Bentley, A. Airway Abnormalities in Adult Mucopolysaccharidosis and Development of Salford Mucopolysaccharidosis Airway Score. *J. Clin. Med.* **2021**, *10*, 3275. [CrossRef]
6. Apfelbaum, J.; Hagberg, C.; Caplan, R.; Blitt, C.; Connis, R.; Nickinovich, D.; Benumof, J.; Berry, F. American Society of Anesthesiologists Task Force on Management of the Difficult Airway Practice guidelines for management of the difficult airway: An updated report by the American Society of Anesthesiologists Task Force on Management of the Difficult Airway. *Anesthesiology* **2013**, *118*, 251–270.
7. Patil, V. Predicting the difficulty of intubation utilizing an intubation gauge. *Anesth. Rev.* **1983**, *10*, 32–33.
8. Braunlin, E.A.; Harmatz, P.R.; Scarpa, M.; Furlanetto, B.; Kampmann, C.; Loehr, J.P.; Ponder, K.P.; Roberts, W.C.; Rosenfeld, H.M.; Giugliani, R. Cardiac disease in patients with mucopolysaccharidosis: Presentation, diagnosis and management. *J. Inherit. Metab. Dis.* **2011**, *34*, 1183–1197. [CrossRef]
9. Neufeld, E.; Muenzer, J. The mucopolysaccharidoses. In *The Metabolic and Molecular Bases of Inherited Diseases*, 8th ed.; Scriver, C.R., Beaudet, A.L., Sly, W.S., Valle, D., Childs, R., Kinzler, K.W., Eds.; McGraw-Hill: New York, NY, USA, 2001; pp. 3421–3452.
10. Valayannopoulos, V.; Nicely, H.; Harmatz, P.; Turbeville, S. Mucopolysaccharidosis vi. *Orphanet J. Rare Dis.* **2010**, *5*, 5. [CrossRef]
11. Berger, K.I.; Fagondes, S.C.; Giugliani, R.; Hardy, K.A.; Lee, K.S.; McArdle, C.; Scarpa, M.; Tobin, M.J.; Ward, S.A.; Rapoport, D.M. Respiratory and sleep disorders in mucopolysaccharidosis. *J. Inherit. Metab. Dis.* **2013**, *36*, 201–210. [CrossRef] [PubMed]
12. Muhlebach, M.S.; Wooten, W.; Muenzer, J. Respiratory manifestations in mucopolysaccharidoses. *Paediatr. Respir. Rev.* **2011**, *12*, 133–138. [CrossRef]
13. Crawley, S.; Dalton, A. Predicting the difficult airway. *BJA Educ.* **2015**, *15*, 253–257. [CrossRef]
14. Frerk, C.; Mitchell, V.S.; McNarry, A.F.; Mendonca, C.; Bhagrath, R.; Patel, A.; O'Sullivan, E.P.; Woodall, N.M.; Ahmad, I. Difficult Airway Society 2015 guidelines for management of unanticipated difficult intubation in adults. *Br. J. Anaesth.* **2015**, *115*, 827–848. [CrossRef]
15. Shiga, T.; Wajima, Z.i.; Inoue, T.; Sakamoto, A. Predicting difficult intubation in apparently normal patients: A meta-analysis of bedside screening test performance. *J. Am. Soc. Anesthesiol.* **2005**, *103*, 429–437. [CrossRef] [PubMed]
16. Mitchell, J.; Berger, K.I.; Borgo, A.; Braunlin, E.A.; Burton, B.K.; Ghotme, K.A.; Kircher, S.G.; Molter, D.; Orchard, P.J.; Palmer, J. Unique medical issues in adult patients with mucopolysaccharidoses. *Eur. J. Intern. Med.* **2016**, *34*, 2–10. [CrossRef]
17. Hendriksz, C.J.; Burton, B.; Fleming, T.R.; Harmatz, P.; Hughes, D.; Jones, S.A.; Lin, S.-P.; Mengel, E.; Scarpa, M.; Valayannopoulos, V. Efficacy and safety of enzyme replacement therapy with BMN 110 (elosulfase alfa) for Morquio A syndrome (mucopolysaccharidosis IVA): A phase 3 randomised placebo-controlled study. *J. Inherit. Metab. Dis.* **2014**, *37*, 979–990. [CrossRef] [PubMed]
18. Clarke, L.A.; Wraith, J.E.; Beck, M.; Kolodny, E.H.; Pastores, G.M.; Muenzer, J.; Rapoport, D.M.; Berger, K.I.; Sidman, M.; Kakkis, E.D. Long-term efficacy and safety of laronidase in the treatment of mucopolysaccharidosis I. *Pediatrics* **2009**, *123*, 229–240. [CrossRef] [PubMed]

19. Harmatz, P.; Giugliani, R.; Schwartz, I.V.D.; Guffon, N.; Teles, E.L.; Miranda, M.C.S.; Wraith, J.E.; Beck, M.; Arash, L.; Scarpa, M. Long-term follow-up of endurance and safety outcomes during enzyme replacement therapy for mucopolysaccharidosis VI: Final results of three clinical studies of recombinant human N-acetylgalactosamine 4-sulfatase. *Mol. Genet. Metab.* **2008**, *94*, 469–475. [CrossRef]
20. Aldenhoven, M.; Wynn, R.F.; Orchard, P.J.; O'Meara, A.; Veys, P.; Fischer, A.; Valayannopoulos, V.; Neven, B.; Rovelli, A.; Prasad, V.K. Long-term outcome of Hurler syndrome patients after hematopoietic cell transplantation: An international multicenter study. *Blood J. Am. Soc. Hematol.* **2015**, *125*, 2164–2172. [CrossRef] [PubMed]
21. Baker, P.; Depuydt, A.; Thompson, J. Thyromental distance measurement–fingers don't rule. *Anaesthesia* **2009**, *64*, 878–882. [CrossRef] [PubMed]
22. Al Ramadhani, S.; Mohamed, L.; Rocke, D.; Gouws, E.; Ramadhani, S. Sternomental distance as the sole predictor of difficult laryngoscopy in obstetric anaesthesia. *Br. J. Anaesth.* **1996**, *77*, 312–316. [CrossRef]
23. Braunlin, E.; Steinberger, J.; DeFor, T.; Orchard, P.; Kelly, A.S. Metabolic syndrome and cardiovascular risk factors after hematopoietic cell transplantation in severe mucopolysaccharidosis type I (Hurler syndrome). *Biol. Blood Marrow Transpl.* **2018**, *24*, 1289–1293. [CrossRef] [PubMed]
24. Lin, H.-Y.; Lee, C.-L.; Chiu, P.C.; Niu, D.-M.; Tsai, F.-J.; Hwu, W.-L.; Lin, S.J.; Lin, J.-L.; Chang, T.-M.; Chuang, C.-K. Relationships among Height, Weight, Body Mass Index, and Age in Taiwanese children with different types of mucopolysaccharidoses. *Diagnostics* **2019**, *9*, 148. [CrossRef]
25. Wilson, M.; Spiegelhalter, D.; Robertson, J.; Lesser, P. Predicting difficult intubation. *Br. J. Anaesth.* **1988**, *61*, 211–216. [CrossRef]
26. Mallampati, S.R.; Gatt, S.P.; Gugino, L.D.; Desai, S.P.; Waraksa, B.; Freiberger, D.; Liu, P.L. A clinical sign to predict difficult tracheal intubation; a prospective study. *Can. Anaesth. Soc. J.* **1985**, *32*, 429–434. [CrossRef]
27. Huang, H.-H.; Lee, M.-S.; Shih, Y.-L.; Chu, H.-C.; Huang, T.-Y.; Hsieh, T.-Y. Modified Mallampati classification as a clinical predictor of peroral esophagogastroduodenoscopy tolerance. *BMC Gastroenterol.* **2011**, *11*, 12. [CrossRef]
28. Dalewski, B.; Kamińska, A.; Syrico, A.; Kałdunska, A.; Pałka, Ł.; Sobolewska, E. The Usefulness of Modified Mallampati Score and CT Upper Airway Volume Measurements in Diagnosing OSA among Patients with Breathing-Related Sleep Disorders. *Appl. Sci.* **2021**, *11*, 3764. [CrossRef]
29. Cormack, R.; Lehane, J. Difficult tracheal intubation in obstetrics. *Anaesthesia* **1984**, *39*, 1105–1111. [CrossRef] [PubMed]
30. Yentis, S. The effects of single-handed and bimanual cricoid pressure on the view at laryngoscopy. *Anaesthesia* **1997**, *52*, 332–335. [CrossRef] [PubMed]
31. Cook, T. A new practical classification of laryngeal view. *Anaesthesia* **2000**, *55*, 274–279. [CrossRef]
32. Jain, K.; Gupta, N.; Yadav, M.; Thulkar, S.; Bhatnagar, S. Radiological evaluation of airway—What an anaesthesiologist needs to know! *Indian J. Anaesth.* **2019**, *63*, 257–264. [PubMed]
33. Hui, C.; Tsui, B. Sublingual ultrasound as an assessment method for predicting difficult intubation: A pilot study. *Anaesthesia* **2014**, *69*, 314–319. [CrossRef]
34. Ezri, T.; Gewürtz, G.; Sessler, D.; Medalion, B.; Szmuk, P.; Hagberg, C.; Susmallian, S. Prediction of difficult laryngoscopy in obese patients by ultrasound quantification of anterior neck soft tissue. *Anaesthesia* **2003**, *58*, 1111–1114. [CrossRef] [PubMed]
35. Sharma, R.; Tol, G.; Stepien, K.; Yadthore, S.; Watson, S.; Samraj, P.; Gadepalli, C. Role of 3-dimensional (3D) reconstruction of radiology images and virtual endoscopy in the assessment of airways in adult mucopolysaccharidosis patients. *Mol. Genet. Metab.* **2020**, *129*, S147–S148. [CrossRef]
36. Gadepalli, C.; Tol, G.; Yadthore, S.; Sharma, R.; Jovanovic, A.; Palmer, J.; Stepien, K.M. Nasendoscopy findings in adult patients with mucopolysaccharidosis: A tertiary UK centre experience. *Mol. Genet. Metab.* **2020**, *129*, S59–S60. [CrossRef]
37. Han, Y.; Tian, Y.; Zhang, H.; Zhao, Y.; Xu, M.; Guo, X. Radiologic indicators for prediction of difficult laryngoscopy in patients with cervical spondylosis. *Acta Anaesthesiol. Scand.* **2018**, *62*, 474–482. [CrossRef] [PubMed]

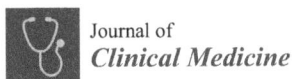

Review

Do Not Miss the (Genetic) Diagnosis of Gaucher Syndrome: A Narrative Review on Diagnostic Clues and Management in Severe Prenatal and Perinatal-Lethal Sporadic Cases

Aleksandra Jezela-Stanek [1,*], Grazina Kleinotiene [2], Karolina Chwialkowska [3] and Anna Tylki-Szymańska [4]

1. Department of Genetics and Clinical Immunology, National Institute of Tuberculosis and Lung Disease, 01-138 Warsaw, Poland
2. Faculty of Medicine, Vilnius University, 01513 Vilnius, Lithuania; grazina.kleinotiene@santa.lt
3. Centre for Bioinformatics and Data Analysis, Medical University of Bialystok, 15-089 Bialystok, Poland; karolina.chwialkowska@umb.edu.pl
4. Department of Pediatrics, Nutrition and Metabolic Diseases, Children's Memorial Health Institute, 04-730 Warsaw, Poland; A.Tylki@ipczd.pl
* Correspondence: jezela@gmail.com

Abstract: With a growing number of proved therapies and clinical trials for many lysosomal storage disorders (LSDs), a lot of hope for many patients and families exists. However, there are sometimes cases with poor prognosis, fatal outcomes when our efforts must be directed towards a prompt and correct genetic diagnosis, which offers the only possibility of providing the family with appropriate prevention and treatment. To address this issue, in this article, we present the clinical and genetic hallmarks of the lethal form of Gaucher disease (PLGD) and discuss the potential management. We hope that this will draw attention to its specific manifestations (such as collodion-baby phenotype, ichthyosis, arthrogryposis), which differ from best-known GD complications and ensure appropriate diagnostic assessment to provide families at risk with reliable counselling and treatment to avoid the medical complication of GD.

Keywords: Gaucher disease; NIHF; perinatal-lethal Gaucher disease; PLGD; ichthyosis; GBA gene

1. Introduction

Gaucher disease (MIM # 230800) is one of the most common lysosomal storage disorders, characterized by an accumulation of glucocerebrosides resulting from mutations in the *GBA* gene (MIM *606463). The gene encodes a lysosomal membrane protein (glucocerebrosidase, GCase) that cleaves the beta-glucosidic linkage of glycosylceramide, an intermediate in glycolipid metabolism [1]. In the GD molecular etiology, a related pseudogene, located approximately 12 kb downstream of *GBA* on chromosome 1, also plays a role [2].

The disease is classically categorized phenotypically into three main types: non-neuronopathic type I, acute neuronopathic type II (GD2; # 230900), and subacute neuronopathic type III (GD3; # 231000). Among the clinical continuum of neuronopathic phenotypes, GD lethal form is also observed, which has a separate phenotype MIM number (# 608013) [2]. It is considered to be a distinct form of type II Gaucher disease. The prognosis for survival is decidedly poor in this GD form. Non-immune hydrops fetalis (NIHF), which is its key characteristic, is associated with death in utero with 90% risk or within two days of birth; in the absence of hydrops, death usually occurs within three months of life [3].

For the sporadic cases (in families with non-remarkable history), the earliest possible recognition of this disease is thus crucial as it allows for carrier screening, reliable genetic counselling and family planning. To facilitate the identification of the most severe types of GD, its perinatal lethal type (PLGD), particularly in the context of genetic testing, we

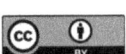

aimed to present its molecular and clinical characteristics based on literature review and our own experience.

2. Materials and Methods

The cases included in our literature review have been identified through a literature (PubMed) search (by phrases: perinatal-lethal Gaucher disease; Gaucher disease AND prenatal) and encompass severe prenatal and perinatal-lethal genetically confirmed diagnoses of Gaucher disease. In the Discussion, we also referred to our cases.

The most recent review on the genetic etiology of non-immune hydrops fetalis (NIFH) has been published this year and included 23 cases of Gaucher disease [4]. Moreover, 10 other papers on the perinatal-lethal form of GD (not mentioned in the latest reviews: from 2008 [5] and from 2003 [6] have been identified.

In all these articles, molecular data have been reported in 2 and 10 papers, respectively, including 12 GBA variants, which were further analyzed for the purpose of our article.

GBA variants

GBA variants provided were classified according to ACMG/AMP guidelines (American College of Medical Genetics and Genomics and the Association for Molecular Pathology, Bethesda, Maryland, USA; Richards et al., 2015) with respect to current ACGS (The Association for Clinical Genomic Science, London, UK) and ClinGen (The Clinical Genome, National Institutes of Health—NIH, Bethesda, Maryland, USA) recommendations.

Variants were analyzed using hg38 human reference genome and MANE Selected transcript (NM_000157.4).

3. Results

Available clinical and molecular data on GD diagnoses performed in pregnancies complicated with non-immune hydrops fetalis (NIHF) and stillbirths and neonates presenting a potentially lethal form of GD are listed in Table 1.

Table 1. *GBA* variants identified in Gaucher disease based on prenatal or perinatal-lethal complication.

Pathogenic Variant (as Presented in the Article)	HGVS cDNA—NM_000157.4 Protein—NP_000148.2	Prenatal/Perinatal Features and Weeks' Gestation (WG)	Outcome	Family History, Ethnicity	Reference
[p.P391L] + [p.L444P]	c.[1319C > T];[1448T > C] p.[(Pro440Leu)]; [(Leu483Pro)]	at 26 WG: hydrops fetalis, no fetal motility, moderate cardiac dysfunction and reduced size of thorax	prenatal NIHF as the main feature hydropic fetus, splenomegaly, pulmonary hypoplasia, micropenis with no malformations	nd	[7]
homozygous deletion: NM_001005741.2: c.(115+1_116−1) _(1616+1_?)del	c.[(115+1_116−1) _(1611+1_?)del];[c.(115+1_116−1) _(1611+1_?)del] p.[(Gly39_Gln536del)]; [(Gly39_Gln536del)]	at 23 WG: microcephaly, ascites, and fetal akinesia; at 24 WG: hydrops fetalis and pontocerebellar hypoplasia in addition to microcephaly	symmetric growth restriction with all biometric parameters < 5th percentile; diffuse cutaneous "collodion-like" edema, nonspecific craniofacialdysmorphism related to microcephaly, macroglossia, arthrogryposis, as well as major hepatosplenomegaly and ascites the brain shows no primary fissures associated with the brainstem and vermis hypoplasia.	the previous child in the family was born to the first-degree consanguineous parents	[8]

Table 1. Cont.

Pathogenic Variant (as Presented in the Article)	HGVS cDNA—NM_000157.4 Protein—NP_000148.2	Prenatal/Perinatal Features and Weeks' Gestation (WG)	Outcome	Family History, Ethnicity	Reference
c.[1505+1_1505+12ins; 1505 A > G]/RecNciI	c.[1505G > A](predicted to disrupt splicing and resulting in: c.1505+1_1505+12ins;1505G > A);[1448T > C;1483G > C;1497G > C] p.[(Arg502His)](predicted to disrupt splicing and resulting in p.Arg502Gln;Gln502ins4); [(Leu483Pro);(Ala495Pro);(Val499=)]	polyhydramnios	perinatal lethal manifestation from birth: non-immune hydrops fetalis and hepatosplenomegaly, collodion skin, dysmorphic features (low-set malformed ears, hypertelorism, narrow palpebral fissures, a flat occipital bone, bell-shaped thorax with extremely thin ribs, short neck, and small scrotum); died at 14 days of life	Greek case	[9]
RecNciI allele (L444P, A456P and V460V); p. R131C (c.508 C > T)	c.[1448T > C;1483G > C;1497G > C];[508C > T] p.[(Leu483Pro);(Ala495Pro); (Val499=)];[(Arg170Cys)]	30 WG: hepatosplenomegaly	at birth: generalized skin edema and extensive peeling of skin cardiomegaly tonic seizures profound and persistent metabolic acidosis; died at 6 h of life	nonconsanguinous Asian mother	[10]
compound heterozygosity for R131C and RecNciI (A456P (cDNA 1483G.C, genomic DNA 7354), and V460V (cDNA 1497G.C, genomic DNA 7368)	c.[508C > T];[1448T > C;1483G > C;1497G > C] p.[Arg170Cys)];[(Leu483Pro); (Ala495Pro);(Val499=)]	18 WG: isolated choroid plexus cysts 30 WG: unremarkable 35 WG: hepatosplenomegaly, with both organs measuring above the 95th percentile 37 WG: also decreased fetal movements	at birth: bradycardia, apnea, and hypertonia generalized edema, ichthyotic and collodion skin, palpable hepatosplenomegaly poor biventricular function with pulmonary hypertension, transverse arch flow reversal, and a large patent ductus arteriosus with a right-to-left shunt; died 6 h after birth	nonconsanguineous couple of Chinese ancestry	[11]
homozygous R463H	c.[1505G > A];[1505G > A](predicted to disrupt splicing and resulting in: c.[1505+1_1505+12ins;1505G > A];[1505+1_1505+12ins;1505G > A]) p.[(Arg502His)];[(Arg502His)] (predicted to disrupt splicing and resulting in p.[Arg502Gln;Gln502ins4)]; [(Arg502Gln_Gln502ins4]		34 WG: cesarian sections, severe neurologic signs with refractory thrombocytopenia, hepatosplenomegaly; tight and shiny skin; desquamating on the wrist and ankle, multiple dysmorphic features, including microphthalmia, a flattened nasal bridge, anteverted nares, a short throat, and a partial Simian crease; seizures did not respond to multiple anticonvulsants therapy; died at 46 days of age from respiratory failure	consanguinity was reported among the parents but there was no pertinent family history related to childhood disease or death	[12]
homozygosity for the RecNciI allele (c.1448T > C, c.1483G > C and c.1497G > C)	c.[1448T > C;1483G > C;1497G > C];c.[1448T > C;1483G > C;1497G > C] p.[(Leu483Pro);(Ala495Pro);(Val499=)]; p.[(Leu483Pro);(Ala495Pro);(Val499=)]	30 WG: foetal akinesias subsequently: progressive hepatosplenomegaly, cerebellar hypoplasia, pulmonary hypoplasia and unusual facial features	at birth: ichthyosis and diffuse purpural rash over most of the body facial dysmorphism (flattened-face, hypertelorism, retrognathia, anteverted nares, everted lips and ankyloblepharon) flexion contractures, thin gracile ribs with occasional gaps and abnormal phalanges in the hands; lungs hypoplasia with features of hepatosplenomegaly hypoplastic cerebellum with atrophic pons atypical macrophages within the brain; died 2 h after birth	parents are second cousins	[13]

Table 1. Cont.

Pathogenic Variant (as Presented in the Article)	HGVS cDNA—NM_000157.4 Protein—NP_000148.2	Prenatal/Perinatal Features and Weeks' Gestation (WG)	Outcome	Family History, Ethnicity	Reference
c.1255G > A leading to the substitution of Aspartic Acid by Asparagine (p.Asp419Asn) [no data on homozygosity]	c.1255G > A p.(Asp419Asn) zygosity unknown	third trimester: severe hydrops fetalis with skin edema, polyhydramnios, hepatomegaly, clustered bowel loops, and fetal hypokinesia.	at birth: apnea shiny and thickened skin, reminiscent of a collodion-baby phenotype died in the first day of life	previous preterm male stillborn and undiagnosed; non-immune hydrops fetalis cases of non-immune hydrops fetalis	[14]
homozygosity for the RecNcil mutation	c.[1448T > C;1483G > C;1497G > C];c.[1448T > C;1483G > C;1497G > C] p.[(Leu483Pro);(Ala495Pro);(Val499=)]; p.[(Leu483Pro);(Ala495Pro);(Val499=)]	27 WG: severe fetal hydrops with increased abdominal circumference due to ascites and elevated Middle Cerebral Artery Peak Systolic Velocity fetal anemia (treated with transfusions) 28 WG: intrauterine death	subtle facial anomalies including a high arched palate with no clefting, flat, broad nose with hypertelorism, and rounded face stiff elbow and knee joints with fixed flexion deformities and pterygia on the flexor surfaces	east Indian ethnic background;previous uninvestigated male stillbirth followed by an uncomplicated pregnancy	[15]
missense G234E and H413P heterozygous mutations	c.[701G > A];[1238A > C] p.[(Gly234Glu)];[(.His413Pro)]	36 WG: oligohydramnios increased cardiothoracic ratio, and a small lung volume, indicating pulmonary hypoplasia	at birth: severe respiratory distress flexion contractures at the elbow and knee joint, hypertonia, akinesiahepatosplenomegalyfacial dysmorphism (hypertelorism, downslanting eyes, an eye movement disorder, ectropion, hypophysis, thickening of the helix, constriction of the auricular rim, curl of the auricle and auricle cartilage, a flat nasal bridge, small nostrils, and everted lips) ichthyotic and collodion skin covered the entire body hypoplastic external genitals myoclonic seizure	Chinese mother (gravida 2, para 2); non-consanguineous parents	[16]
c.667T > C p.W223R; c. 1448C > T p. L483P (RecNcI)	c.[667T > C];[1488C > T] p.[(Trp223Arg)];[(Leu483Arg)]	28 WG: NIHF, hepatosplenomegaly	29–30 WG: intrauterine fetal demise—NIHF, facial dysmorphism, hepatosplenomegaly, cerebellum and pons hypoplasia	GI—miscarriage GII—fetal edema (NIHF), splenomegaly at 29 WG; boy died 15 min after birth	[17]
p. Asp448His (NM_000157.3:c.1342G > C) and p.Tyr531Ter (NM_000157.3:c.1593C > A).	c.[1342G > C];[1593C > A] p.[(Asp448His)];[(Tyr531Ter)]	polyhydramnios	at birth: widespread blueberry muffin skin lesion s and respiratory distress hepatosplenomegaly and cardiomegalyanemia and thrombocytopenia prompt initiation of enzyme replacement therapy clinical condition progressively worsened, leading to death at 3 months of age due to hepato-renal insufficiency	nd	[18]

4. Discussion

4.1. Genetic of Gaucher Disease

Up to date, more than 400 genetic mutations have been found to be associated with Gaucher disease (Gaucher Registry—International Collaborative Gaucher Group, Naarden, The Netherlands, 2021, accessed on 5 August 2021). Some of the variants are causing mild disease symptoms, while others are connected to very severe clinical phenotypes, characterized by the presence of primary neurologic disease.

The most common pathogenic genetic variant in *GBA* is NM_000157.4(NP_000148.2):p.(Asn409Ser), followed by c.84dupG, c.115+1G > A, and p.Leu483Pro. These four variants account for 50–60% of mutated alleles in non-Jewish individuals with type 1, non-neuronopathic GD. Homozygous individuals for p.Asn409Ser have a milder form of GD than people with just one copy plus another mutation or those having other pathogenic mutations. Individuals who are homozygous for the p.Leu483Pro variant tend to have disease connected to neurologic complications, which is a consequence of mutated protein dysfunctionality/residual glucocerebroside activity, and which may impact secondary protein structure as these residues differ in some properties. Functional studies of L483P indicate that it is poorly activated by phosphatidylserine, has a residual enzyme activity of 5–10% of wild type, and is unstable [19,20].

4.2. Genetic Characteristics of Provided Cases

Within the probands with prenatal or perinatal-lethal complications, presented in Table 1, none had any of the three most common mutations associated with GD: p.Asn409Ser, c.84dupG and c.115+1G > A. Variant p.Leu483Pro has been identified in one individual, however with compound heterozygosity with very rare pathogenic variant p.Pro440Leu (NC_000001.11:g.155235750G > A (dbSNP rsID: rs74598136) NM_000157.4:c.1319C > T NP_000148.2:p.(Pro440Leu)0. This variant can be found in the literature also as P440L, P391L, P353L and P401L.

Variant p.Pro440Leu was classified according to ACMG/AMP guidelines as pathogenic (criteria applied: PS4 + PM3 + PM1 + PM2_Supporting + PP3 + PP4). That is specifically based on the fact that it is:

- located in a mutational hot-spot in functional protein domain: Glycosyl hydrolase family 30 TIM-barrel domain (pfam; PM1),
- affected nucleotide position is conserved (GERP RS = 4.0399),
- predicted to affect protein function based on numerous in-silico predictors: metapredictor REVEL—Pathogenic (0.896); MutationTaster—Disease causing (1.0); SIFT—Damaging (0.001); PolyPhen-2 HumVar—Probably damaging (0.997); FATHMM-MKL—Damaging (0.9902); EIGEN—Pathogenic (0.7286) (PP3),
- absent from population controls (based on GnomAD v2.1.1 controls; PM2_Supporting)
- identified in multiple probands with GD clinical phenotype in trans with other pathogenic variant (PP4, PM3; PS4).

For comparison, the most frequent *GBA* pathogenic variant—p.(Leu483Pro (NC_000001.11:g.155235252A > G (dbSNP rsID: rs421016) NM_000157.4:c.1448T > C NP_000148.2:p.(Leu483Pro)) can be found in the literature as: L483P, L396P, L434P, L444P. It was classified according to ACMG/AMP guidelines as pathogenic, based on criteria applied: PS3 + PM1 + PM3 + PM5 + PP3 + PP4):

- change at amino acid residue where a different missense change (p.Leu483Arg) was determined to be pathogenic accordingly to ACMG guidelines (PM5),
- functional studies show a damaging effect on the protein function; PS3 [21,22]—has a residual enzyme activity of 13% of wild type, unstable, poorly activated by phosphatidylserine ([20]),
- located in a mutational hot-spot in functional protein domain: Glycosyl hydrolase family 30 beta-sandwich domain (pfam; PM1),
- affected nucleotide position is semi-conserved (GERP RS = 3.16),
- predicted to affect protein function based on numerous in-silico predictors: metapredictor REVEL—Pathogenic (0.8579); MutationTaster—Disease causing (1.0); SIFT—Damaging (0.002); PolyPhen-2 HumVar—Probably damaging (0.976); FATHMM-MKL—Damaging (0.9181) (PP3),
- present in reasonably low frequency in population controls (0.12% based on GnomAD v2.1.1 controls; PM2 not applicable),
- identified in multiple probands with GD clinical phenotype in the homozygous or compound heterozygous state with another pathogenic variant (PP4; PM3; PS4 not applicable due to frequency in the population).

Considering the severe, pre- and perinatal manifestation of Gaucher disease, the most interesting is another *GBA* variant—Rec*Nci*I allele, which is most frequently observed in the analyzed group. It is a name for a variant NC_000001.11:g.155235252A > G; 155235217C > G;155235203C > G (dbSNP rsIDs: rs421016, rs368060, rs1135675) NM_000157.4:c.1448T

> C;1483G > C;1497G > C NP_000148.2:p.(Leu483Pro);(Ala495Pro);(Val499=) that can be classified according to ACMG/AMP guidelines as pathogenic because being a haplotype contains NM_000157.4:c.1448T > C NP_000148.2:p.(Leu483Pro) already classified as pathogenic (described above). Rec*Nci*I allele is a recombinant allele covering a complex triply mutant haplotype. This variant results from a gene conversion event between the functional *GBA* gene and its pseudogene *GBAP* located downstream [23]. Recombination is possible because *GBA* and its pseudogene are highly homologous—*GBAP* has 96% exonic sequence homology to the *GBA* coding region [24,25]. Close localization of such similar homologous regions increases the risk for recombination events giving rise to complex alleles. The homology between the *GBA* gene and its pseudogene is highest between exons 8 and 11, and thus most of the pathogenic mutations have been accumulated in this location [25]. Díaz-Font et al. [23] have proved that Rec*Nci*I alleles are generated by gene conversion, and they mapped the precise crossover site on the rearranged alleles [23]. Rec*Nci*I haplotype has been identified in multiple individuals with GD clinical phenotype in the homozygous or compound heterozygous state with another pathogenic variant [25], Table 1.

The patient described by Sudrié-Arnaud et al. [8] had homozygous deletion p.[(Gly39_G ln536del)] resulting in the complete loss of the region encoding exons from 3 to the 11—up to the protein end. The remaining gene part encoded properly only the first 38 amino acids; however, due to the absence of the rest of the native transcript, it can be supposed that mRNA is subjected to nonsense-mediated decay (NMD). Nonetheless, as the precise breakpoints are not known, the effect cannot be precisely predicted. In this patient, glucosylceramidase activity should have been completely absent.

Patient characterized by Akdag et al. [12] had homozygous c.1505G > A variant potentially resulting in simple missense p.Arg502His change; however in silico analyses revealed that this G > A change causes 5′ splicing donor loss and creation of a cryptic site 12 nucleotides downstream (VarSEAK, SpliceAI, dbscSNV ADA and RF scores). This is predicted to result in Arg502Gln and insertion of codons for 4 amino acids, preserving the reading frame. The resultant protein is 4 amino acids longer and has an insertion in the glycosyl hydrolase family 30 beta-sandwich domain, affecting its functioning.

4.3. Perinatal Lethal GD Complications and Management Options

Unfortunately, there is no definitive treatment available now for perinatal lethal complications when fetal ascites, hydrops, and/or hepatomegaly are prenatally diagnosed. Only symptomatic management can be considered, i.e., in fetal anemia (suspected based on middle cerebral artery peak systolic velocity, MCA-PSV and placentomegaly), transfusions are an option [15]; occasionally, in case of poly- or oligohydramnios (mentioned in Table 1) only symptomatic treatment is available. Otherwise, the pregnancy needs to be monitored, and optimal delivery time has to be planed. Depending on the legal regulations in the given country concerned, parents must be presented with options on how to proceed with the pregnancy so that they can make individual decisions. However, regardless of their decisions, during an obstetric assessment, the crucial step is to isolate fetal DNA (during amniocentesis, cordocentesis or from formalin-fixed paraffin-embedded (FFPE) blocks) to enable a genetic diagnosis to be made. The recommendation refers to every unexplained potentially lethal situation, especially in families with positive history (previous stillbirths, fetal edema, parents' consanguinity). When, e.g., fetal hydrops is observed, we are unable to make any clinical diagnosis. Considering only inherited metabolic disease, it may be a feature of several, such as mucopolysaccharidosis (especially type VII, type IVA), galactosialidosis, infantile sialic acid storage disease, Gaucher disease 2 and 3, GM1 gangliosidosis, sialidosis or Niemann–Pick disease [4].

As presented in Table 1, the severe GD form usually manifests in the neonatal period with small birth weight, massive hepatosplenomegaly and ascites. In many cases, akinesia or joints contractures were described [8,13,15,16]. Decreased spontaneous movements at birth, followed by hypertonia and progressive neurologic deterioration, can be expected. The prognosis is now considered to be very poor, even in the attempt of early enzymatic therapy [18]. The neonates manifest significant respiratory distress, especially when lung hypoplasia and cardiomegaly are present, which altogether is unresponsive to any medical interventions. Maybe children with GD lethal form will benefit from chaperone therapy? To our knowledge, it has not yet been described. We can speculate that, as chaperones were proved to assist in the refolding of a mutated enzyme (i.e., GCase), significantly increased GCase activity in cultured macrophages derived from patient blood monocytic cell (PBMC) [26] and may pass through the blood-brain barrier thus restoring GCase activity in neurons [27].

Notably, the very characteristic and frequent feature is dermatological manifestations of PLGD, encompassing collodion-baby phenotype, sometimes accompanied by recognizable facial features (ectropion, everted lips), ichthyosis or ichthyosiform erythroderma (see Table 1). Its exact mechanism is still to be elucidated, but clinically these are unique and sporadic features that are certainly memorable. We can draw on our own experience here, when two cases were diagnosed with GD mainly because of severe skin manifestation (ichthyosis and subcutaneous hydrops). The presence of arthrogryposis and ichthyosis in newborns with hepatosplenomegaly should raise suspicion of GD. Therefore, we recommend that any biological material be stored to perform genetic tests or enzymes studies, necessary for genetic counselling regarding following pregnancies and family risk. Carriership of the disease in the parents can, in turn, only be confirmed by genetic testing; the results of enzyme analyses are not reliable.

4.4. Pre- and Perinatal Diagnostics of Lethal GD

Unfortunately, the available data concerning family histories, shown in Table 1, is limited, but we can note that even in consanguineous couples or history of pregnancy complications, the parents' carriership has not been mentioned, and was established following the diagnosis of GD in an affected child. Yet, the options of prenatal diagnostics depend on the family history and genetic status of the parents. In a pregnancy at increased risk, when both pathogenic variants in a family are known, prenatal diagnosis is possible using molecular genetic testing. Otherwise, if only one or neither pathogenic variant in the family at risk is known, an assay of glucocerebrosidase enzymatic activity in the amniotic fluid can be performed. The use of prenatal testing is a personal decision of the parent(s), and discussion of these issues should always be offered. When the family history of GD is negative, the disease can only be diagnosed based on clinical suspicion and necessitates glucocerebrosidase enzymatic measurement and/or molecular testing of the entire *GBA* gene. The biochemical analyses allow the establishment of the diagnosis of GD but are, however, of no value for the parents as far as carriership is concerned.

Unfortunately, there is no definitive treatment available now for perinatal lethal complications when fetal ascites, hydrops, and/or hepatomegaly are prenatally diagnosed. Only symptomatic management can be considered, i.e., in fetal anemia (suspected based on middle cerebral artery peak systolic velocity, MCA-PSV and placentomegaly), transfusions are an option [15]; occasionally, in case of poly- or oligohydramnios (mentioned in Table 1) only symptomatic treatment is available. Otherwise, the pregnancy needs to be monitored, and optimal delivery time has to be planed. Depending on the legal regulations in the given country concerned, parents must be presented with options on how to proceed with the pregnancy so that they can make individual decisions. However, regardless of their decisions, during an obstetric assessment, the crucial step is to isolate fetal DNA (during amniocentesis, cordocentesis or from formalin-fixed paraffin-embedded (FFPE) blocks) to enable a genetic diagnosis to be made. The recommendation refers to every unexplained potentially lethal situation, especially in families with positive history (previous stillbirths, fetal edema, parents' consanguinity). When, e.g., fetal hydrops is observed, we are unable to make any clinical diagnosis. Considering only inherited metabolic disease, it may be a feature of several, such as mucopolysaccharidosis (especially type VII, type IVA), galactosialidosis, infantile sialic acid storage disease, Gaucher disease 2 and 3, GM1 gangliosidosis, sialidosis or Niemann–Pick disease [4].

The genetic diagnosis of GD is complicated by the presence of a highly homologous pseudogene, *GBAP*; thus, the appropriate genetic test must be considered; PCR-based methods have to be designed to differentiate *GBA* from the pseudogene. Some diagnostic gene panels may possibly not include the *GBA* gene. Moreover, testing for the p.Leu483Pro variant alone will not distinguish its isolated presence from Rec alleles [28].

Another concern is the fact that the number of rare genetic variants known to date in the *GBA* gene is very high, and none of the most frequent variants has been identified in fetal cases presented in Table 1 fatal GD cases. Thus, because the probability that these variants are present in the proband with pre- and perinatal characteristics of Gaucher disease is extremely low, the laboratory analyses should not be limited only to the most popular mutations present in a given population. At that point, without doubt, the Rec*Nci*I recombinant allele should be taken into account, as noted in half of our reviewed cases (6/12).

Author Contributions: Conceptualization A.J.-S. and A.T.-S.; formal analysis A.J.-S. and K.C.; investigation G.K. and A.T.-S.; writing—original draft preparation A.J.-S. and K.C.; writing—review and editing A.J.-S. and A.T.-S.; supervision A.J.-S. All authors have read and agreed to the published version of the manuscript.

Funding: This research received no external funding.

Institutional Review Board Statement: Not applicable.

Informed Consent Statement: Not applicable.

Conflicts of Interest: The authors declare no conflict of interest.

References

1. Dandana, A.; Ben Khelifa, S.; Chahed, H.; Miled, A.; Ferchichi, S. Gaucher Disease: Clinical, Biological and Therapeutic Aspects. *Pathobiology* **2016**, *83*, 13–23. [CrossRef]
2. OMIM. GBA. Available online: https://omim.org/entry/606463 (accessed on 11 October 2021).
3. OMIM. GD Perinatal Lethal. Available online: https://omim.org/entry/608013 (accessed on 11 October 2021).
4. Iyer, N.S.; Gimovsky, A.C.; Ferreira, C.R.; Critchlow, E.; Al-Kouatly, H.B. Lysosomal storage disorders as an etiology of nonimmune hydrops fetalis: A systematic review. *Clin. Genet.* **2021**, *100*, 493–503. [CrossRef]
5. Zay, A.; Choy, F.Y.; Macleod, P.; Tan-Dy, C.R. Perinatal lethal Gaucher's disease without prenatal complications. *Clin. Genet.* **2008**, *73*, 191–195. [CrossRef]
6. Mignot, C.; Gelot, A.; Bessières, B.; Daffos, F.; Voyer, M.; Menez, F.; Fallet Bianco, C.; Odent, S.; Le Duff, D.; Loget, P.; et al. Perinatal-lethal Gaucher disease. *Am. J. Med. Genet. A* **2003**, *120a*, 338–344. [CrossRef] [PubMed]
7. Gort, L.; Quintana, E.; Moliner, S.; González-Quereda, L.; López-Hernández, T.; Briones, P. An update on the molecular analysis of classical galactosaemia patients diagnosed in Spain and Portugal: 7 new mutations in 17 new families. *Med. Clin.* **2009**, *132*, 709–711. [CrossRef]
8. Sudrié-Arnaud, B.; Marguet, F.; Patrier, S.; Martinovic, J.; Louillet, F.; Broux, F.; Charbonnier, F.; Dranguet, H.; Coutant, S.; Vezain, M.; et al. Metabolic causes of nonimmune hydrops fetalis: A next-generation sequencing panel as a first-line investigation. *Clin. Chim. Acta* **2018**, *481*, 1–8. [CrossRef] [PubMed]
9. Michelakakis, H.; Dimitriou, E.; Moraitou, M.; Valari, M.; Yatrakou, E.; Mitsiadi, V.; Cozar, M.; Vilageliu, L.; Grinberg, D.; Karachristou, K. Perinatal lethal form of Gaucher disease. Clinical and molecular characterization of a Greek case. *Blood Cells Mol. Dis.* **2010**, *44*, 82–83. [CrossRef] [PubMed]
10. Plakkal, N.; Soraisham, A.S.; Jirapradittha, J.; Pinto-Rojas, A. Perinatal lethal Gaucher disease. *Indian J. Pediatr.* **2011**, *78*, 106–108. [CrossRef] [PubMed]
11. Goebl, A.; Ferrier, R.A.; Ferreira, P.; Pinto-Rojas, A.; Matshes, E.; Choy, F.Y. Gaucher disease with prenatal onset and perinatal death due to compound heterozygosity for the missense R131C and null Rec Nci I GBA mutations. *Pediatr. Dev. Pathol.* **2011**, *14*, 240–243. [CrossRef]
12. Akdag, A.; Oğuz, S.S.; Ezgü, F.; Erdeve, O.; Uraş, N.; Dilmen, U. A newborn case with perinatal-lethal Gaucher disease due to R463H homozygosity complicated by C677T homozygosity in the MTHFR gene. *J. Pediatr. Endocrinol. Metab.* **2011**, *24*, 381–383. [CrossRef]
13. Frosk, P.; Phillips, S.M.; Del Bigio, M.R.; Chodirker, B.N. Atypical features in a case of lethal perinatal Gaucher disease. *Neuropathol. Appl. Neurobiol.* **2014**, *40*, 946–950. [CrossRef]
14. BenHamida, E.; Ayadi, I.; Ouertani, I.; Chammem, M.; Bezzine, A.; BenTmime, R.; Attia, L.; Mrad, R.; Marrakchi, Z. Perinatal-lethal Gaucher disease presenting as hydrops fetalis. *Pan Afr. Med. J.* **2015**, *21*, 110. [CrossRef]

15. Bhutada, E.; Pyragius, T.; Petersen, S.G.; Niemann, F.; Matsika, A. Perinatal Lethal Gaucher Disease due to RecNciI Recombinant Mutation in the GBA Gene Presenting with Hydrops Fetalis and Severe Congenital Anemia. *Case Rep. Pathol.* **2018**, *2018*, 2549451. [CrossRef] [PubMed]
16. Wei, M.; Han, A.; Wei, L.; Ma, L. A Neonatal Case With Perinatal Lethal Gaucher Disease Associated With Missense G234E and H413P Heterozygous Mutations. *Front. Pediatr.* **2019**, *7*, 201. [CrossRef]
17. Voloshchuk, I.N.; Barinova, I.V.; Andreeva, E.N.; Fattakhov, A.R.; Baydakova, G.V.; Zakharova, E.Y. [Perinatal lethal Gaucher disease. Case report]. *Arkh. Patol.* **2021**, *83*, 56–60. [CrossRef]
18. Rosanio, F.M.; D'Acunzo, I.; Mozzillo, F.; Di Pinto, R.; Tornincasa, C.; Amabile, S.; Piccirillo, A.; Roma, V.; Giordano, L. Perinatal-lethal Gaucher disease presenting with blueberry muffin lesions. *Pediatr. Dermatol.* **2021**. [CrossRef] [PubMed]
19. Grace, M.E.; Newman, K.M.; Scheinker, V.; Berg-Fussman, A.; Grabowski, G.A. Analysis of human acid beta-glucosidase by site-directed mutagenesis and heterologous expression. *J. Biol. Chem.* **1994**, *269*, 2283–2291. [CrossRef]
20. Malini, E.; Grossi, S.; Deganuto, M.; Rosano, C.; Parini, R.; Dominisini, S.; Cariati, R.; Zampieri, S.; Bembi, B.; Filocamo, M.; et al. Functional analysis of 11 novel GBA alleles. *Eur. J. Hum. Genet.* **2014**, *22*, 511–516. [CrossRef]
21. Migdalska-Richards, A.; Wegrzynowicz, M.; Rusconi, R.; Deangeli, G.; Di Monte, D.A.; Spillantini, M.G.; Schapira, A.H.V. The L444P Gba1 mutation enhances alpha-synuclein induced loss of nigral dopaminergic neurons in mice. *Brain* **2017**, *140*, 2706–2721. [CrossRef]
22. Sheth, J.; Pancholi, D.; Mistri, M.; Nath, P.; Ankleshwaria, C.; Bhavsar, R.; Puri, R.; Phadke, S.; Sheth, F. Biochemical and molecular characterization of adult patients with type I Gaucher disease and carrier frequency analysis of Leu444Pro—A common Gaucher disease mutation in India. *BMC Med. Genet.* **2018**, *19*, 178. [CrossRef]
23. Díaz-Font, A.; Cormand, B.; Blanco, M.; Chamoles, N.; Chabás, A.; Grinberg, D.; Vilageliu, L. Gene rearrangements in the glucocerebrosidase-metaxin region giving rise to disease-causing mutations and polymorphisms. Analysis of 25 Rec NciI alleles in Gaucher disease patients. *Hum. Genet.* **2003**, *112*, 426–429. [CrossRef] [PubMed]
24. Hruska, K.S.; LaMarca, M.E.; Scott, C.R.; Sidransky, E. Gaucher disease: Mutation and polymorphism spectrum in the glucocerebrosidase gene (GBA). *Hum. Mutat.* **2008**, *29*, 567–583. [CrossRef] [PubMed]
25. Leija-Salazar, M.; Sedlazeck, F.J.; Toffoli, M.; Mullin, S.; Mokretar, K.; Athanasopoulou, M.; Donald, A.; Sharma, R.; Hughes, D.; Schapira, A.H.V.; et al. Evaluation of the detection of GBA missense mutations and other variants using the Oxford Nanopore MinION. *Mol. Genet. Genom. Med.* **2019**, *7*, e564. [CrossRef] [PubMed]
26. Kopytova, A.E.; Rychkov, G.N.; Nikolaev, M.A.; Baydakova, G.V.; Cheblokov, A.A.; Senkevich, K.A.; Bogdanova, D.A.; Bolshakova, O.I.; Miliukhina, I.V.; Bezrukikh, V.A.; et al. Ambroxol increases glucocerebrosidase (GCase) activity and restores GCase translocation in primary patient-derived macrophages in Gaucher disease and Parkinsonism. *Parkinsonism Relat. Disord.* **2021**, *84*, 112–121. [CrossRef]
27. Aflaki, E.; Borger, D.K.; Moaven, N.; Stubblefield, B.K.; Rogers, S.A.; Patnaik, S.; Schoenen, F.J.; Westbroek, W.; Zheng, W.; Sullivan, P.; et al. A New Glucocerebrosidase Chaperone Reduces α-Synuclein and Glycolipid Levels in iPSC-Derived Dopaminergic Neurons from Patients with Gaucher Disease and Parkinsonism. *J. Neurosci.* **2016**, *36*, 7441–7452. [CrossRef]
28. Tayebi, N.; Stubblefield, B.K.; Park, J.K.; Orvisky, E.; Walker, J.M.; LaMarca, M.E.; Sidransky, E. Reciprocal and nonreciprocal recombination at the glucocerebrosidase gene region: Implications for complexity in Gaucher disease. *Am. J. Hum. Genet.* **2003**, *72*, 519–534. [CrossRef]

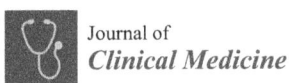

Article

Anaesthesia-Relevant Disease Manifestations and Perianaesthetic Complications in Patients with Mucolipidosis—A Retrospective Analysis of 44 Anaesthetic Cases in 12 Patients

Luise Sophie Ammer [1,*], Nicole Maria Muschol [1], René Santer [1], Annika Lang [1,2], Sandra Rafaela Breyer [1], Phillip Brenya Sasu [2], Martin Petzoldt [2] and Thorsten Dohrmann [2]

[1] International Center for Lysosomal Disorders (ICLD), Department of Paediatrics, University Medical Centre Hamburg-Eppendorf, 20246 Hamburg, Germany; muschol@uke.de (N.M.M.); r.santer.ext@uke.de (R.S.); annika.lang@stud.uke.uni-hamburg.de (A.L.); s.breyer@uke.de (S.R.B.)

[2] Department of Anaesthesiology, University Medical Centre Hamburg-Eppendorf, 20246 Hamburg, Germany; p.sasu@uke.de (P.B.S.); m.petzoldt@uke.de (M.P.); t.dohrmann@uke.de (T.D.)

* Correspondence: l.ammer.ext@uke.de; Tel.: +49-40-7410-53714

Citation: Ammer, L.S.; Muschol, N.M.; Santer, R.; Lang, A.; Breyer, S.R.; Sasu, P.B.; Petzoldt, M.; Dohrmann, T. Anaesthesia-Relevant Disease Manifestations and Perianaesthetic Complications in Patients with Mucolipidosis—A Retrospective Analysis of 44 Anaesthetic Cases in 12 Patients. *J. Clin. Med.* 2022, 11, 3650. https://doi.org/10.3390/jcm11133650

Academic Editors: Karolina M. Stepien, Christian J. Hendriksz and Gregory M Pastores

Received: 18 May 2022
Accepted: 17 June 2022
Published: 24 June 2022

Publisher's Note: MDPI stays neutral with regard to jurisdictional claims in published maps and institutional affiliations.

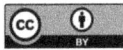

Copyright: © 2022 by the authors. Licensee MDPI, Basel, Switzerland. This article is an open access article distributed under the terms and conditions of the Creative Commons Attribution (CC BY) license (https://creativecommons.org/licenses/by/4.0/).

Abstract: Mucolipidosis (ML) type II, intermediate, and III are lysosomal storage disorders with progressive multiorgan manifestations predisposing patients to a high risk of perioperative morbidity. The aims of the study were to systematically assess disease manifestations relevant to anaesthesia as well as anaesthesia-related complications. This retrospective study includes ML patients who underwent anaesthesia in two centres between 2008 and 2022. We reviewed patients' demographics, medical history, disease manifestations, as well as procedure- and outcome-related data. A total of 12 patients (7 MLII, 2 ML intermediate, 3 MLIII) underwent 44 anaesthesia procedures (per patient: median 3, range 1–11). The median age was 3.3 years (range 0.1–19.1). At least one complication occurred in 27.3% of the anaesthesia procedures. The vast majority of complications (94%) occurred in children with MLII and ML intermediate. A predicted difficult airway was found in 100% and 80% of the MLII and ML intermediate patients, respectively. Accordingly, most complications (59%) occurred during the induction of anaesthesia. Altogether, respiratory complications were the most frequent (18%), followed by difficult airway management (14%). The risk for anaesthesia-related complications is alarmingly high in patients with ML, particularly in those with MLII and ML intermediate. Multidisciplinary risk–benefit analysis and thoughtful anaesthesia planning are crucial in these patients.

Keywords: mucolipidosis; ML; MLII; disease manifestations; symptoms; morbidity; anaesthesia; airway; perioperative complications; surgery

1. Introduction

Mucolipidosis type II (OMIM 252500; MLII), type III alpha/beta (OMIM 252600; MLIII alpha/beta), and type III gamma (OMIM 252605; MLIII gamma) are caused by pathogenic variants in the *GNPTAB*- and *GNPTG*-genes encoding for the N-acetylglucosamine (GlcNAc)-1-phosphotransferase [1]. This enzyme is involved in the intracellular trafficking of lysosomal enzymes by catalysing the first step of tagging a mannose-6-phosphate (M6P) recognition marker on newly synthesized lysosomal enzymes [2,3]. M6P-markers are required by most soluble lysosomal enzymes for their receptor-mediated transport over the Golgi network to the lysosomes. In MLII and III, an absent or reduced GlcNAc-1-phosphotransferase activity results in global mis-sorting of lysosomal enzymes and subsequent secretion into the extracellular compartment. Consecutively, partially degraded macromolecules (i.e., glycosaminoglycans, phospholipids, cholesterol) accumulate in the lysosomes impairing cellular function [4].

MLII is a rapidly progressing multi-systemic disease form with a fatal outcome, usually due to cardiorespiratory complications, within the first decade of life. Patients with MLIII commonly reach adulthood [5]. They present a later onset of symptoms, slower disease progression, and predominant skeletal symptoms [6,7]. ML patients who clinically cannot be attributed to either MLII or III are classified as ML intermediate. These patients are characterized by somatic findings similar to but slightly milder than MLII. The estimated incidence of MLII and III globally ranges from 0.22 to 2.70 per 100,000 live births [5]. No curative therapy is yet available [4].

Clinical features in ML overlap with those of patients with mucopolysaccharidosis (MPS), another more frequent lysosomal storage disorder. The overlapping progressive symptoms comprise craniofacial dysmorphism (i.e., flat face, shallow orbits, depressed nasal bridge, macroglossia), a short neck, respiratory insufficiency and upper airway obstruction, sleep apnoea, cardiac dysfunction, skeletal deformities (e.g., growth impairment, spine and chest deformity), and neurocognitive delay. Radiological features are subsumed as dysostosis multiplex [4–6,8,9]. For patients with MPS, these symptoms are known to be associated with a high risk of morbidity and mortality when undergoing general anaesthesia [10]. Direct laryngoscopy is especially challenging in these patient groups, causing high rates of failed airway management and cardiorespiratory events [11,12].

Thus far, anaesthesia-related complications have only been explored in single case reports [13,14] and small case series [12,15,16] of ML patients. Despite a suspected high incidence of complications in ML, a comprehensive analysis has not yet been performed. A clear understanding of the anaesthesia-relevant manifestations in different ML types and their effect on the anaesthetic risk is vital to improve clinical management and to avoid fatal outcomes related to difficult airway management. This study aims to ascertain the extent of anaesthesia-relevant disease manifestations as well as of perianaesthetic complications in patients with MLII, ML intermediate, and MLIII and to promote anaesthesia management recommendations.

2. Materials and Methods

2.1. Study Site and Patients

This cross-sectional study was conducted by retrospective chart review of patients of the International Centre for Lysosomal Disorders (ICLD) of the University Medical Center Hamburg-Eppendorf (UKE), Hamburg, Germany. Inclusion criteria were clinically and biochemically or molecular genetically confirmed diagnosis either of MLII, ML intermediate, or MLIII and at least one anaesthesia procedure (general anaesthesia; sedation; regional anaesthesia; monitored anaesthesia care) performed within the framework of the clinical routine between November 2008 and January 2022. The study cohort comprises cases from two centres, the UKE and the Children's Hospital Altona (AKK), Hamburg, Germany.

2.2. Data Acquisition

The following information was extracted by systematic review of anaesthesia charts and analogue and electronic health records (Soarian Health Archive, Release 3.04 SP12, Siemens Healthcare, Erlangen, Germany): baseline characteristics, anaesthesia-relevant symptoms, and procedure- and outcome-related data. Baseline characteristics comprise the patients' demographics and the medical history, including, amongst others, the underlying subtype (by clinical phenotype) and whether experimental hematopoietic stem cell transplantation (HSCT) or frequent respiratory infections was recorded.

As part of the standard of care, the patients underwent a multidisciplinary evaluation and diagnostic workup before elective anaesthesia. The following medical preconditions were considered anaesthesia-relevant and gathered by the time of anaesthesia (case): age, height, and weight; craniofacial dysmorphia; gingival hyperplasia; macroglossia; tonsil hyperplasia; short neck; cervical spinal stenosis; dens hypoplasia with atlantoaxial instability; spinal deformities; thorax deformities; sleep apnoea (as per polysomnography); obstructive lung disease; apparent dysphagia; cardiac pathologies; organomegaly (as per standard deviation of the index for body length); and growth retardation (as per body length and age- and gender-adapted Z-scores). Cardiac pathologies were described by the time of each anaesthesia procedure and categorized as recently published [10] as unremarkable, mild (plump valves; valvular defects Grades I/I–II, minor septum defects, atrioventricular block Grade I, left bundle branch block, arterial hypertension), moderate (valvular heart defects Grade II, discrete cardiac hypertrophy or dilative cardiomyopathy), or severe (valvular heart defects Grade III/IV, any manifestation requiring cardiac medication or intervention). In case of multiple anaesthesia procedures in one patient, the most pathologic finding determined the patient's characteristics. As patients with ML intermediate present with severe and multi-systemic disease manifestations, we grouped patients with MLII and ML intermediate for descriptive analysis.

The following procedure-related data were collected for each study case: indication for anaesthesia; number of procedures during anaesthesia; duration; type of anaesthesia; primary airway approach; whether postoperative intensive care unit (ICU) care had been provided.

The outcome parameters for perioperative complications were subdivided into four distinct entities: (1) difficult airway management, (2) respiratory, (3) cardiocirculatory, and (4) other intraoperative and postoperative complications documented until hospital discharge. Airway management and cardiorespiratory complications were defined as previously published [11].

2.3. Statistics

Data were collected in Microsoft Excel (Version 2011, Microsoft Corporation, Redmond, WA, USA) and analysed in R 4.0.3 (R core team, Vienna, Austria). Demographic data, disease manifestations, procedure-related factors, and outcome data were stratified by disease type and summarized as frequencies and percentages for categorical variables and as medians and ranges or means and standard deviations (SD) for continuous variables, as appropriate. The body metrics were collected at each patient contact, thus introducing a cluster structure. We used a mixed-effects linear model to correct for the repeated measurements within each patient using the lme4 package in R [17]. The use of natural cubic splines facilitated a non-linear relationship. Marginal means with corresponding 95% confidence intervals were calculated for the disease subtypes at different ages.

3. Results

3.1. Data Acquisition and Quality

We identified 22 patients with ML (13 MLII, 2 ML intermediate, 7 MLIII), of whom a subset of 12 (55%) had undergone at least 1 anaesthesia procedure in our centres during the study period of 13.3 years. The 12 enrolled patients underwent a total of 44 anaesthesia procedures. For all anaesthesia procedures, the protocols were available and readable. With a missing rate of 1%, the data quality is sufficient.

3.2. Patient Characteristics

3.2.1. Patient Baseline Characteristics

The predominant phenotype in our study population was MLII ($n = 7$), followed by MLIII ($n = 3$) and, lastly, ML intermediate ($n = 2$). Two of the three MLIII patients were siblings. The median overall age at anaesthesia was 3.3 years (range 0.1–19.1). Patients with MLII and intermediate underwent intervention at a younger age than patients with MLIII. Among all, sex was even. One MLII patient underwent haematopoietic stem cell transplantation (HSCT) at nine months of age [18]. Altogether, the burden of anaesthesia-relevant symptoms was more pronounced in MLII and ML intermediate than in MLIII (Table 1).

Table 1. Characteristics and anaesthesia-relevant symptoms of patients with mucolipidosis.

Characteristic	Overall, N = 12	MLII, N = 7	MLII/III, N = 2	MLIII, N = 3
Demographics				
Male sex [2]	6 (50)	4 (57)	1 (50)	1 (33)
Minimum age at anaesthesia [1]	1.7 (0.1–19.0)	0.9 (0.1–5.1)	4.4 (2.4–6.4)	14.4 (5.1–19.0)
Maximum age at anaesthesia [1]	5.9 (0.8–19.1)	3.7 (0.8–6.6)	6.5 (6.4–6.7)	15.4 (8.4–19.0)
Medical history				
Number of anaesthesias [1]	4 (1–11)	4 (2–11)	2 (1–4)	3 (1–5)
HSCT [2]	1 (8)	1 (14)	-	-
History of recurrent infections [2]	2 (17)	2 (29)	-	1 (33)
Upper airway and respiratory tract pathology				
Craniofacial dysmorphia [2]	10 (83)	7 (100)	2 (100)	1 (33)
Gingival hyperplasia [2]	9 (75)	7 (100)	2 (100)	-
Macroglossia [2]	6 (50)	5 (71)	1 (50)	-
Tonsil hyperplasia [2]	6 (50)	2 (29)	2 (100)	2 (67)
Sleep apnoea [2]				
No	3 (25)	1 (14)	-	2 (67)
Yes	5 (42)	2 (29)	2 (100)	1 (33)
NIV-treated	4 (33)	4 (57)	-	-
Obstructive lung disease [2]				
Yes	5 (42)	4 (57)	-	1 (33)
Antiobstructive medication	2 (17)	1 (14)	1 (50)	-
Thorax deformities [2]				
Pectus carinatum	5 (42)	4 (57)	1 (50)	-
Narrow thorax	1 (8.3)	1 (14)	-	-
Cardiovascular manifestations				
Severity of cardiac pathologies [2]				
Mild	3 (25)	1 (14)	1 (50)	1 (33)
Moderate	3 (25)	2 (29)	-	1 (33)
Severe	5 (42)	4 (57)	1 (50)	-
Cardiac pathology [2]				
Valve insufficiency	9 (75)	5 (71)	2 (100)	2 (67)
ASD type II	5 (42)	5 (71)	-	-
LVH	4 (33)	4 (57)	-	-
PFO	2 (17)	2 (29)	-	-
PA stenosis	2 (17)	2 (29)	-	-
Heart failure	2 (17)	1 (14)	1 (50)	-
LV dilatation	1 (8)	1 (14)	-	-
Hypertension	1 (8)	1 (14)	-	-
Tachycardia	1 (8)	-	-	1 (33)
Gastrointestinal manifestations				
Organomegaly [2]				
Hepatomegaly	4 (33)	4 (57)	-	-
Hepatosplenomegaly	1 (8)	1 (14)	-	-
Dysphagia [2]				
Yes	4 (33)	3 (43)	1 (50)	-
Gastric tube	1 (8)	1 (14)	-	-
Spine disease				
Short neck [2]	12 (100)	7 (100)	2 (100)	3 (100)
Cervical spinal stenosis [2]				
Stenosis	5 (42)	4 (57)	1 (50)	-
Stenosis + myelopathy	1 (8)	1 (14)	-	-
State after surgical decompression	1 (8)	-	1 (50)	-
Cervical spinal instability [2]	6 (50)	4 (57)	2 (100)	-
Spinal deformities [2]				
Thoracolumbar kyphosis	5 (42)	4 (57)	1 (50)	-
Lumbar hyperlordosis	1 (8)	-	-	1 (33)
Kyphoscoliosis	1 (8)	-	1 (50)	-

Abbreviations: ASD type II, atrial septal defect type II; NIV, non-invasive ventilation; LVH, left ventricular hypertrophy; PA stenosis, pulmonary artery stenosis; PFO, patent foramen ovale. [1] median (range), [2] n (%).

3.2.2. Growth

All of the MLII and intermediate patients presented severe growth failure. In MLII, vertical growth was only observed in infancy and in ML intermediate within the first three years of life (Figures 1 and S1). Marginal means calculated from the mixed model showed a substantial height difference at the age of five years. Patients with MLII reached a mean, presumably maximum height of 73 cm (CI 69.4–76.6), and those with ML intermediate, a mean, presumably maximum height of 88.4 cm (CI 81.8–95). In contrast, the growth velocity of MLIII patients slowed down during childhood but did not cease. The mean height of MLIII patients was 104 cm (CI 97.5–111) at five years and 143 cm (CI 137.8–148.9) at 18 years of age.

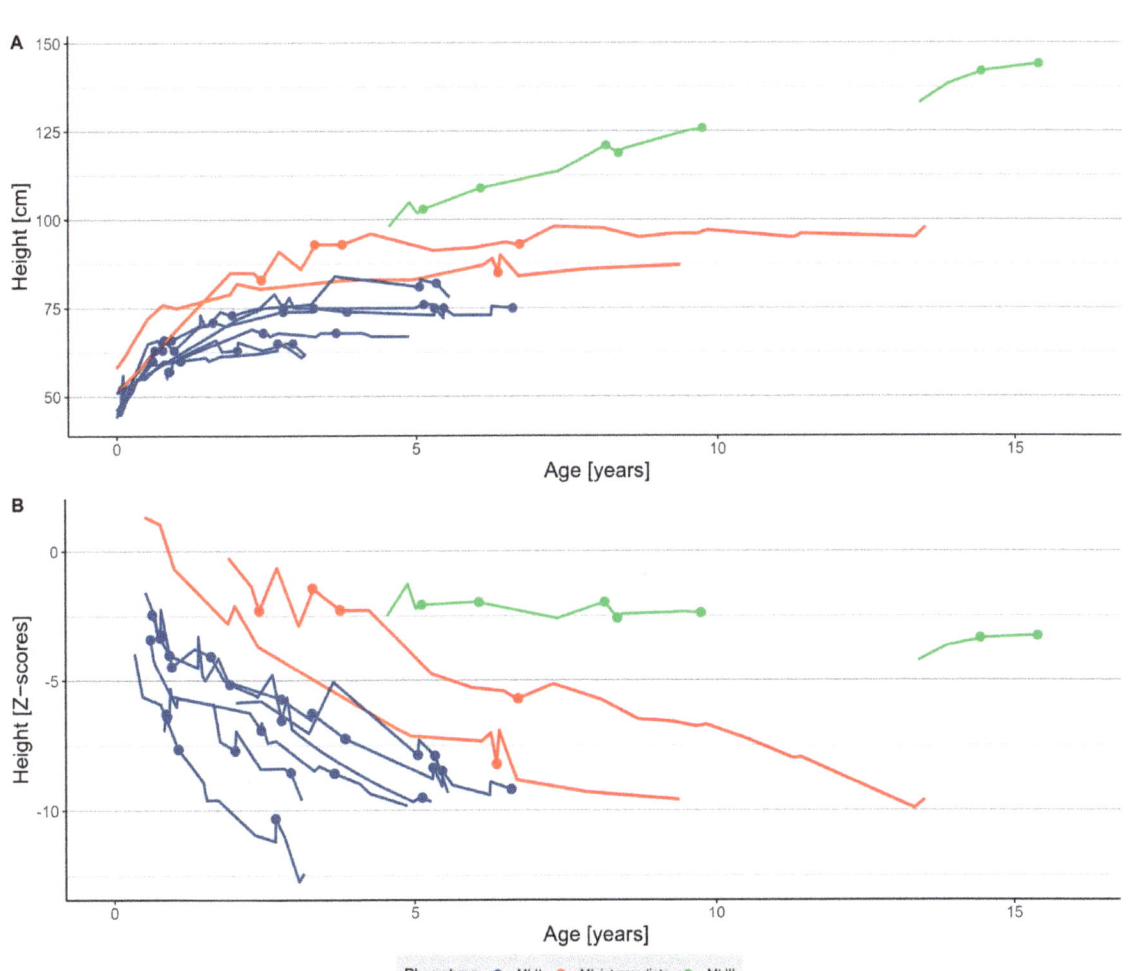

Figure 1. Growth in mucolipidosis. (**A**) Absolute height and (**B**) Z-scores [19] of patients with mucolipidosis type II (MLII, n = 7), intermediate (ML intermediate, n = 2), and III (MLIII, n = 3). Dots indicate the timepoints of anaesthesia procedures.

3.2.3. Upper Airway and Respiratory Tract Pathologies

Considering the severe growth retardation, patients with MLII and ML intermediate keep small thoraces and airways lifelong. Additional thorax deformities were documented in six MLII/intermediate patients, precisely an extremely narrow thorax (1/9; 11%) and pectus carinatum (5/9; 56%). Besides macroglossia, tonsil hyperplasia, and obstructive lung disease, the vast majority (8/9; 88%) of MLII/intermediate patients suffered from (obstructive or central) sleep apnoea, of which half (4/8) required non-invasive ventilation (NIV). NIV was initiated between one and six years of age.

3.2.4. Cardiovascular Manifestations

All nine MLII/intermediate patients presented at least one cardiac pathology, 56% (5/9) of them even severe ones. Progressive valve insufficiency prevailed in all ML patients (9/12; 75%; mitral insufficiency $n = 9$, aortic insufficiency $n = 6$, tricuspid insufficiency $n = 5$). Septum defects were solely observed in MLII. One MLII patient suffering from a hemodynamically relevant atrial septal defect (ASD) type II was treated by catheter intervention at 4.9 years of age. A patent foramen ovale (PFO) and pulmonary artery stenosis were seen in the very young and heart failure rather in the longer-surviving children. The cardiac manifestations of the MLIII patients of this study were limited to mild to moderate valve insufficiency and sinus tachycardia.

3.2.5. Gastrointestinal Manifestations

Dysphagia was manifested in 44% (4/9) of the MLII/intermediate patients, one MLII patient required enteral feeding, and 56% (5/9) of the MLII/intermediate patients had at least one relevant organomegaly.

3.2.6. Spine Disease

Most of the MLII/intermediate children presented atlantoaxial instability (6/9; 67%) or stenosis of the craniocervical junction (7/9; 78%). One MLII patient even had cervical stenosis with myelopathy, and one ML intermediate patient had undergone cervical spine decompression surgery at the age of 2.8 years.

3.3. Characteristics of Anaesthesia Procedures

3.3.1. Frequency of Anaesthesias and Technical Information

Anaesthesia care was provided for 12 patients with ML, accounting for 44 anaesthesia procedures (MLII $n = 30$; ML intermediate $n = 5$; MLIII $n = 9$). The majority of patients (83%) underwent more than one anaesthesia procedure (median 3, range 1–11). Anaesthesia procedures of MLII/intermediate patients (35/44; 80%) outnumbered those of MLIII patients (9/44; 20%). General anaesthesia was the preferred type of anaesthesia (33/44; 75%). In seven anaesthesia cases (7/44; 16%), procedural sedation was performed for diagnostics (primarily magnetic resonance imaging, MRI). Regional anaesthesia (2/44) was rarely applied. Tracheal intubation was carried out in 73% of the general anaesthesia cases (24/33) and a laryngeal mask airway in 27% (9/33). For most of the MLII/ML intermediate cases who were intubated, intubation was facilitated either by videolaryngoscopy (5/21; 24%) or fibreoptic intubation through a laryngeal mask (13/21; 62%). Therefore, in 86% (18/21) of the MLII/intermediate cases, an indirect intubation technique was used as the first-line airway approach. This was in contrast to patients with MLIII, for whom the laryngeal mask was the preferred primary airway approach for general anaesthesia (4/7; 57%).

The most frequently used anaesthesia regime was total intravenous anaesthesia with Propofol for induction and the maintenance of anaesthesia. Inhalative induction was only used in six cases (15%). Sufentanil and Remifentanil were the preferred analgesics for general anaesthesia. Detailed information about the anaesthesia procedures and drug combinations is presented in Table 2 and Supplementary Figure S2.

Table 2. Characteristics of anaesthesia procedures.

Characteristic	Overall, N = 44	MLII, N = 30	MLII/III, N = 5	MLIII, N = 9
	Cases			
Age (years) [1]	3.3 (0.1; 19.1)	2.2 (0.1; 6.6)	3.8 (2.4; 6.7)	9.7 (5.1; 19.1)
Weight (Z-score) [1]	−3.6 (−13.1; 0.3)	−4.8 (−13.1; −0.6)	−1.7 (−4.6; −0.7)	−0.8 (−2.5; −0.3)
Height (Z-score) [1]	−5.7 (−10.3; −1.4)	−6.6 (−10.3; −2.4)	−2.3 (−8.2; −1.4)	−2.37 (−3.3; −2.0)
Present respiratory infection [2]	6 (14)	4 (13)	2 (40)	-
ASA score [2]				
2	8 (18)	-	1 (20)	7 (78)
3	32 (73)	27 (90)	3 (60)	2 (22)
4	4 (9)	3 (10)	1 (20)	0 (0)
	Procedural information			
Number of procedures during anaesthesia [2]	1.0 (1.0; 6.0)	1.0 (1.0; 6.0)	2.0 (1.0; 3.0)	1.0 (1.0; 2.0)
Duration (minutes) [1]	120 (55; 405)	122 (55; 270)	270 (90; 405)	105 (60; 240)
Postoperative ICU care [2]	24 (56)	19 (63)	5 (100)	-
	Technical information			
Type of anaesthesia [2]				
Standby	2 (5)	1 (3)	-	1 (11)
Sedation	7 (16)	7 (23)	-	-
Regional only	2 (5)	1 (3)	-	1 (11)
General anaesthesia	33 (75)	21 (70)	5 (100)	7 (78)
Total intravenous anaesthesia	29 (66)	17 (57)	5 (100)	7 (78)
Balanced anaesthesia	4 (9)	4 (13)	-	-
Induction of anaesthesia				
Intravenous (Propofol)	34 (85)	25 (89)	3 (60)	6 (86)
Inhalative (Sevoflurane)	6 (15)	3 (11)	2 (40)	1 (14)
Primary airway approach [2]				
No airway	11 (25)	9 (30)	-	2 (22)
Laryngeal mask	9 (20)	5 (17)	-	4 (44)
Tracheal intubation	24 (55)	16 (53)	5 (100)	3 (33)
Direct laryngoscopy	3 (7)	2 (7)	1 (20)	-
Videolaryngoscopy	8 (18)	5 (17)	-	3 (33)
FOI-SGA	13 (30)	9 (30)	4 (80)	-

Abbreviations: ASA score, American Society of Anesthesiology score; FOI-SGA, fiberoptic through a supraglottic airway; ICU, intensive care unit; TIVA, total intravenous anaesthesia. Z-Score derived from Kromeyer-Hauschild et al. [19]. [1] median (range), [2] n (%).

3.3.2. Indication for Anaesthesia

Two or more procedures were frequently combined within one anaesthesia. Anaesthesia was mainly performed for diagnostics (27/60; 45%; i.e., MRI n = 18; BERA n = 6; CT n = 1; ophthalmological and neurophysiological examinations n = 2). The most common surgical indications for anaesthesia were ear, nose, and throat (ENT) surgeries (11/60; 18%), carpal tunnel release (6/60; 10%), and hernia repair (3/60; 5%). Three quarters (9/12) of all ML patients underwent at least one ENT surgery. Carpal tunnel release was mainly performed in MLIII and hernia repair exclusively in MLII (Figure 2).

3.4. Outcome

Anaesthesia-related complications were common among ML patients. At least one anaesthesia-related complication occurred in 27.3% (12/44) of the anaesthesia procedures (Table 3). Altogether, 17 complications associated with anaesthesia occurred until discharge. Almost all complications (16/17; 94%) occurred in MLII/intermediate cases, in which the complication rate hence was increased compared to MLIII (31.4% vs. 11.1%).

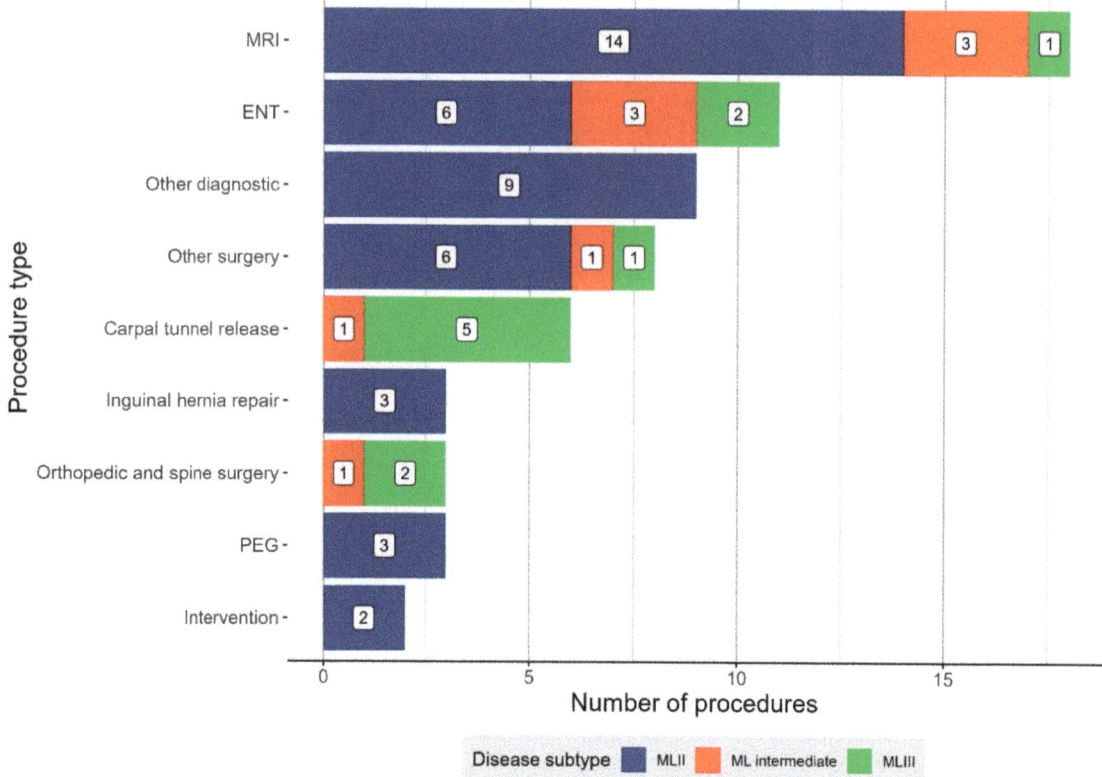

Figure 2. Indication for anaesthesia in all cases of patients with mucolipidosis. "Other diagnostic" sums up brainstem evoked response audiometry (BERA), ophthalmological, and neurophysiological assessments. "Other surgery" denotes all surgeries not represented in any other category and includes gingivectomy, dental, cardiac, and oncologic surgeries, and "intervention" indicates one lumbar puncture and one skin biopsy. Abbreviation: ENT, ear, nose, and throat surgery; MRI, magnetic resonance imaging; PEG, percutaneous endoscopic gastrostomy placement or exchange.

Table 3. Anaesthesia-related complications subdivided by ML types.

Characteristic, n (%)	Overall, N = 44	MLII, N = 30	MLII/III, N = 5	MLIII, N = 9
Anaesthesias with at least one complication	12 (27)	8 (27)	3 (60)	1 (11)
Difficult airway management	6 (14)	5 (17)	1 (20)	-
Difficult facemask ventilation	5 (14)	4 (18)	1 (20)	-
Difficult laryngeal mask airway	1 (4)	1 (6.2)	-	-
Difficult tracheal intubation	6 (23)	5 (29)	1 (20)	-
Respiratory complications	8 (18)	6 (20)	2 (40)	-
Cardiocirculatory complications	-	-	-	-
Other complications	3 (7)	1 (3)	1 (20)	1 (11)

More than half (10/17; 59%) of the complications arose during induction of anaesthesia, only 12% (2/17) during anaesthesia or extubation, and 29% (5/17) after anaesthesia. The most frequently experienced complications were respiratory complications (8/44; 18%) and difficult airway management (6/44; 14%). Respiratory complications, especially hypoxia, prevailed during the challenging airway management and extubation (5/8; 62.5% of the respiratory events). A predicted difficult airway was found in 100%, 80%, and 0% of the MLII, ML intermediate, and MLIII patients, respectively.

Success rates were 33% for direct laryngoscopy, 100% for videolaryngoscopy, and 92% for fibreoptic intubation through a laryngeal mask. Awake intubation was not performed. Facemask ventilation was difficult or impossible in five cases (14%). The laryngeal mask airway was difficult in only one case (4%). One child suffered from severe bradycardia with consecutive cardiac arrest due to hypoxia during difficult airway management. The placement of a laryngeal mask re-established sufficient oxygenation during critical events in all of the cases, at least temporarily. Subsequent rescue techniques comprised videolaryngoscopy and intubation via flexible optic with or without guidance via a laryngeal mask. Airway management was eventually successful in all cases so that no emergency tracheotomy or anaesthesia-related death occurred. None of the children experienced anaesthesia-related sequels. Individual case descriptions are presented in Table 4.

Of note, the data show a trend towards higher numbers of anaesthesia procedures over the study period of 13.3 years, while the number of complications remained relatively stable (Figure S3); hence, the risk of complications decreased over time.

Table 4. Details of perianaesthetic complications in patients with ML.

Pat.	Sex	Subtype	Year	Age	Procedure	Airway Management	Anaesthesia Procedure	Event Categories	Detailed Descriptions
1	Female	MLII	2020	3 years	PEG exchange	VL → FOI-LM	TIVA: Propofol, Remifentanil	DiffAir, RESP	Videolaryngoscopy: failed, C/L 4 view; FOI-LM: passage of 4.0 tube failed, successful placement of 3.5 uncuffed tube; tube exchange because of significant air leak (3.5 cuffed tube via exchange catheter); hypoxemia with SpO$_2$ 75%; unplanned ICU admission
1	Female	MLII	2019	2 years	MRI, BERA	No airway	Sedation: Propofol, Esketamine	RESP	Fever, bronchopneumonia treated with i.v. antibiotics
1	Female	MLII	2017	10 months	MRI, lumbar puncture	No airway → LM → VL → FOI-LM	Sedation: Propofol, Esketamine	DiffAir, RESP, other	Sedation: failed due to insufficient spontaneous breathing; difficult face mask ventilation; tracheal intubation: failed (conventional and videolaryngoscopy VL: C/L 3; hypoxemia and consecutive severe bradycardia requiring CPR; LM (rescue manoeuvre) facilitated oxygenation, ROSC, massive hypercapnia; FOI-LM: finally successful; postoperative respiratory insufficiency with prolonged ventilation on ICU; sepsis on ICU
2	Male	MLII/III	2008	6 years	ENT surgery	FOI-LM	TIVA: Propofol, Sufentanil	RESP	Postoperative tube dislocation into the main bronchus with atelectasis
3	Male	MLIII	2020	8 years	hip osteotomy	VL	Sevoflurane, TIVA: Propofol, Remifentanil	Other	Postoperative fever
4	Male	MLII	2021	2 years	ENT surgery	FOI-LM → VL → FOI	TIVA: Propofol, Remifentanil	DiffAir, RESP	Impossible face mask ventilation; FOI-LM: failed due to secretion and unfavourable angle; VL failed (C/L 3). Finally, tracheal intubation was secured by oral FOI. Hypoxemia with minimal SpO$_2$ 58%
5	Male	MLII	2017	1 year	MRI	FOI-LM	TIVA: Propofol, Remifentanil	RESP	Hypoxemia with minimal SpO$_2$ of 70% during intubation

Table 4. Cont.

Pat.	Sex	Subtype	Year	Age	Procedure	Airway Management	Anaesthesia Procedure	Event Categories	Detailed Descriptions
5	Male	MLII	2016	11 months	ENT surgery	DL	TIVA: Propofol, Sufentanil	DiffAir	Impossible face mask ventilation, LM; tracheal intubation via direct laryngoscopy
6	Female	MLII	2014	7 months	Quinton catheter implantation	DL → other	Balanced: Propofol, Sufentanil, Sevoflurane	DiffAir	Difficult intubation; conventional laryngoscopy C/L 3; successful intubation with a rigid bronchoscope
7	Female	MLII/III	2015	6 years	ENT surgery, MRI	FOI-LM	TIVA: Propofol, Sufentanil	Other	Postoperative fever
7	Female	MLII/III	2012	3 years	Atlantooccipital decompression	DL → VL → other	Sevoflurane TIVA: Propofol, Sufentanil	DiffAir, RESP	Difficult mask ventilation; VL: C/L 3; intubation with a McCoy blade and rigid bronchoscope, hypoxemia
8	Male	MLII	2021	5 years	ENT surgery, MRI, other diagnostics	VL	TIVA: Propofol, Remifentanil	RESP	Postextubation airway obstruction with severe hypoxemia (SpO_2 8%)

Abbreviations: BERA, brainstem electric response audiometry; C/L, Cormack/Lehane; CPR, cardiopulmonary resuscitation; DiffAir, difficult airway management; DL, direct laryngoscopy; ENT, ear, nose, and throat; FOI, fibreoptic intubation; LM, laryngeal mask; FOI-LM, fibreoptic intubation guided by laryngeal mask; GA, general anaesthesia; ICU, intensive care unit; MRI, magnetic resonance imaging; PEG, percutaneous endoscopic gastrostomy; RESP, respiratory event; ROSC, return of spontaneous circulation; VL, videolaryngoscopy; TIVA, total intravenous anaesthesia.

4. Discussion

The present study is the largest published case series of patients with ML undergoing anaesthesia [11,12]. Furthermore, it is the first study to assess the full extent of anaesthesia-relevant multiorgan manifestations in this particularly rare disease. At least one complication arose during or after anaesthesia in more than a quarter of anaesthesia procedures. According to our data, difficult airway management and respiratory complications form the most alarming anaesthesia-relevant complications in patients with ML. Almost all complications occurred in patients with MLII and ML intermediate, even though indirect intubation techniques were favoured, as recommended in patients with skeletal dysplasia [20] and suggested in ML [11]. This correlates with the wide phenotypical spectrum between MLII and MLIII, with a much more pronounced anaesthesia-relevant disease burden in MLII and ML intermediate than in MLIII.

As pointed out recently [18], the natural history of ML is not yet described in detail. The present study specifies various disease manifestations relevant for anaesthesia planning. Although cardiorespiratory complications are widely known to be the leading cause of death in MLII [5], detailed data on the cardiac manifestations are sparse in the current literature [6,7]. Our study found frequent valve insufficiency and hypertrophic and dilated cardiomyopathy in the longer-surviving children, which is in agreement with previous reports [21,22]. In the sense of a continuum, similar cardiac manifestations may be present in MLIII as in MLII, but usually less severe or later in life. Interestingly, relevant cardiocirculatory complications have not been found in our case series.

The vast majority (89%) of the MLII and intermediate patients of this cohort suffered from sleep apnoea, which is in line with two case series [16,23] on sleep-disordered breathing in patients with MLII or intermediate, of whom 100% were documented to have obstructive sleep apnoea (OSA). The OSA turned out to be progressive with the eventual need for NIV in all children, which was inevitable with upper airway surgery (adenotonsillectomy). This can be explained by the multiple-level airway obstruction by the accumulation of undigested substrates in various body tissues leading to a hypertrophic tongue base, adenotonsillar hypertrophy, a thickened and retroflexed epiglottis, a thickened and anteriorly placed larynx, subglottic stenosis and a generally narrow and possibly curved trachea [12,15,24,25]. The craniofacial abnormalities, particularly the flat face and the depressed nasal bridge, also predispose patients to OSA, and cervical spine stenosis may precipitate central apnoea [26]. The high prevalence of OSA, as early as in infancy [23], fortifies the need for a systematic polysomnographic follow-up program in ML patients, as recommended for other lysosomal storage disorders [27]. Restrictive lung disease due to profound growth retardation, chest and spine deformities, and decreased thoracic elasticity may additionally contribute to respiratory insufficiency [8] and reduce the respiratory reserve during apnoeic episodes such as during airway management [28]. Pre-planned ICU monitoring may hence be beneficial for ML patients with severe disease forms. Of note, tonsil hyperplasia, sleep apnoea, and obstructive lung disease were also found in MLIII. All these symptoms lead to a high risk of perianaesthetic respiratory complications.

This is the first study to provide frequencies of different spinal pathologies in ML. Our study revealed a strikingly high percentage of stenosis of the craniocervical junction (78%) and atlantoaxial instability (67%) in patients with MLII and ML intermediate. Progressive cervical spinal cord compression with resulting respiratory failure and death has been described before [26]. However, not only patients with cervical spine pathologies need special attention, but also those with lower vertebral column abnormalities, which are also common in ML. The frequency of MLII children with thoracolumbar gibbus abnormality in this study (57%) roughly equals the percentage reported by Alegra et al. (50%) [29]. The literature contains a number of reports on children with MPS with neurological sequels after anaesthesia [10], such as an MPS IH patient with a 76° thoracic kyphosis and irreversible paraplegia after extremity surgery [30]. According to Farley et al., the spinal cord intramedullar pressure increases significantly in thoracic kyphosis exceeding 63° [31]. Cervical spinal stenosis and instability and thoracolumbar kyphosis may not be the predominant symptoms in MLIII. However, MLIII patients should also be handled with particular caution, considering that they may also present severe scoliosis and signs of spinal cord compression with possible loss of ambulation [6,7]. The high burden of spine disease highlights the importance of the careful positioning of all anaesthetized ML patients. Following this, we did not observe any neurological sequels in our patient cohort.

Due to their multiorgan morbidity, patients with ML frequently require anaesthesia for diagnostic or surgical interventions [7,11,12]. The patients in our study cohort had a median of three anaesthesias at our centres. We found a higher complication rate in MLII and intermediate than in MLIII (31.4% vs. 11.1%). Therefore, a more severe disease burden of patients with MLII and ML intermediate correlates with an increased risk for morbidity during and after anaesthesia. As indicated by Dohrmann et al. [11], the event rate in MLII (25%) is increased compared to MPSIII (9.1%) and certainly dramatically increased compared to the healthy paediatric population (0.14–5.2%) [32,33]. The majority of the anaesthesia procedures in case series of patients with MLII and III [12,15,16] published so far were described as challenging. However, several of these reported cases required emergency intubations because of acute respiratory distress associated with an infection [15,16]. One of the emergency intubations in a non-specialized hospital failed altogether with subsequent death [16]. Two other patients eventually required tracheotomy [15]. Considering the poor outcome of MLII patients intubated during respiratory distress, a restriction of elective anaesthesia to infection-free periods might be advisable. Furthermore, preoperative diagnostics allow for a multidisciplinary risk–benefit analysis of the planned intervention and improved counselling of the parents or patients. The event rate decreased over the study period of 13.3 years, and the anaesthesia management hence tendentially became safer. This underlines the importance of elective anaesthesias to be performed in tertiary hospitals with an ICU and a multidisciplinary team well-acquainted with a number of advanced airway management techniques. Nonetheless, the event rate should be interpreted with caution as the study population may have changed with improved disease detection and supportive clinical management.

The case number of this study remains too low to analyse perioperative management factors in order to deduce a standard of intraoperative care. We hence can only make suggestions based on the results of this study and a review of the literature [11,12,15,16]. ML patients have complex airways with predicted difficult airway management in 100% of MLII and 80% of ML intermediate patients. Indirect intubation methods such as videolaryngoscopy or fibreoptic intubation with guidance through a supraglottic conduit had the highest success rate in a previous study from our institution [11] and should be favoured for a first-line airway approach. With both methods, hyperextension of the head can be avoided [34]. However, our data indicate that, even with these prerequisites, a high risk for respiratory complications during airway management persists. A laryngeal mask airway can be used temporarily to re-establish stable ventilation during critical events [15]. Taking into account the severe growth retardation in patients with MLII and ML intermediate, anaesthesiologists should consider a smaller tube size than standard for the child's age [12]. After all, the airway techniques should be chosen individually, depending on each patient's complex manifestations and the distinct experience of the handling of anaesthesiologists and the institution.

This study has a few limitations. It is a retrospective study, so the documentation, including the anaesthesia-relevant complications, may have been incomplete. The small case number, especially of patients with MLIII, is based on limited patient availability: firstly, because ML is an extremely rare disease and, secondly, because preoperative risk–benefit considerations frequently trigger a decision against anaesthesia, and thus only patients with a mandatory indication for anaesthesia or an appealing risk–benefit ratio might have been selected for anaesthesia. Therefore, the true anaesthesia-relevant disease burden might even be higher. This centre's experience may have caused a selection bias, so our results should only be generalized with caution.

5. Conclusions

Featuring 12 ML patients who underwent anaesthesia on 44 occasions, the present study is currently the largest study published on anaesthetic risk in ML. Moreover, it is the first to give full particulars on anaesthesia-relevant disease manifestations among the different ML types. At least one complication occurred in 27.3% of the anaesthesia procedures, almost all (94%) in patients with MLII or ML intermediate. This finding corresponds with a much more pronounced anaesthesia-relevant disease burden in MLII and ML intermediate than in MLIII. Most complications (59%) occurred during critical airway management. Hence, we suggest indirect intubation techniques (i.e., videolaryngoscopy and fibreoptic intubation through a supraglottic airway) to be routinely used for the a priori airway approach in these children. This study highlights the necessity of individualized preoperative risk–benefit analysis, shared and multidisciplinary decision-making, and thoughtful anaesthesia planning in patients with ML.

Supplementary Materials: The following supporting information can be downloaded at: https://www.mdpi.com/article/10.3390/jcm11133650/s1, Figure S1: Estimated marginal means of the height of patients with mucolipidosis; Figure S2: Frequency of drug combinations used during general anaesthesia and sedation; Figure S3: Centre experience.

Author Contributions: Conceptualization, L.S.A., T.D., N.M.M.; formal analysis, L.S.A., T.D.; data acquisition, L.S.A., T.D., A.L., S.R.B.; statistical analysis, T.D.; writing—original draft preparation, L.S.A., T.D.; writing—review and editing, L.S.A., T.D., M.P., N.M.M., R.S., S.R.B., P.B.S.; visualization and editing, L.S.A., T.D.; supervision, M.P., N.M.M. All authors have read and agreed to the published version of the manuscript.

Funding: This research received no external funding.

Institutional Review Board Statement: According to the ethical committee of the medical board Hamburg, Germany, ethical review and approval were waived for this study as it is a retrospective analysis of anonymised data (ethical consultation number WF-056/18, 30 October 2018).

Informed Consent Statement: Patient consent was waived as this is a retrospective chart analysis of anonymized data acquired during clinical routine visits.

Data Availability Statement: The data that support the findings of this study are available from the corresponding author upon reasonable request. The data are not publicly available to ensure that the privacy of the study patients with rare diseases is not compromised.

Conflicts of Interest: The authors declare no conflict of interest.

References

1. Tiede, S.; Storch, S.; Lubke, T.; Henrissat, B.; Bargal, R.; Raas-Rothschild, A.; Braulke, T. Mucolipidosis II is caused by mutations in GNPTA encoding the alpha/beta GlcNAc-1-phosphotransferase. *Nat. Med.* **2005**, *11*, 1109–1112. [CrossRef]
2. Braulke, T.; Bonifacino, J.S. Sorting of lysosomal proteins. *Biochim. Biophys. Acta* **2009**, *1793*, 605–614. [CrossRef]
3. Kollmann, K.; Pohl, S.; Marschner, K.; Encarnacao, M.; Sakwa, I.; Tiede, S.; Poorthuis, B.J.; Lübke, T.; Müller-Loennies, S.; Storch, S.; et al. Mannose phosphorylation in health and disease. *Eur. J. Cell Biol.* **2010**, *89*, 117–123. [CrossRef]
4. Khan, S.A.; Tomatsu, S.C. Mucolipidoses Overview: Past, Present, and Future. *Int. J. Mol. Sci.* **2020**, *21*, 6812. [CrossRef]
5. Dogterom, E.J.; Wagenmakers, M.; Wilke, M.; Demirdas, S.; Muschol, N.M.; Pohl, S.; van der Meijden, J.C.; Rizopoulos, D.; van der Ploeg, A.T.; Oussoren, E. Mucolipidosis type II and type III: A systematic review of 843 published cases. *Genet. Med. Off. J. Am. Coll. Med. Genet.* **2021**, *23*, 2047–2056. [CrossRef]
6. Cathey, S.S.; Leroy, J.G.; Wood, T.; Eaves, K.; Simensen, R.J.; Kudo, M.; Stevenson, R.E.; Friez, M.J. Phenotype and genotype in mucolipidoses II and III alpha/beta: A study of 61 probands. *J. Med. Genet.* **2010**, *47*, 38–48. [CrossRef]
7. Oussoren, E.; van Eerd, D.; Murphy, E.; Lachmann, R.; van der Meijden, J.C.; Hoefsloot, L.H.; Verdijk, R.; Ruijter, G.J.G.; Maas, M.; Hollak, C.E.M.; et al. Mucolipidosis type III, a series of adult patients. *J. Inherit. Metab. Dis.* **2018**, *41*, 839–848. [CrossRef]
8. Velho, R.V.; Harms, F.L.; Danyukova, T.; Ludwig, N.F.; Friez, M.J.; Cathey, S.S.; Filocamo, M.; Tappino, B.; Güneş, N.; Tüysüz, B.; et al. The lysosomal storage disorders mucolipidosis type II, type III alpha/beta, and type III gamma: Update on GNPTAB and GNPTG mutations. *Hum. Mutat.* **2019**, *40*, 842–864.
9. Ammer, L.S.; Oussoren, E.; Muschol, N.M.; Pohl, S.; Rubio-Gozalbo, M.E.; Santer, R.; Stuecker, R.; Vettorazzi, E.; Breyer, S.R. Hip Morphology in Mucolipidosis Type II. *J. Clin. Med.* **2020**, *9*, 728. [CrossRef]

10. Ammer, L.S.; Dohrmann, T.; Muschol, N.M.; Lang, A.; Breyer, S.R.; Ozga, A.K.; Petzoldt, M. Disease Manifestations in Mucopolysaccharidoses and Their Impact on Anaesthesia-Related Complications—A Retrospective Analysis of 99 Patients. *J. Clin. Med.* 2021, *10*, 3518. [CrossRef]
11. Dohrmann, T.; Muschol, N.M.; Sehner, S.; Punke, M.A.; Haas, S.A.; Roeher, K.; Breyer, S.; Koehn, A.F.; Ullrich, K.; Zöllner, C.; et al. Airway management and perioperative adverse events in children with mucopolysaccharidoses and mucolipidoses: A retrospective cohort study. *Paediatr. Anaesth.* 2020, *30*, 181–190. [CrossRef]
12. Scott-Warren, V.L.; Walker, R. Perioperative management of patients with Mucolipidosis II and III: Lessons from a case series. *Paediatr. Anaesth.* 2021, *31*, 260–267. [CrossRef]
13. Mahfouz, A.K.; George, G. Anesthesia for gingivectomy and dental extractions in a child with I-cell disease—A case report. *Middle East J. Anaesthesiol.* 2011, *21*, 121–124.
14. Mahfouz, A.K.; George, G.; Al-Bahlani, S.S.; Al Nabhani, M.Z. Difficult intubation management in a child with I-cell disease. *Saudi J. Anaesth.* 2010, *4*, 105–107. [CrossRef]
15. Mallen, J.; Highstein, M.; Smith, L.; Cheng, J. Airway management considerations in children with I-cell disease. *Int. J. Pediatric Otorhinolaryngol.* 2015, *79*, 760–762. [CrossRef]
16. Edmiston, R.; Wilkinson, S.; Jones, S.; Tylee, K.; Broomfield, A.; Bruce, I.A. I-Cell Disease (Mucolipidosis II): A Case Series from a Tertiary Paediatric Centre Reviewing the Airway and Respiratory Consequences of the Disease. *JIMD Rep.* 2019, *45*, 1–8.
17. Bates, D.; Maechler, M.; Bolker, B.; Walker, S. Fitting Linear Mixed-Effects Models Using lme4. *J. Stat. Softw.* 2015, *67*, 1–48. [CrossRef]
18. Ammer, L.S.; Pohl, S.; Breyer, S.; Aries, C.; Denecke, J.; Perez, A.; Petzoldt, M.; Schrum, J.; Müller, I.; Muschol, N.M. Is hematopoietic stem cell transplantation a therapeutic option for mucolipidosis type II? *Mol. Genet. Metab. Rep.* 2021, *26*, 100704. [CrossRef]
19. Kromeyer-Hauschild, K.; Wabitsch, M.; Kunze, D.; Geller, F.; Geiß, H.C.; Hesse, V.; Von Hippel, A.; Jaeger, U.; Johnsen, D.; Korte, W.; et al. Perzentile für den Body-mass-Index für das Kindes- und Jugendalter unter Heranziehung verschiedener deutscher Stichproben. *Mon. Kinderheilkd.* 2001, *149*, 807–818. [CrossRef]
20. White, K.K.; Bompadre, V.; Goldberg, M.J.; Bober, M.B.; Cho, T.J.; Hoover-Fong, J.E.; Irving, M.; Mackenzie, W.G.; Kamps, S.E.; Raggio, C.; et al. Best practices in peri-operative management of patients with skeletal dysplasias. *Am. J. Med. Genet. Part A* 2017, *173*, 2584–2595. [CrossRef]
21. Dangel, J.H. Cardiovascular changes in children with mucopolysaccharide storage diseases and related disorders—Clinical and echocardiographic findings in 64 patients. *Eur. J. Pediatrics* 1998, *157*, 534–538. [CrossRef]
22. Carboni, E.; Sestito, S.; Lucente, M.; Morrone, A.; Zampini, L.; Chimenz, R.; Ceravolo, M.D.; De Sarro, R.; Ceravolo, G.; Calabrò, M.P. Dilated cardiomyopathy in mucolipidosis type 2. *J. Biol. Regul. Homeost. Agents* 2020, *34* (Suppl. 2), 71–77.
23. Tabone, L.; Caillaud, C.; Amaddeo, A.; Khirani, S.; Michot, C.; Couloigner, V.; Brassier, A.; Cormier-Daire, V.; Baujat, G.; Fauroux, B. Sleep-disordered breathing in children with mucolipidosis. *Am. J. Med. Genet. Part A* 2019, *179*, 1196–1204. [CrossRef]
24. Peters, M.E.; Arya, S.; Langer, L.O.; Gilbert, E.F.; Carlson, R.; Adkins, W. Narrow trachea in mucopolysaccharidoses. *Pediatr. Radiol.* 1985, *15*, 225–228. [CrossRef]
25. Poore, T.S.; Prager, J.; Weinman, J.P.; Larson, A.; Houin, P. Tracheal and lower airway changes in a patient with mucolipidosis type II. *Pediatr. Pulmonol.* 2020, *55*, 1843–1845. [CrossRef]
26. Nakaoka, S.; Kondo, H.; Matsuoka, K.; Shibuya, T.; Otomo, T.; Hamada, Y.; Sakamoto, K.; Ozono, K.; Sakai, N. Mucolipidosis II and III with neurological symptoms due to spinal cord compression. *Brain Dev.* 2021, *43*, 867–872. [CrossRef]
27. Scarpa, M.; Almássy, Z.; Beck, M.; Bodamer, O.; Bruce, I.A.; De Meirleir, L.; Guffon, N.; Guillén-Navarro, E.; Hensman, P.; Jones, S.; et al. Mucopolysaccharidosis type II: European recommendations for the diagnosis and multidisciplinary management of a rare disease. *Orphanet J. Rare Dis.* 2011, *6*, 72. [CrossRef]
28. Wooten, W.I., 3rd; Muhlebach, M.S.; Muenzer, J.; Loughlin, C.E.; Vaughn, B.V. Progression of Polysomnographic Abnormalities in Mucolipidosis II (I-Cell Disease). *J. Clin. Sleep Med.* 2016, *12*, 1695–1696. [CrossRef]
29. Alegra, T.; Sperb-Ludwig, F.; Guarany, N.R.; Ribeiro, E.M.; Lourenco, C.M.; Kim, C.A.; Valadares, E.R.; Galera, M.F.; Acosta, A.X.; Horovitz, D.D.G.; et al. Clinical Characterization of Mucolipidoses II and III: A Multicenter Study. *J. Pediatric Genet.* 2019, *8*, 198–204. [CrossRef]
30. Pruszczynski, B.; Mackenzie, W.G.; Rogers, K.; White, K.K. Spinal Cord Injury After Extremity Surgery in Children with Thoracic Kyphosis. *Clin. Orthop. Relat. Res.* 2015, *473*, 3315–3320. [CrossRef]
31. Farley, C.W.; Curt, B.A.; Pettigrew, D.B.; Holtz, J.R.; Dollin, N.; Kuntz, C., IV. Spinal cord intramedullary pressure in thoracic kyphotic deformity: A cadaveric study. *Spine* 2012, *37*, E224–E230. [CrossRef]
32. Habre, W.; Disma, N.; Virag, K.; Becke, K.; Hansen, T.G.; Jöhr, M.; Leva, B.; Morton, N.S.; Vermeulen, P.M.; Zielinska, M.; et al. Incidence of severe critical events in paediatric anaesthesia (APRICOT): A prospective multicentre observational study in 261 hospitals in Europe. *Lancet Respir. Med.* 2017, *5*, 412–425. [CrossRef]
33. Kurth, C.D.; Tyler, D.; Heitmiller, E.; Tosone, S.R.; Martin, L.; Deshpande, J.K. National pediatric anesthesia safety quality improvement program in the United States. *Anesth. Analg.* 2014, *119*, 112–121. [CrossRef]
34. Lee, J.J.; Lim, B.G.; Lee, M.K.; Kong, M.H.; Kim, K.J.; Lee, J.Y. Fiberoptic intubation through a laryngeal mask airway as a management of difficult airway due to the fusion of the entire cervical spine—A report of two cases. *Korean J. Anesthesiol.* 2012, *62*, 272–276. [CrossRef]

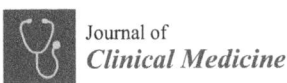

Review

Healthcare Transition in Inherited Metabolic Disorders—Is a Collaborative Approach between US and European Centers Possible?

Jessica I. Gold [1],* and Karolina M. Stepien [2,3],*

1 Division of Human Genetics, Children's Hospital of Philadelphia, Philadelphia, PA 19104, USA
2 Inherited Metabolic Disorders Department, Salford Royal NHS Foundation Trust, Salford H6 8HD, UK
3 Division of Diabetes, Endocrinology and Gastroenterology, University of Manchester, Manchester M13 9PL, UK
* Correspondence: goldj@chop.edu (J.I.G.); kstepien@doctors.org.uk (K.M.S.)

Abstract: Inherited metabolic diseases (IMDs) are rare heterogenous genetic conditions. Advanced technology and novel therapeutic developments have led to the improved life expectancy of patients with IMDs. Long-term, they require close surveillance from specialist adult metabolic providers. Healthcare transition (HCT) is the planned, purposeful process of preparing adolescents for adult-centered medical care and has been recognized globally as a necessary component of care for IMDs. Two recent surveys outlined barriers to the HCT in the US and the UK. The limited knowledge of IMDs among adult physicians was one of the barriers. Some work on specialty curriculum has started and aims to improve the structured training and awareness of rare diseases. Other barriers included social and legal aspects of adulthood, social, vocational and educational support for young adults, care fragmentation and insurance coverage. Although various HCT tools are available, they cannot always be standardized for IMDs. Despite the remarkable differences in the healthcare systems and physicians' training, collaboration among metabolic centers is possible. International rare disease alliance may enhance the patients' management via guidelines development and standardized training for adult metabolic providers.

Keywords: transition service; adult metabolic medicine; collaboration; challenges; inherited metabolic diseases; healthcare systems

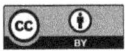

1. Introduction

Inherited Metabolic Diseases (IMDs) encompass an expanding group of rare diseases caused by inherited defects in various biochemical pathways [1]. Although the individual incidence is low (from 1 in 10,000 to 1 in 1 million), the overall incidence of all IMDs ranges from 1 in 800 to 1 in 2500 newborns [1,2].

Recent advances in screening, diagnosis, and management of IMDs have resulted in improved clinical and patient-reported outcomes, increased life expectancy, and new recognition of adult-onset phenotypes [3,4]. Latest estimates suggest that over 90% of patients with IMD now survive past 20 years old and that adults (16–80 years) comprise nearly 50% of those with IMD [3–5]. Despite this rapidly growing population, adult phenotypes remain underdefined and often diverge from pediatric ones. Specific challenges exist for metabolic providers—historically, this field was entirely within the purview of pediatricians and adult physicians have limited familiarity with these diagnoses or their management. Given the progressive and complex nature of many IMDs, adult age-related health problems, and multi-specialty support systems, these young adults require long-term surveillance of adult metabolic providers.

Healthcare transition (HCT)—the planned, purposeful process of preparing adolescents for adult-centered medical care—has been recognized globally as a necessary component of care for IMD [1,6,7]. HCT for youths with IMD must recognize these unique barriers to optimize adult well-being. This report compares and contrasts barriers to HCT in two different healthcare systems.

2. Report

Two recent surveys answer the growing call to define HCT practice among metabolic providers in the United States (US) and European Union (EU) [1,8]. Both surveys assessed current facilitators and barriers to HCT, identifying several similarities among the US and EU responses. HCT is universally recognized as a critical component of IMD healthcare, yet few providers use validated tools to assess transition readiness. A significant barrier globally is the lack of knowledgeable adult providers in all areas of medicine, especially metabolic and psychology/psychiatry, leading to fragmented care. Limited training opportunities in adolescent and adult metabolic medicine are acknowledged by both groups. Despite the perceived importance of HCT, greater efforts need to be directed toward educating providers and standardizing transition practices.

How can metabolic providers in the US and EU collaborate on IMD-specific HCT tools? At first glance, bridging the wide gap between the nationalized health systems of the EU and the disjointed US amalgam of private and governmental health services seems challenging. However, similar initiatives for creation and dissemination of standardized HCT instruments are needed on both sides of the Atlantic. As an example, the 'Ready, Steady, Go' document has been translated into several languages and could be potentially adopted by many countries [9].

Lack of specific adult services or healthcare providers trained to care for rare metabolic diseases results in poor HCT transition program [10] Subspecialty providers are increasingly hailed as critical to HCT efforts due to their sphere of knowledge and strong longitudinal family relationships [11]. These initial steps are medical institution-independent and can be enhanced by integration of global methods. To identify the strengths in our differences, we visit several aspects of metabolic care and HCT in the US and the UK.

A common thread through both surveys was the predominance of pediatrically trained metabolic providers and general challenges with physician recruitment. In the US, metabolic physicians first complete a genetics residency coupled with a more general residency. In total, 67.2% of geneticists in the US are dual-certified in pediatrics and genetics while only 11.4% are dual certified in internal medical/family medicine and genetics [12]. An optional year of accredited training in medical biochemical genetics is gaining popularity and is increasingly required for employment. In total, most metabolic providers receive 4–5 years of post-graduate training in the field of genetics and metabolism.

The UK has a specific pathway for adult metabolic medicine through their Royal College of Pathologists. Physicians receive training in internal medicine or surgery followed by training in Chemical Pathology and Metabolic Medicine. Together, metabolic training in the UK occurs over 10 years. New diagnostic and therapeutic developments in the field of rare diseases has increased an interest among clinicians, but the current training pathway with difficult FRCPath examinations had a negative impact on recruitment. A new accredited curriculum on acute management of IMD is under development. It aims to attract clinicians from different specialties, e.g., neurology, renal medicine or cardiology to develop a special interest in this field [13,14]. Given the diversity of the specialty training backgrounds of clinicians in adult metabolic medicine, the training curriculum requires some flexibility to meet their training needs [15]. In addition, there is overlap of the knowledge-based competencies between the UK adult metabolic medicine training curriculum [13,15] and pediatric biochemical genetics [15].

Nearly 98.9% of US respondents take care of pediatric and adult patients compared to 84.1% of European centers [1,8]. European centers, mainly the UK, are more likely to have a separate adult metabolic clinic, which may vary in clinical scope from only lysosomal storage disorders to only intermediary disorders of metabolism. In contrast, US centers, where adults predominantly receive care in pediatric clinics, tend to offer wide-ranging IMD care, engaging a multidisciplinary team of dietitians, social workers and genetic counselors. Continuity of care at pediatric metabolic clinics likely improves patient adherence to follow-up. The implementation of separate adult metabolic medicine clinics in the UK achieved similar goals. Prior to 2005, all patients were discharged from pediatric IMD clinics at 16 years old. The creation of adult-specific IMD clinics introduced a new medical home for these adolescents, ensuring continual care. It resulted in many childhood-onset cases being re-referred to adult services after many years of no follow up, no treatment or special diets.

Care fragmentation occurs in both health systems. The UK's National Health Service (NHS) provides government-funding (through taxation) for consultation, investigations, and follow-up appointments. There is little involvement from the private sector. However, while pediatric and adult patients are seen within the same health system, visits occur at different hospitals with separate non-integrated electronic health records. The US system of private and government-funded health insurance leads to greater splintering of healthcare delivery. Many tertiary pediatric hospitals are stand-alone institutions, unaffiliated with any local adult institution. IMD patients who received centralized pediatric medical care may be forced to seek care at several different adult institutions due to limitations of their medical insurance. Adult hospitals that are not affiliated with pediatric institutions rarely have genetic or metabolic specialists. They are unlikely to carry metabolic formula, medications for acute IMD care, or run IMD-specific laboratories [8]. For many American institutions, this prevents adults from receiving acute metabolic care in adult hospitals.

US health insurance coverage changes as patients age. Adolescents must apply for adult Medicaid, the public aid-based insurance, even if previously receiving pediatric Medicaid. Private health insurance is usually employment-based, though 2010's Affordable Care Act allows youth to remain on their parent's health insurance through age 26 and created marketplaces to purchase independent plans. Regardless of insurance, many states do not mandate coverage of metabolic formula, medical food, or supplements for adults [16]. In contrast, every employed patient in the UK pays monthly into the National Insurance Scheme, which covers universal healthcare for everyone. Unemployed patients are not required to make these monthly payments, but still receive free medical care. Refugees and certain other citizen groups are also treated for free with access to a General Practitioner, acute medical care and social services support.

Optimal HCT should prepare youth for social and legal aspects of adulthood. The age of majority is 16 in the UK and 18 in the US. At this age, adolescents automatically become their own legal decision-maker, regardless of comorbidities. Youth should receive counseling on decision-making supports, such as guardianship or healthcare power of attorney, prior to this birthday. Guardianship, the legal process to become the primary decision-maker for a young adult, is very complex in the UK. While youths reach adulthood at 16, they do not receive all legal rights until 18 years of age. Thus, a guardian cannot be assigned before 18 years old. Between the ages of 16–18, there is a void for a designated decision-maker, which is especially apparent for patients lacking capacity [17]. For complex options, court involvement may be required [17]. Discussing capacity prior to age 16–18 is crucial for avoiding confusion during medical emergencies or to protect patients from predatory behavior.

Education, vocation, and income supports factor largely into HCT planning. Many youths receive healthcare support, such as physical therapy, through their school system. At the completion of schooling (in the US at 21 and the UK at 18), these supports are discontinued, forcing patients to pay out of pocket or through insurance. Day programs or vocational programs exist for those over 21 but can be expensive and usually have limited availability. Income support in the UK is administered at the national level. For many youths with IMD, their caregivers are also able to register for benefits, allowing them to be compensated for full-time care. In the US, income support is administered at the state level with each state setting their own application criteria. Some states will use a medical diagnosis for approval, while others require documented intellectual disability [18]. This inequity can be harmful for young adults with IMD who may have complex medical needs but normal IQs.

3. Discussion

Despite systemic differences, the basic tenets of HCT permit international collaboration. Emphasizing HCT research and training is timely—expanded newborn screening via tandem mass spectroscopy began nearly twenty years ago in many countries [19], leading to a growing population of adolescents with IMD requiring transition to adult-centered medical care. International collaboration has been critical in other HCT-related fields, such as long-term follow-up for survivors of childhood cancer to determine rare late sequalae and compile surveillance recommendations [20]. Rare disease alliances, including the Europe Union's International Rare Disease Research Consortium (IRDiRC) and the US's National Organization for Rare Disorders (NORD), illustrate the greater impact of collective research efforts and data sharing [21]. The main HCT principles are consistent throughout these medical systems. Adolescents need preparation for adult-centered medical care, education and vocational opportunities, income support, and assistance with decision-making. Defining measurable outcomes for young adults with IMD is also necessary, permitting evaluation and refinement of HCT programs [5,7]. Some parameters will vary by country—such as insurance lapses or care fragmentation. However, creating unified measures to track and assess HCT internationally is beneficial for all. Here, collaboration between international IMD societies on HCT is a necessary first step. Since these disorders are rare and there is a limited pool of metabolic specialists, international collaboration is necessary to implement full-scale HCT planning including best practice recommendations.

One imperative for designing international IMD-related instruments is that current standardized HCT tools, such as "Ready, Steady, Go" are not comprehensive enough for IMD and IMD-specific assessments have not been validated [22]. Managing a rare disease is challenging in adult-centered healthcare. HCT requires a partnership between pediatric and adult providers. Yet, commitment to HCT is skewed toward greater participation and knowledge from pediatric providers and greater disinterest from adult providers. Many adult clinicians have no knowledge of the clinical care of IMD [23]. Adults are likely to see several care teams due to the multisystemic complications. For patients with intermediary disorder of metabolism, self-management is complex and there is an underlying risk of presenting for acute care in a state of transient encephalopathy [24]. Adults with IMD commonly need to educate their own physicians and act as strong advocates for their care. Providing young adults with the educational tools to accomplish this level of self-care is important [5,7]. Disease-specific guidelines will be necessary to properly inform adult-trained clinicians of current management, long-term complications, and surveillance recommendations. A collaborative approach to develop and disseminate these tools would be beneficial for the international IMD community.

Globally, recruitment of adult metabolic physicians and engagement of local clinicians about IMD are critical barriers to successful HCT and transfer. A stronger international alliance of professional societies and patient support groups could lead to greater promotion of adult metabolic medicine and resource curation. Together, IMD societies could partner with general internal medicine or adolescent medicine organizations to increase IMD representation, for example—by expanding the SSIEM Adult IMD course [15]. As both societies have active adult IMD sections, joint meetings are possible. Additionally, institution-based transition coordinators are instrumental in preparing young adults for this process [7]. Employing a transition coordinator may alleviate HCT barriers due to workforce limitations and clinician knowledge and has been shown to improve health outcomes [25,26]. International IMD societies should lead in developing guidelines that include a job description for transition coordinators. Representatives from many countries should be solicited to collaborate on HCT. The current report is limited by the comparison of two developed countries with individualistic attitudes to health care. Our HCT experience may not be generalizable to nations with more community-based health care.

Last, we must reiterate the difference between healthcare transition and healthcare transfer. HCT is the process of preparing adolescents for medical, social, and fiscal autonomy. Transfer, when a young adult leaves a pediatric practice and initiates care with an adult practice occurs more commonly in the EU (90%) than the US (25%) [1,8]. HCT is required for all adolescents with IMD, even those who will receive from the same IMD provider through adulthood. Metabolic physicians are well poised to promote HCT. International collaboration on HCT will strengthen its delivery.

4. Conclusions

Despite the differences in the health systems and physicians' training, collaboration between metabolic centers is possible. International rare disease alliance may enhance the patients' management via guidelines development and standardized training for adult metabolic providers. Further research and careful planning of coordination of transition care is required to ensure a smooth patients' transfer to adult metabolic services and empower them in decision making and improve their adherence to follow-up. The successful transfer of care will result in better patients' engagement with healthcare system.

Author Contributions: J.I.G. and K.M.S.—Concept, design, data acquisition, revision. All authors have read and agreed to the published version of the manuscript.

Funding: J.I.G. is supported by NIH T32 GM008638.

Institutional Review Board Statement: Not applicable.

Informed Consent Statement: Not applicable.

Data Availability Statement: Not applicable.

Acknowledgments: The authors would like to thank all patients with inherited metabolic disorders who inspired us to write this article.

Conflicts of Interest: The authors declare no conflict of interest.

References

1. Stepien, K.M.; Kieć-Wilk, B.; Lampe, C.; Tangeraas, T.; Cefalo, G.; Belmatoug, N.; Francisco, R.; Del Toro, M.; Wagner, L.; Lauridsen, A.G.; et al. Challenges in Transition From Childhood to AdulthoodCare in Rare Metabolic Diseases: Results From the First Multi-Center European Survey. *Front. Med.* **2021**, *8*, 652358. [CrossRef] [PubMed]
2. Waters, D.; Adeloye, D.; Woolham, D.; Wastnedge, E.; Patel, S.; Rudan, I. Global birth prevalence and mortality from inborn errors of metabolism: A systematic analysis of the evidence. *J. Global Health* **2018**, *8*, 021102. [CrossRef] [PubMed]
3. Schwarz, M.; Wendel, U. Inborn errors of metabolism (IEM) in adults. A new challenge to internal medicine. *Med. Klin.* **2005**, *100*, 547–552. [CrossRef] [PubMed]
4. Gariani, K.; Nascimento, M.; Superti-Furga, A.; Tran, C. Clouds over IMD? Perspectives for inherited metabolic diseases in adults from a retrospective cohort study in two Swiss adult metabolic clinics. *Orphan. J. Rare Dis.* **2020**, *15*, 210. [CrossRef] [PubMed]
5. Sirrs, S.; Hollak, C.; Merkel, M.; Sechi, A.; Glamuzina, E.; Janssen, M.C.; Lachmann, R.; Langendonk, J.; Scarpelli, M.; Ben Omran, T.; et al. The Frequencies of Different Inborn Errors of Metabolism in Adult Metabolic Centres: Report from the SSIEM Adult Metabolic Physicians Group. *JIMD Rep.* **2016**, *27*, 85–91. [CrossRef] [PubMed]
6. Stępień, K.M.; Hendriksz, C.J. The principles of the transition process from paediatric to adult services in inborn errors of metabolism—own experience. *Dev. Period Med.* **2015**, *19*, 523–527. [PubMed]
7. Lampe, C.; McNelly, B.; Gevorkian, A.K.; Hendriksz, C.J.; Lobzhanidze, T.V.; Pérez-López, J.; Stepien, K.M.; Vashakmadze, N.D.; Del Toro, M. Transition of patients with mucopolysaccharidosis from paediatric to adult care. *Mol. Genet. Metab. Rep.* **2019**, *21*, 100508. [CrossRef] [PubMed]
8. Gold, J.I.; Gold, N.B.; Strong, A.; Tully, E.; Xiao, R.; Schwartz, L.A.; Ficicioglu, C. The current state of adult metabolic medicine in the United States: Results of a nationwide survey. *Genet Med.* **2022**, *24*, 1722–1731. [CrossRef] [PubMed]
9. Graham-Rowe, D. Ready, Steady, Go. New Scientist. 1999. Available online: https://www.nice.org.uk/sharedlearning/implementing-transition-care-locally-and-nationally-using-the-ready-steady-go-programme (accessed on 15 April 2022).
10. Schrander-Stumpel, C.T.; Sinnema, M.; Van Den Hout, L.; Maaskant, M.A.; van Schrojenstein Lantman-de Valk, H.M.; Wagemans, A.; Schrander, J.J.; Curfs, L.M. Healthcare transition in persons with intellectual disabilities: General issues, the Maastricht model, and Prader-Willi syndrome. *Am. J. Med. Genet. C Semin. Med. Genet.* **2007**, *145C*, 241–247. [CrossRef] [PubMed]

11. Fair, C.; Cuttance, J.; Sharma, N.; Maslow, G.; Wiener, L.; Betz, C.; Porter, J.; McLaughlin, S.; Gilleland-Marchak, J.; Renwick, A.; et al. International and Interdisciplinary Identification of Health Care Transition Outcomes. *JAMA Pediatr.* **2016**, *170*, 205–211. [CrossRef] [PubMed]
12. Cross-Certification of Diplomates of AMBGG and Other ABMS Member Boards. Available online: http://www.abmgg.org/pdf/Cross-CertificationSummarywithOtherABMSBoards.pdf (accessed on 13 January 2022).
13. Joint Royal Colleges of Physicians Training Board. Training Curriculum for the Sub-Specialty of Metabolic Medicine (August 2010). Available online: https://www.jrcptb.org.uk/specialties/metabolic-medicine-sub-specialty (accessed on 13 December 2021).
14. Royal College of Pathologists United Kingdom. Curriculum for Specialty Training in Chemical Pathology: Appendix A. 2021. Available online: https://www.gmc-uk.org/education/standards-guidance-and-curricula/curricula/chemical-pathology-curriculum (accessed on 22 July 2022).
15. Sechi, A.; Fabbro, E.; Sirrs, S. The right tool for the job-Fit for purpose training programs in adult metabolic medicine. *J. Inherit. Metab. Dis.* **2022**, *45*, 864–865. [CrossRef] [PubMed]
16. NORD State Report Card-Medical Nutrition. Available online: https://rarediseases.org/policy-issues/medical-nutrition (accessed on 15 February 2022).
17. Mental Capacity Act. 2005. Available online: https://www.nhs.uk/conditions/social-care-and-support-guide/making-decisions-for-someone-else/mental-capacity-act/ (accessed on 22 July 2022).
18. Steinway, C.; Gable, J.L.; Jan, S. Transitioning to Adult Care: Supporting Youth with Special Health Care Needs. 2017. Available online: https://policylab.chop.edu/sites/default/files/pdf/publications/Transitions_Of_Care.pdf (accessed on 22 July 2022).
19. Chace, D.H. Mass spectrometry in newborn and metabolic screening: Historical perspective and future directions. *J. Mass. Spectrom.* **2009**, *44*, 163–170. [CrossRef] [PubMed]
20. Gebauer, J.; Skinner, R.; Haupt, R.; Kremer, L.; van der Pal, H.; Michel, G.; Armstrong, G.T.; Hudson, M.M.; Hjorth, L.; Lehnert, H.; et al. The chance of transition: Strategies for multidisciplinary collaboration. *Endocr. Connect.* **2022**, *11*, e220083. [CrossRef] [PubMed]
21. Julkowska, D.; Austin, C.P.; Cutillo, C.M.; Gancberg, D.; Hager, C.; Halftermeyer, J.; Jonker, A.H.; Lau, L.P.L.; Norstedt, I.; Rath, A.; et al. The importance of international collaboration for rare diseases research: A European perspective. *Gene. Ther.* **2017**, *24*, 562–571. [CrossRef] [PubMed]
22. New England Consortium of Metabolic Program Transition to Adult Care. Available online: https://www.newenglandconsortium.org/transition-to-adult (accessed on 31 August 2022).
23. Segal, S.; Roth, K.S. Inborn errors of metabolism: A new purview of internal medicine. *Ann. Intern. Med.* **1994**, *120*, 245–246. [CrossRef] [PubMed]
24. Lee, P.J.; Lachmann, R.H. Acute presentations of inherited metabolic disease in adulthood. *Clin. Med.* **2008**, *8*, 621–624. [CrossRef] [PubMed]
25. Morton, B.; Damato, E.G.; Ciccarelli, M.R.; Currie, J. Care Coordination for Children with Special Healthcare Needs Anticipating Transition: A Program Evaluation. *J. Pediatr. Nurs.* **2021**, *61*, 7–14. [CrossRef] [PubMed]
26. Samuel, S.; Dimitropoulos, G.; Schraeder, K.; Klarenbach, S.; Nettel-Aguirre, A.; Guilcher, G.; Pacaud, D.; Pinzon, J.; Lang, E.; Andrew, G.; et al. Pragmatic trial evaluating the effectiveness of a patient navigator to decrease emergency room utilisation in transition age youth with chronic conditions: The Transition Navigator Trial protocol. *BMJ Open* **2019**, *9*, e034309. [CrossRef] [PubMed]

MDPI
St. Alban-Anlage 66
4052 Basel
Switzerland
www.mdpi.com

Journal of Clinical Medicine Editorial Office
E-mail: jcm@mdpi.com
www.mdpi.com/journal/jcm

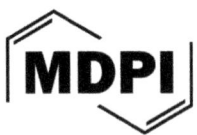

Disclaimer/Publisher's Note: The statements, opinions and data contained in all publications are solely those of the individual author(s) and contributor(s) and not of MDPI and/or the editor(s). MDPI and/or the editor(s) disclaim responsibility for any injury to people or property resulting from any ideas, methods, instructions or products referred to in the content.

www.ingramcontent.com/pod-product-compliance
Lightning Source LLC
LaVergne TN
LVHW070500100526
838202LV00014B/1758